New Aspects of Nuclear Dynamics

NATO ASI Series

Advanced Science Institutes Series

A series presenting the results of activities sponsored by the NATO Science Committee, which aims at the dissemination of advanced scientific and technological knowledge, with a view to strengthening links between scientific communities.

The series is published by an international board of publishers in conjunction with the NATO Scientific Affairs Division

A	**Life Sciences**	Plenum Publishing Corporation
B	**Physics**	New York and London
C	**Mathematical and Physical Sciences**	Kluwer Academic Publishers Dordrecht, Boston, and London
D	**Behavioral and Social Sciences**	
E	**Applied Sciences**	
F	**Computer and Systems Sciences**	Springer-Verlag
G	**Ecological Sciences**	Berlin, Heidelberg, New York, London,
H	**Cell Biology**	Paris, and Tokyo

Recent Volumes in this Series

Volume 204—Techniques and Concepts of High-Energy Physics V
edited by Thomas Ferbel

Volume 205—Nuclear Matter and Heavy Ion Collisions
edited by Madeleine Soyeur, Hubert Flocard, Bernard Tamain, and Madeleine Porneuf

Volume 206—Spectroscopy of Semiconductor Microstructures
edited by Gerhard Fasol, Annalisa Fasolino, and Paolo Lugli

Volume 207—Reduced Thermal Processing for ULSI
edited by Roland A. Levy

Volume 208—Measures of Complexity and Chaos
edited by Neal B. Abraham, Alfonso M. Albano, Anthony Passamante, and Paul E. Rapp

Volume 209—New Aspects of Nuclear Dynamics
edited by J. H. Koch and P. K. A. de Witt Huberts

Volume 210—Crystal Growth in Science and Technology
edited by H. Arend and J. Hulliger

Volume 211—Phase Transitions in Soft Condensed Matter
edited by Tormod Riste and David Sherrington

Series B: Physics

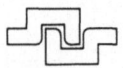

New Aspects of Nuclear Dynamics

Edited by

J. H. Koch

National Institute for Nuclear Physics and High-Energy Physics
Amsterdam, The Netherlands
and University of Amsterdam
Amsterdam, The Netherlands

and

P. K. A. de Witt Huberts

National Institute for Nuclear Physics and High-Energy Physics
Amsterdam, The Netherlands
and University of Utrecht
Utrecht, The Netherlands

Plenum Press
New York and London
Published in cooperation with NATO Scientific Affairs Division

Proceedings of a NATO Advanced Study Institute on
New Aspects of Nuclear Dynamics,
held August 8-21, 1988
in Dronten, The Netherlands

Library of Congress Cataloging-in-Publication Data

NATO Advanced Study Institute on New Aspects of Nuclear Dynamics (1988 Dronten, Netherlands)
New aspects of nuclear dynamics / edited by J.H. Koch and P.K.A. de Witt Huberts.
p. cm. -- (NATO ASI series. Series B, Physics ; vol. 209)
"Proceedings of a NATO Advanced Study Institute on New Aspects of Nuclear Dynamics, held August 8-21, 1988, in Dronten, The Netherlands"--T.p. verso.
Includes bibliographical references.
ISBN-13:978-1-4612-7860-3 e-ISBN-13:978-1-4613-0547-7
DOI: 10.1007/978-1-4613-0547-7

1. Nuclear reactions--Congresses. 2. Nuclear matter--Congresses. I. Koch, J. H. II. Witt Huberts, P. K. A. de. III. Title. IV. Title: Nuclear dynamics. V. Series: NATO ASI series. Series B, Physics ; v. 209.
QC793.9.N38 1988
539.7'5--dc20 89-25521
CIP

Softcover reprint of the hardcover 1st edition 1989

A Division of Plenum Publishing Corporation
233 Spring Street, New York, N.Y. 10013

SCIENTIFIC ORGANIZING COMMITTEE

P.K.A. de Witt Huberts, Chairman
J.H. Koch, Secretary
J. Konijn, Treasurer
A.E.L. Dieperink
M.N. Harakeh
R. Kamermans

PREFACE

The 1988 Summer School on New Aspects of Nuclear Dynamics took place in the style that by now has become a tradition: a series of lectures by well known scientists on modern topics of nuclear physics, where special emphasis is placed on the didactic aspects of the lectures.

In the past few years, we have witnessed a rapid evolution of the field of nuclear physics towards novel directions of research. This development is accompanied by the construction of some of the largest experimental facilities ever built for nuclear research. The subjects covered by the Summer School focussed on two main issues currently under active investigation and which will be pursued with the new facilities: the transition from nucleonic to quark degrees of freedom in the decription of nuclear reactions, and the behavior of nuclear matter as one approaches extreme densities and temperatures. These topics in many respects go beyond traditional nuclear physics and the speakers therefore also included high energy physicists. From the response of the participants it was clear that the program of the school filled a gap in the curriculum of many students. We wish to thank all the speakers for their well organized lectures, which were nicely geared to the level of the school, and for spending extra time on problem sessions and extensive discussions.

The organization of this Summer School was made possible by substantial support from the Science Committee of the North Atlantic Treaty Organization. In addition, assistance was obtained from the Netherland's Physical Society.

By now also a tradition was the pleasant collaboration with the management of the College of Agriculture in Dronten, where the school was held. Furthermore, the organizers wish to thank Marijke Oskam-Tamboezer for her skilled help in the preparation of the Summer School. She and Monique Fokke also made sure that the Summer School ran smoothly and took care of all those unforeseen problems that needed to be taken care of immediately.

J.H. Koch

P.K.A. de Witt Huberts

CONTENTS

DEEP INELASTIC SCALING IN NUCLEAR AND PARTICLE PHYSICS

Geoffrey B. West

Theoretical Division, T-8, MS B285
Los Alamos National Laboratory
Los Alamos, NM 87545

I INTRODUCTION

These lectures are intended to be a pedagogical introduction to some of the ideas and concepts concerning scaling phenomena which arise in nuclear and particle physics. The level will be fairly modest and is aimed at the graduate student who has some familiarity with Feynman diagrams and the rudiments of quantum field theory. In actual fact, the first two-thirds of these lectures really only requires a standard background in non-relativistic quantum mechanics.

In spite of the fact that scaling and the closely related subject of dimensional analysis have been an integral part of the language of physics for almost a century, it is really only in the past 15 years or so that these ideas have found their way into nuclear and particle physics. In particle physics the observation of scaling phenomena was absolutely critical in changing our ideas about the fundamental constituents of matter.

Indeed, until the discovery almost twenty years ago that the structure functions of nucleons, as measured in deep-inelastic electron scattering exhibited a point-like scaling behavior, the idea that hadrons really were bound states of quarks was not generally taken seriously.[1] Quarks somehow were thought of as fictitious objects carrying certain quantum numbers which could explain the general features of the hadronic spectrum.[2] In spite of the great success of this "naïve" quark model, quarks as real hard objects which could be "seen" in electron scattering were not given much credence by the cognoscenti. Indeed the "real" nucleon was still thought of as a "bare" nucleon surrounded by a mesonic cloud and so was expected to respond as a soft spongy object when probed by a hard scattering. Thus the observation of a point-like scaling behavior in deep-inelastic electron scattering played a crucial rôle in establishing quarks as "real" objects from which all hadronic matter is constructed.[1,3]

Indeed these experiments completely re-oriented our thinking about strong interactions and opened the way to re-establishing quantum field theory as the paradigm for describing all fundamental interactions. Since that time enormous progress has been made and it is fair to say that we now have an almost universally accepted realistic quantum field theory describing all the fundamental interactions with the possible exception of gravity.[4] Quarks enter as a fundamental fermionic field with strong interactions mediated by massless vector bosons, called gluons. This strong interaction part of the theory is called quantum chromodynamics (QCD) because it closely mimics QED. The crucial difference is that the gluons, as well as the quarks, carry the fundamental "charge" of the theory, here called color. In QED, the photons are not, of course, electrically charged (unlike the electrons) and so do not directly interact with each other. It is generally believed that it is this curious complexity, namely that gluons are colored (and therefore self-interact) that ultimately leads to the confinement of quarks (and more generally of color itself). For, the great paradox surrounding the quark model is that even though quarks are undoubtedly the fundamental constituents of hadrons and, as already emphasized, have in fact been "seen" in deep inelastic experiments, it seems impossible to isolate them in the laboratory. Over the years many arguments based on QCD have been proposed for explaining this apparent paradox. Although none are truly convincing and we await the ultimate rigorous proof that "infrared slavery" can co-exist with "asymptotic freedom" most believe that such a proof is indeed a consequence of QCD.[4]

Prior to the development of QCD there was no serious framework allowing one to address the sorts of questions raised by confinement and scaling. In the naïve quark model a nucleon was typically thought of much like a nucleus, namely as non- relativistic constituents bound by some potential. This actually gives a remarkably good description of the hadronic spectrum, as well as other low energy phenomena such as decay rates.[5] It is therefore not unreasonable to address the scaling vs. confinement paradox within this theoretical lab. of non-relativistic many-body theory. It is as if we were to suppose that the nucleons in a nucleus were bound to each other by a confining potential such as an harmonic oscillator, for example, and were to ask whether the non-relativistic structure functions, as measured in deep inelastic electron scattering, scale; and, if so, how would the confinement mechanism manifest itself? It was out of considerations such as these that the phenomenon of y-scaling in non-relativistic systems such as nuclei and liquids arose.[3]

It is ironic that, although much of the intuition for interpreting the high energy data as scattering from structureless constituents came from nuclear physics (and to a lesser extent atomic physics) virtually no data existed for nuclear targets in the non-relativistic regime until relatively recently. It is therefore not so surprising that, in spite of the fact that the basic nuclear physics has been well understood for a very long time, the corresponding non-relativistic scaling law was not written down until <u>after</u> the relativistic one, relevant to particle physics, had been explored.[3] Of course, to the extent that these scaling laws simply reflect quasi-elastic scattering of the probe from the constituents, they contain little new physics once the nature of the constituents is known and understood. On the other hand, <u>deviations from scaling</u> represent corrections to the impulse approximation and can reflect important dynamical and coherent features of the system. Furthermore, as will be discussed in detail below, the scaling curve itself represents the single particle momentum distribution of constituents inside the target. *It is therefore prudent to plot the data in terms of a suitable scaling variable since this immediately focuses attention on the dominant physics.* Extraneous physics, such as Rutherford scattering in the case of electrons, or magnetic scattering in the case of thermal neutrons is factored out and the use of a scaling variable (such as y) automatically takes into account the fact that the target is a bound state of well-defined constituents.

The first part of these lectures will be devoted to scaling in non-relativistic systems. Although the formalism developed applies equally well to both electron scattering from nuclei and thermal neutron scattering from liquids, I shall usually be thinking of the former. On the other hand I shall completely ignore spin considerations (as well as relativistic corrections) so, ironically, the results actually apply more to the latter case!

I shall show how the classic sum rules of Bethe and Heisenberg[6] already suggest the possibility of scaling. In order for scaling to be a useful tool, one must clearly have some idea as to how it is approached as one increases $\underline{q}^2$. To this end we carry out a dynamical calculation to show how corrections can be evaluated in terms of the basic inter-nucleon potential. Indeed, as a byproduct of this I shall show that scaling follows even if the potential is confining; that is, the system behaves in a free manner even though the constituents are forever bound. This is not, of course, relevant for nuclei but may have some bearing on the relativistic hadronic problem. Apart from these potential corrections to scaling there is also the very physical effect of correlations; i.e., the system will not behave in a quasi-free fashion until $|\underline{q}|$ exceeds the coherence length in the system. Finally, there is a further constraint to scaling from nuclear systems and that is the eventual effect of meson production. By the time q is large enough for scaling to dominate, it may also be large enough for pions to be produced. Since we shall consider only nucleon degrees of freedom and remain in the non-relativistic domain our calculations ignore this contribution. Thus our "predictions" are only useful provided one remains in a region where pion production is negligible.

In particle physics, the analog to pion production is gluon production (radiative corrections) and in QCD these are responsible for the phenomenon of asymptotic freedom[7]. In the last part of these lectures I shall show that, up to logarithms, exact scaling results as if the proton were made simply of point-like objects which can be identified with quarks. It is, in fact, the radiation of soft gluons which, analogous to the radiation of soft photons in QED, is the origin of the lograrithmic violation of exact scaling, predicted by a naïve impulse approximation. The experimental observation of these violations is one of the basic reasons that QCD is believed to be the correct theory of the strong interactions. An important ingredient in the derivation of asymptotic freedom is the renormalization group[4,8]. This expresses the fact that physics cannot depend upon the scale at which the theory is renormalized. Recall that in quantum field theory infinities arise from the ultra-violet divergences inherent in the perturbation expansion. These can be controlled by renormalizing coupling constants and masses so that the physical parameters of the theory now depend upon some arbitrary scale. I shall try to show that this invariance to scale can be viewed as a generalization of ordinary dimensional analysis so that classical scaling and the scaling associated with quantum field theory can be incorporated in a unified picture.

Thus, to set the scene I shall begin by first reviewing classical scaling and dimensional analysis. Although this is all "well-known" there are some novel features which are usually suppressed but which play a central rôle in relating the results to asymptotic freedom[9].

I Classical Scaling and Dimensional Analysis

The physical content of scaling is very often formulated in terms of the language of dimensional analysis. The seminal idea seems to be due to Fourier. He is, of course, most famous for the invention of "Fourier analysis," introduced in his great treatise *Theorie Analytique de la Chaleur*, first published in Paris in 1822. However, it is generally not appreciated that this same book contains another great contribution, namely, the use of dimensions for physical quantities. It is the ghost of Fourier that is the scourge of all freshman physics majors, for it was he who first realized that every physical quantity "has one *dimension* proper to itself, and that the terms of one and the same equation could not be compared, if they had not the same *exponent of dimension.*" He goes on: "We have introduced this consideration ··· to verify the analysis ··· it is the equivalent of the fundamental lemmas which the Greeks have left us without proof." Indeed it is! Check the dimensions!–the rallying call of all physicists (and, hopefully, all engineers).

A Drag Force on a Ship

As a simple example, consider the classic problem of the drag force F on a ship moving through a viscous fluid of density ρ. We shall choose F , ρ, the velocity ν, the viscosity of the fluid μ, some length parameter of the ship l, and the acceleration due to gravity g as our variables. Notice that we exclude other variables, such as the wind velocity and the amplitude of the sea waves because, under calm conditions, these are of secondary importance. Our conclusions may therefore not be valid for sailing ships!

The physics of the problem is governed by the Navier-Stokes equation (which incorporates Newton's law of viscous drag, telling us the dimensions of μ) and the gravitational force law (telling us the dimensions of g). Using these dimensions automatically incorporates the appropriate physics. Since we have limited the variables to a set of six, which must be expressible in terms of three basic units (mass M, length L, and time T), there will only be three independent dimensionless combinations. These are chosen to be $P \equiv F/\rho\nu^2 l^2$ (the pressure coefficient), $R \equiv \nu l\rho/\mu$ (Reynold's number), and $N_F \equiv \nu^2/lg$(Froude's number). *Although any three similar combinations could have been chosen, these three are special because they delineate the physics.* For example, Reynold's number R relates to the viscous drag on a body moving through a fluid, whereas Froude's number N_F relates to the forces involved with waves and eddies generated on the surface of the fluid by the movement. Thus the rationale for the combinations R and N_F is to separate the role of the viscous forces from that of the gravitational: R does not depend on g, and F does not depend on μ. Furthermore, P does not depend on either!

Dimensional analysis now requires that the solution for the pressure coefficient, whatever it is, must be expressible in the dimensionless form

$$P = f(R, N_F). \tag{1}$$

The actual drag force F can easily be obtained from this equation by re-expressing it in terms of the dimensional variables (see Eq. 3 below).

First, however, consider a situation where surface waves generated by the moving object are *un*important (an extreme example is a submarine). In this case g will not enter the solution since it is manifested as the restoring force for surface waves. N_F can then be dropped from the solution, reducing Eq. 1 to the simple form

$$P = f(R). \tag{2}$$

In terms of the original dimensional variables, this is equivalent to

$$F = \rho v^2 l^2 f(vl\rho/\mu). \tag{3}$$

Historically, these last equations have been well tested by measuring the speed of different sizes and types of balls moving through different liquids. If the data are plotted using the dimensionless variables, that is P versus R, then *all* the data should lie on just *one* curve regardless of the size of the ball or the nature of the liquid. Such a curve is called a *scaling curve*, a wonderful example of which is shown in Fig. 1 where one sees a scaling phenomenon that varies over seven orders of magnitude! It is important to recognize that if one had used dimensional variables and plotted F versus l, for example, then, instead of a single curve, there would have been *many* different and apparently unrelated curves for the different liquids. Using carefully chosen dimensionless variables (such as Reynold's number) is not only physically more sound but usually greatly simplifies the task of representing the data.

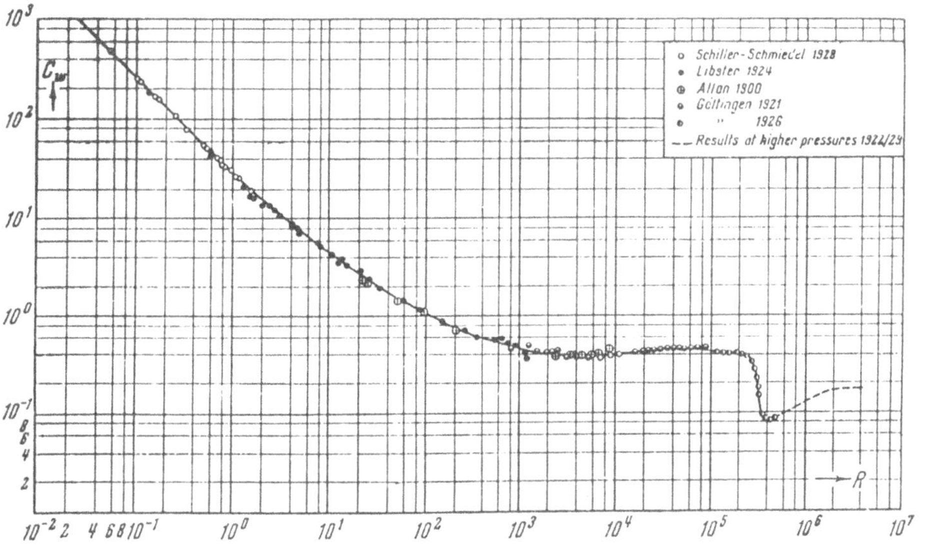

Figure 1. The scaling curve for the motion of a sphere through a fluid that results when data from a variety of experiments are plotted in terms of two dimensionless variables: the pressure or drag coefficient P versus Reynolds number R. (Figure adapted from AIP Handbook of Physics, 2 nd edition (1963): section II, p. 253.)

A remarkable consequence of this analysis is that, for similar bodies, the ratio of drag force to weight *decreases* as the size of the structure increases. From Archimedes' principle the volume of water displaced by a ship is proportional to its weight, that is, $W \propto l^3$ (this, incidentally, is why there is no need to include W as an independent variable in deriving these equations). Combined with Eq. 3 this leads to the conclusion that

$$\frac{F}{W} \propto \frac{1}{l}. \tag{4}$$

This scaling law was extremely important in the 19th century because it showed that *it was cost effective to build bigger ships*, thereby justifying the use of large iron steamboats!

The great usefulness of scaling laws is also illustrated by the observation that the behavior of P for large ships ($l \to \infty$) can be derived from the behavior of small ships moving very fast ($\nu \to \infty$). This is so because both limits are controlled by the same asymptotic behavior of $f(R) = F(\nu l \rho/\mu)$. Such observations form the basis of *modeling* theory so crucial in the design of aircraft, ships, buildings, and so forth.

McMahon, in an article in *Science*[10], has pointed out another, somewhat more amusing, consequence to the drag force equation. He was interested in how the speed of a rowing boat scales with the number of oarsmen n and argued that, at a steady velocity, the power expended by the oarsmen E to overcome the drag force is given by $F\nu$. Thus

$$E = F\nu = \rho\nu^3 l^2 f(R). \tag{5}$$

Using Archimedes' principle again and the fact that both E and W should be directly proportional to n leads to the remarkable scaling law

$$\nu \propto n^{1/9}, \tag{6}$$

which shows a *very* slow growth with n. Figure 2 exhibits data collected by McMahon from various rowing events for the time $t(\propto 1/\nu)$ taken to cover a fixed 2000-meter course under calm conditions. One can see quite plainly the verification of his predicted law–a most satisfying result!

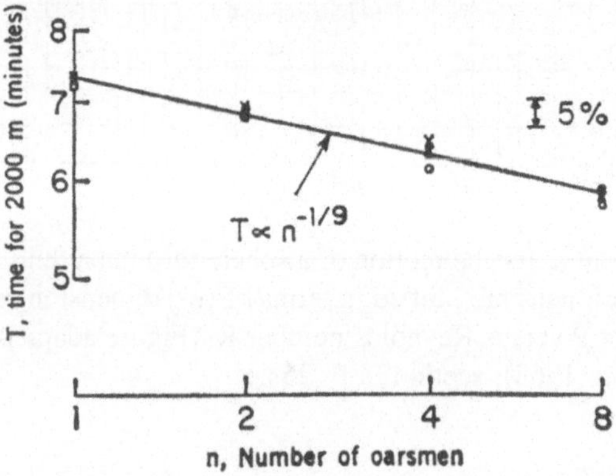

Figure 2. The time needed for a rowing boat to complete a 2000-meter course in calm conditions as a function of the number of oarsmen. Data were taken from several international rowing championship events and illustrate the surprisingly slow dropoff predicted by modeling theory.

B Run-off From a Watershed (Conservation Laws)

There are many other fascinating and exotic examples of the power of dimensional analysis. However, rather than belaboring the point, I would like to mention a slightly different example of scaling before I turn to the mathematical formulation. This example nicely illustrates the rôle that a conservation law can play in deriving a scaling result.

I want to consider the run-off of rainwater from a watershed. Every river has a watershed: this is a geographical region (normally hilly or mountainous) through which a river flows and from which all of the water it carries emanates. It is therefore simply the area (A) drained by the river. Geographers have devised reliable ways of estimating A; thus the Colorado river has a drainage area of approximately $7 \times 10^5 \text{km}^2$ whereas for the Nile it is roughly $4 \times 10^6 \text{km}^2$

Interestingly enough there is an almost linear relationship between A and l^2, l being the river's length, exemplifying a simple form of geometric scaling.

Let us imagine that during some short period of time (less than a day, say) there is a rainstorm which deposits h cms. of water on the watershed. This represents a total volume of water $V = Ah$. We want to investigate the behavior of the flow rate of water (Q) in the river during the ensuing days. This is obviously a very complicated problem and depends on many variables; however suppose we are interested in comparing flow-rates in different watersheds with similar geography and geology. To keep things simple we might limit the variables to Q, A, L, t*(time)*, g *(the acceleration due to gravity))*, ρ *(the density of water) and* μ *(its viscosity)*. It is worth giving some thought as to what other variables might be relevant and what is being assumed by using only this limited set. Generally speaking it is the choice of the pertinent variables and their grouping into appropriate dimensionless combinations that the "hard" work of dimensional analysis is involved. Progress in science depends crucially on choosing interesting, relevant variables.

With the above choice of variables we can form the following four dimensionless combinations:

$$\begin{aligned} q &= \frac{Q}{g^{1/2}A^{3/4}h} \\ x &= \frac{tg^{1/2}}{A^{1/4}} \\ y &= \frac{\mu^2}{\rho^2 g A^{3/2}} \\ z &= \frac{A}{h^2} \end{aligned} \tag{7}$$

It must therefore be that Q can be expressed in the form

$$Q \equiv g^{1/2}A^{3/4}hq(x, y, z) \tag{8}$$

This is as far as we can go with conventional dimensional analysis. However there is a presumed conservation constraint that must be imposed, namely that <u>all</u> the water that fell during the rainstorm eventually flows down the river, i.e.

$$\int_0^\infty Q dt = Ah \tag{9}$$

[The time $t=0$ is defined as the day the rain fell]. In terms of the dimensionless variables this reads

$$\int_0^\infty q(x,y,z)\,dx = 1 \tag{10}$$

This is a sum rule and, as already stated, simply reflects the conservation of water. Notice the remarkable structure of this sum rule: an integral which "should" be a function of y and z is constrained by the conservation law to be a constant (namely, unity). Furthermore since $q \geq 0$, one might guess that the way this is accomplished is that q itself is independent of y and z, i.e.

$$q(x,y,z) = f(x) \text{ only} \tag{11}$$

This is a remarkable prediction which is, in fact, borne out by the data as illustrated, for

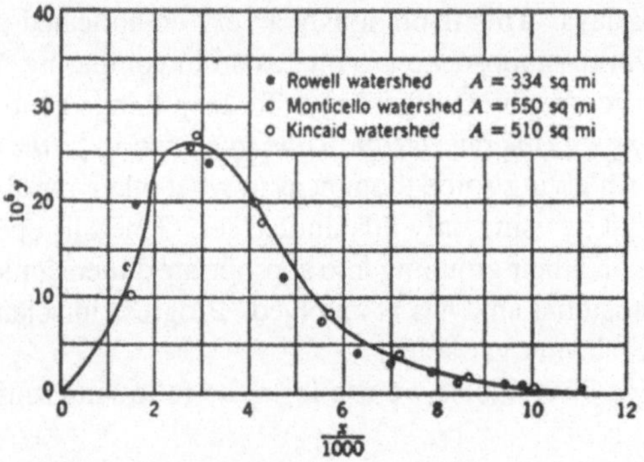

Figure 3. Graph of $10^6 q$ vs. $10^{-3}x$ for three different watersheds in Illinois. Notice that data from different watersheds and different rainfalls all lie on a single curve.

example, in Fig. 3. Data from various run-offs from different watersheds are plotted in a q-x plane and, as can be readily seen from the figure, they all lie on a single curve. Furthermore it is easy to verify that the sum rule, Eq. (10), is indeed verified. In terms of the original physical variables, Eq. (11) reads

$$Q = g^{1/2} A^{3/4} h f\left(\frac{tg^{1/2}}{A^{1/4}}\right) \tag{12}$$

which predicts the simple linear relationship $Q \propto h$ for a given watershed. Again, this is empirically correct.

As promised this example nicely illustrates the power of conservation laws and their relationship to scaling. It should be pointed out that the deduction from the sum rule that

q is independent of y and z is in no way a proof, but, rather is suggestive. To prove such a result would require showing that every moment of q is independent of y and z. As we shall see below, the original suggestion of Bjorken scaling rested on an argument which is the exact analogue of the one given above; the corresponding conserved quantity being electric charge. It was indeed the attempts to prove this by extending it to all moments that eventually revealed the logarithmic violations associated with asymptotic freedom and QCD.

C Mathematical Formulation (Scale Invariance)

Let us now turn our attention to a slightly more abstract mathematical formulation that clarifies the relationship of dimensional analysis to *scale invariance*. By scale invariance we simply mean that the structure of physical laws cannot depend on the choice of units. As already intimated, this is automatically accomplished simply by employing dimensionless variables since these clearly do not change when the system of units changes. However, it may not be immediately obvious that this is equivalent to the *form invariance* of physical equations. Since physical laws are usually expressed in terms of dimensional variables, this is an important point to consider: namely, what are the general constraints that follow from the requirement that the laws of physics look the same regardless of the chosen units. The crucial observation here is that implicit in any equation written in terms of dimensional variables are the "hidden" fundamental scales of mass M, length L, time T, and so forth that are relevant to the problem. Of course, one never actually makes these scale parameters explicit precisely because of form invariance.

Our motivation for investigating this question is to develop a language that can be generalized in a natural way to include the subtleties of quantum field theory. Hopefully classical dimensional analysis and scaling will be sufficiently familiar that its generalization to the more complicated case will be relatively smooth! This generalization has been named the *renormalization group* since its origins lie in the renormalization program used to make sense out of the infinities inherent in quantum field theory[4,8]. It turns out that renormalization requires the introduction of a new arbitrary "hidden" scale that plays a role similar to the role of the scale parameters implicit in any dimensional equation. Thus any equation derived in quantum field theory that represents a physical quantity must not depend upon this choice of hidden scale. The resulting constraint will simply represent a generalization of ordinary dimensional analysis: the only reason that it is different is that variables in quantum field theory, such as fields, change in a much more complicated fashion with scale than do their classical counterparts.

Nevertheless, just as dimensional analysis allows one to learn much about the behavior of a system without actually solving the dynamical equations, so the analogous constraints of the renormalization group lead to powerful conclusions about the behavior of a quantum field theory during the past decade or so. Before describing how this comes about, I shall discuss the simpler and more familiar case of scale change in ordinary classical systems.

To begin, consider some physical quantity F that has dimensions; it will, of course, be a function of various dimensional variables x_l : $F(x_1, x_2 \cdots, x_n)$.

Each of these variables, including F itself, is always expressible in terms of some standard set of independent units, which can be chosen to be mass M, length L, and time T. These are the hidden scale parameters. Obviously, other combinations could be used. There could even be other independent units, such as temperature, or more than one independent length (say, transverse and longitudinal). In this discussion, we shall simply use the conventional M, L and T. Any generalization is straightforward.

In terms of this standard set of units, the magnitude of each x_l is given by

$$x_i = M^{\alpha_i} L^{\beta_i} T^{\gamma_i} \tag{13}$$

The numbers α_i, β_i, and γ_i will be recognized as "the dimensions" of x_i. Now suppose we change the system of units by some scale transformation of the form

$$\begin{aligned} M \rightarrow M' &= \lambda_M M, \\ L \rightarrow L' &= \lambda_L L, \end{aligned}$$

and (14)

$$T \rightarrow T' = \lambda_T T. \tag{15}$$

Each variable then responds as follows:

$$x_i \rightarrow x_i' = Z_i(\lambda)\, x_i, \tag{16}$$

where

$$Z_i(\lambda) = \lambda_M^{\alpha_i} \lambda_L^{\beta_i} \lambda_T^{\gamma_i}, \tag{17}$$

and λ is shorthand for λ_M, λ_L, and λ_T. Since F is itself a dimensional physical quantity, it transforms in an identical fashion under this scale change:

$$F \rightarrow F' = Z(\lambda) F(x_1, x_2, \cdots, x_n), \tag{18}$$

where

$$Z(\lambda) = \lambda_M^{\alpha} \lambda_L^{\beta} \lambda_T^{\gamma}. \tag{19}$$

Here α, β, and γ are the dimensions of F.

There is, however, an alternate but equivalent way to transform from F to F', namely by transforming each of the variables separately. Explicitly we therefore also have

$$F \rightarrow F' = F(Z_1(\lambda) x_1, Z_2(\lambda) x_2 \cdots, Z_n(\lambda) x_n). \tag{20}$$

Equating these two different ways of effecting a scale change leads to the identity

$$F(Z_1(\lambda) x_1, Z_2(\lambda) x_2, \cdots, Z_n(\lambda) x_n) = Z(\lambda) F(x_1, x_2, \cdots, x_n). \tag{21}$$

As a concrete example, consider the equation $E = mc^2$. To change scale one can either transform E directly or transform m and c separately and multiply the results appropriately – obviously the final result must be the same.

We now want to ensure that the resulting form of the equation does not depend on λ. This is best accomplished using Euler's trick of taking $\partial/\partial\lambda$ and then setting $\lambda = 1$. For example, if we were to consider changes in the mass scale, we would use $\partial/\partial\lambda_M$ and the chain rule for partial differentiation to arrive at

$$\sum_{i=1}^{n} x_i \frac{\partial Z_i}{\partial \lambda_M} \frac{\partial F}{\partial x_i'} = \frac{\partial Z}{\partial \lambda_M} F. \tag{22}$$

When we set $\lambda_M = 1$, differentiation of Eqs. (16) and (18) yields

$$\left(\frac{\partial Z_i}{\partial \lambda_M}\right)_{\lambda_M=1} = \alpha_i, \qquad \left(\frac{\partial Z}{\partial \lambda_M}\right)_{\lambda_M=1} = \alpha, \tag{23}$$

and $x_i' = x_i$, so that Eq. (21) reduces to

$$\alpha_1 X_1 \frac{\partial F}{\partial X_1} + \alpha_2 X_2 \frac{\partial F}{\partial X_2} + \alpha_3 X_3 \frac{\partial F}{\partial X_3} + \cdots + \alpha_n X_n \frac{\partial F}{\partial X_n} = \alpha F. \tag{24}$$

Obviously this can be repeated with λ_L and λ_T to obtain a set of three coupled partial differential equations expressing the fundamental *scale invariance of physical laws (that is, the invariance of the physics to the choice of units)* implicit in Fourier's original work. These equations can be solved without too much difficulty; their solution is, in fact, a special case of the solution to the renormalization group equation (given explicitly). Not too surprisingly, one finds that the solution is precisely equivalent to the constraints of dimensional analysis. Thus there is never any explicit need to use these rather cumbersome equations: ordinary dimensional analysis takes care of it for you!

II Non-Relativistic Treatment

In the following few sections, we shall study the non-relativistic theory of electron scattering from composite systems with emphasis upon the asymptotic region. In order to minimize the algebra, we shall limit the discussion to the case of spinless particles and keep only the conventional electric (Coulomb) interaction. Generalizations to spinning particles and magnetic interactions are straightforward and will be dealt with in a relativistic way in later sections. For a non-relativistic discussion, the reader is referred to the literature.

A Cross-Section Formulae

We begin by considering spinless non-relativistic scattering from a target composed of $\mathcal{Z}$ scattering centers such as is the case of a nucleus or of a macroscopic liquid. The formalism that I shall review applies in fact almost precisely to the case of thermal neutron scattering from liquids. In general, the process to be discussed is illustrated in Fig. 1: the scattered probe particle (an electron, say) is detected without regard to the fate of the target final states. In terms of the energy loss (ν) and momentum transfer (q) it is convenient to introduce the structure function (appropriate to Coulomb scattering).

$$W(\nu, q^2) \equiv \frac{(d^2\sigma/d\Omega dE)}{(d\sigma/d\Omega)_{\text{Ruth}}}$$

$$\text{where} \quad \left(\frac{d\sigma}{d\Omega'}\right)_{\text{Ruth}} = \left(\frac{e^2}{2mv^2 \sin^2 \frac{1}{2}\theta}\right)^2 \tag{25}$$

is the classical Rutherford scattering cross-section for structureless particles. [For liquids one factors out the cross-section for the magnetic interaction of the neutron probe with the constituent atoms; for such cases the symbol S is used for W and ω for ν][11]. From the Fermi golden rule W is given by

$$W(\nu,q^2) = \sum_f |< \Psi_f|\sum_{i=1}^{z} Q_i e^{iq.\underline{r}_i}|\Psi_0 > |^2 \delta(E_f - E_o + \nu) \tag{26}$$

where Q_i is the charge of the i'th constituent whose position is $\underline{r}_i$. $\Psi_{0(f)}$ is the initial (final) state of the target. [For the moment I shall assume that the constituent is structureless; to include its structure, one simply replaces Q_i by the relevant elastic form factor][3].

As has already been emphasized in the Introduction all of the interesting physics is contained in the structure function W which can be extracted from the data by simply observing deviations from point Rutherford scattering. The special power of electron scattering is that it allows one to trace out W as a function of both of its variables, in contrast to photoabsorption, say, where one is restricted to teh $\nu = |q|$ plane. It should be noted, however, that in electron scattering

$$q^2 \cong \nu^2 + 4EE'\sin^2\frac{1}{2}\theta \tag{27}$$

which restricts $|q| \geq \nu$. The structure function W is, in fact, closely related to the generalized oscillator strengths introduced over 40 years ago by Bethe[6] and still extensively used in atomic physics.

There is a trick that can be used to eliminate the sum over final states (f) and express W as a ground state expectation value. The point to notice is that if the δ-function were absent in Eq. (26) then the completeness of final states allows one to replace the sum $\sum_f |\Psi_f >< \Psi_f|$ by unity. So, the first step is to replace the delta function by

$$\delta[E_f - E_o + \nu] = \int_{-\infty}^{\infty} \frac{dt}{2\pi} e^{i(E_f - E_o + \nu)t} \tag{28}$$

The phase factors $e^{iE_f t}$ and $e^{-iE_o t}$ can be moved so that they stand next to their corresponding wave functions $|\Psi_o >$ and $< \Psi_f|$. Since E_o and E_f are eigenvalues of the target Hamiltonian H we end up requiring the product of operators $e^{iHt}e^{-iq.\underline{r}_i(o)}e^{-iHt}$ which, by virtue of the Heisenberg equations of motion (or, equivalently, time translation) is $e^{-iq.\underline{r}_i(t)}$. Identifying $t = o$ in the original equation is clearly arbitrary. Putting all of this together allows one to re-express Eq. (26) in the form

$$W(\nu,q^2) = \int_{-\infty}^{\infty} \frac{dt}{2\pi} e^{i\nu t} < \Psi_0|\sum_{i,j} Q_i Q_j e^{iq.\underline{r}(t)} e^{-iq.\underline{r}(o)}|\Psi_0 > \tag{29}$$

The price paid for eliminating the sum over final states is the need for knowledge of the time development of $\underline{r}_i(t)$. This, of course, is governed by the Hamiltonian of the system whose general structure is taken to be

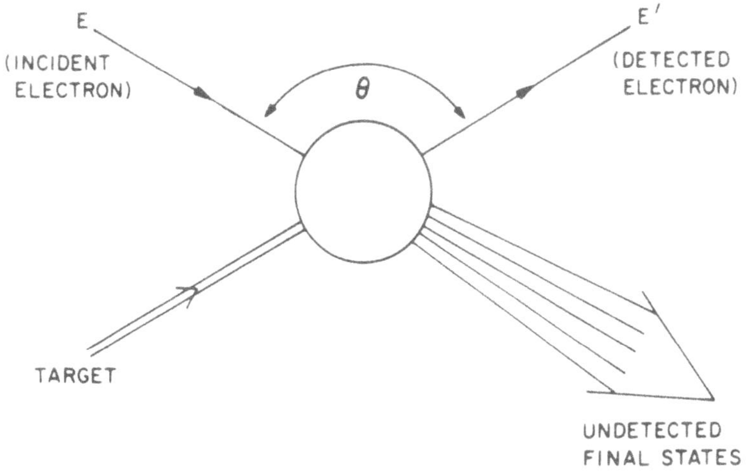

Figure 4. General graph illustrating inclusive scattering from an arbitrary target.

$$H = -\sum_i \frac{\nabla_i^2}{2\mu} + \mathsf{V}(\underline{r}_1, \cdots\cdots, \underline{r}_Z) \tag{30}$$

where μ is the mass of the constituents. Although we will not need to do this in what follows, it is usually assumed that the potential V can be expressed as a sum of 2-body potentials.

$$\mathsf{V}(\underline{r}_1 \cdots \underline{r}_Z) = \sum_{i<j} v(\underline{r}_i - \underline{r}_j) \tag{31}$$

Indeed this usually leads to a 2nd quantized many-body description in terms of creation-destruction operators $a_{\underline{k}}$:

$$W(\nu, q^2) = \int_{-\infty}^{\infty} \frac{dt}{2\pi} e^{i\nu t} < \Psi_0 | [\rho_q(t), \rho_q(o)] | \Psi_0 > \tag{32}$$

The density operator is given by

$$\rho_q \equiv \sum_{\underline{k}} a^{+}_{\underline{k}+q} a_{\underline{k}} \tag{33}$$

Its time development is controlled by the Hamiltonian, Eq. (30) which, in this formalism, can be expressed as

$$H = \sum_{\underline{k}} \frac{\underline{k}^2}{2\mu} a^{+}_{k} a_k + \frac{1}{2} \sum_{k} v(\underline{k}) \rho^{+}_{\underline{k}} \rho_{\underline{k}} \tag{34}$$

$v(\underline{k})$ is just the Fourier transform of the 2-body potential $v(r)$ defined through Eq. (31). This

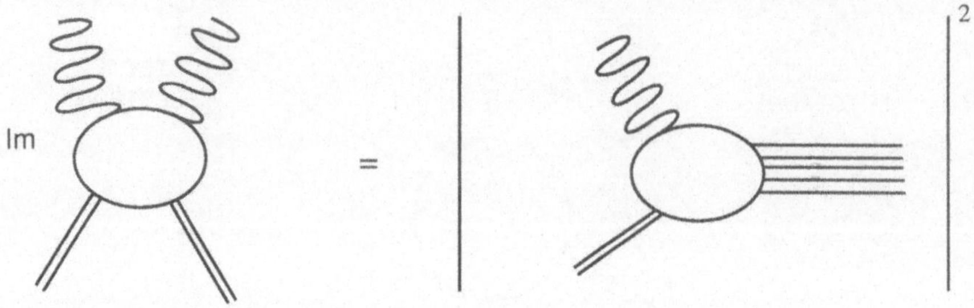

Figure 5. The Optical Theorem relating W to the imaginary past of the forward virtual Compton amplitude.

field theoretic description of Eqs. (26) and (29) allows one to think of W as the imaginary part of the corresponding (virtual) photon, forward Compton scattering amplitude as illustrated in Fig. 5. The question we wish to address is what is the behaviour of W when q becomes very large?

B Elastic Scattering

As an interesting example we shall first consider the case of elastic scattering which is defined by the constraint that $\Psi_f = \Psi_o$, i.e., the target remains in its ground state. In this case, θ and E' are no longer independent variables and the cross-section reduces to a singly differential form:

$$\frac{d\sigma}{d\Omega'} = \left(\frac{d\sigma}{d\Omega'}\right)_{\text{Ruth}} |F(q)|^2 \tag{35}$$

The function $F(q)$ is usually called the *elastic form factor* of the target.

$$F(q) \equiv \langle \Psi_0 | \sum_i Q_i \exp\,(iq.r_i) | \Psi_0 \rangle \tag{36}$$

Notice that it is normalized to the total static charge of the target:

$$F(0) = \langle \Psi_0 | \sum_i Q_i | \Psi_0 \rangle = \sum_i Q_i. \tag{37}$$

In terms of the coordinate space representation of the wave function $\langle r_1, \cdots, r_i, \cdots, r_N | \Psi_0 \rangle$, Eq. (36) reads

$$F(q) = \sum_i Q_i \int d^3 r_1 \cdots d^3 r_N \exp\,(iq.r_i) |\langle r_1, \cdots, r_N | \Psi_0 \rangle|^2. \tag{38}$$

We can, of course, also write a momentum space representation

$$F(q) = \sum_i \int \frac{d^3 k_1}{(2\pi)^3} \cdots \frac{d^3 k_N}{(2\pi)^3} Q_i \langle \Psi_0 | k_1, \cdots, k_i + q, \cdots, k_N \rangle \langle k_1, \cdots, k_N | \Psi_0 \rangle. \tag{39}$$

In the special case where all of the constituents are identical and the wave function is symmetric, (39) simplifies to read

$$F(q) = \mathcal{Z} \int d^3 r \rho(r) \exp{(iq.r)} \tag{40}$$

where

$$\rho(r) = \int d^3 r_2 \cdots d^3 r_N |\langle \Psi_0 | r, r_2, \cdots, r_N \rangle|^2 \tag{41}$$

$\rho(r)$ represents the single particle density distribution where in the last line we have assumed a spherically symmetric charge distribution. This was used extensively by nuclear experimentalists in interpreting their data [12] and it is worthwhile briefly discussing some of its implications:

i)The small q^2 behavior of $F_B(q)$ reflects the large r behavior of $\rho(r)$ [and vice-versa as emphasized in (iii) below]. Now, outside of the effective nuclear well seen by a single constituent the wave function must be of the form $\psi(r) \sim e^{-\alpha r}/r$ where $\alpha = \sqrt{2\mu\epsilon}$ and ϵ is the single particle binding energy. Taking the standard value of $\sim 15\,MeV$ for ϵ leads to $\alpha \cong 170\,MeV$. The large r behavior of $\rho(r)$ is usually parametrized by the experimentalists in terms of a skin depth [12] which in this notation is $1/2\ \alpha$. Using the value of *170 MeV* for α leads to a skin depth of *0.58 fm* in remarkably good agreement with the data.

ii) The saturation of nuclear forces implies that the size of this effective well, $a \propto N^{1/3}$ again in good agreement with experiment. The constant of proportionality is found to be $\sim 1.08\,fm$[12].

iii) For smaller values of r we might intuitively expect $\rho(r)$ to flatten out and remain relatively smooth; in particular, we would not expect it to develop a singular structure, and thus look like Fig. (6). This kind of behavior of $\rho(r)$ is, of course, the origin of the diffractive phenomena exhibited by $F(q)$ and illustrated so nicely in Fig. (7). The dips can be expected at values of q given approximately by $|q|a \sim \pi/2$. For the data shown in Fig.(7) this leads to $a \sim 3.5\,fm$ in agreement with the fit mentioned in (ii) above. As was emphasized in the Introduction, diffractive effects depend upon the existence of an "edge" in the distribution. For few body systems, such an edge many not be well defined as in the case, for example, of the hydrogen atom or molecule, where the wave function is of the form $\exp(-r/a_0)$, a_0 being the equivalent Bohr radius. The form factor corresponding to this type of wave function is generally smooth; for example, for a hydrogen-like wave function, it is of the dipole form

$$F(q) = \left(\frac{1}{1 + q^2 a_0^2}\right)^2 . \tag{42}$$

This gives an excellent fit to the hydrogen data.

iv) Another interesting property of $F(q)$ is its asymptotic form which is clearly sensitive to the short distance behavior of $\rho(r)$. By repeated integration by parts (Riemann – Lebesgue lemma) we can derive the following asymptotic series

$$F_B(q)^2 \ {}^{q^2} \overset{\to \infty}{\to} \ 4\pi \sum_{m=1}^{\infty} \frac{(-1)^m}{(q^2)^m} \left(\frac{d}{dr}\right)^{2(m-1)} [r\rho(r)]_{r=0} . \tag{43}$$

From this, it immediately follows that if $\rho(r)$ is sufficiently smooth at the origin (i.e., it is not singular there), then

$$F_B(q^2) \ {}^{q^2} \overset{\to \infty}{\to} \ 1/q^4 . \tag{44}$$

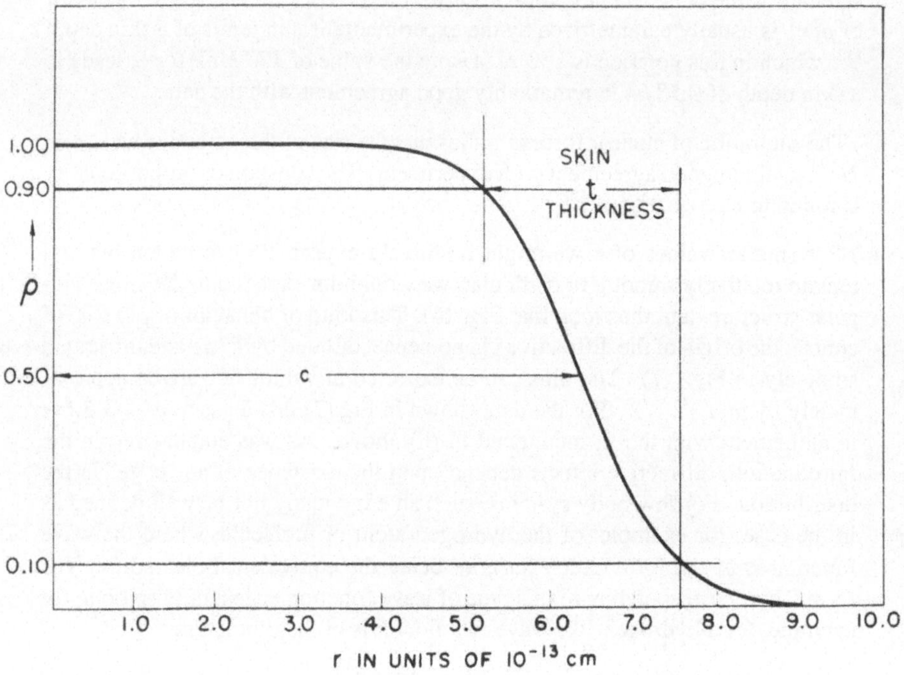

Figure 6. Typical nuclear single particle density distribution $\rho(r)$ versus r (in fm), arbitrarily normalized. This illustrates the radius c and surface thickness t (see ref. [12]).

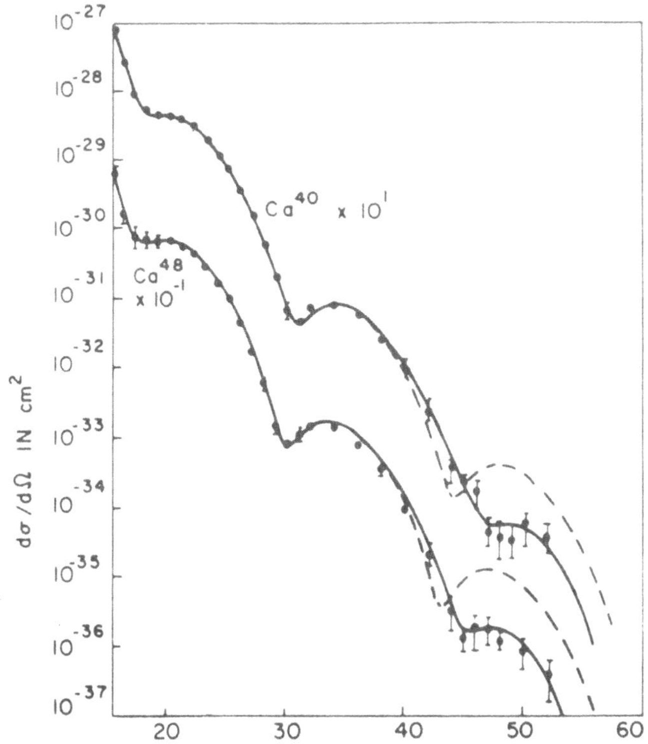

Figure 7. Differential cross-section (in cm^2 versus angle (in degrees) for elastic scattering of 757 MeV incident electrons from ^{40}Ca and ^{48}Ca illustrating diffraction phenomena (taken from ref. [12]; the dashed curve is a theoretical prediction).

In other words, if the probability for finding a particle at the origin remains finite, then the elastic form factor falls off at least as fast as $1/q^4$. We shall refer to this as the natural asymptotic behavior of the form factor. The data discussed in the Introduction is consistent with this result. Perhaps the most fascinating aspect of that data is the fact that the nucleon form factor also falls like $1/q^4$ where q is now the four- momentum transferred. This is suggestive of the idea that a relativistic analogue of the above argument can be made to show that $1/q^4$ is the "natural" behavior of a relativistic bound state system. One might expect such an argument to involve a smoothness postulate for the covariant charge density near the light cone; we shall briefly return to this problem in section 8. Meanwhile, it is worth reiterating the observation that from this point of view the nucleon is somewhat paradoxical since its form factors are so smooth. Indeed, the elastic form factor can be fitted with the dipole form, used for the hydrogen molecule!

$$F(q^2) = \left(\frac{1}{1 - q^2/0.71 GeV^2/c^2}\right)^2 \tag{45}$$

This fit, incidentally, corresponds to a binding energy of $\sim 350\,MeV$, which is not an unreasonable number! It would seem difficult, therefore, to construct a model of the nucleon which contains more than, at most, three constituents if we are to constrain the form factor to be so smooth.

C Sum rules and x-scaling

In this section, we shall focus attention upon some general model-independent aspects of the scattering by discussing the derivation of certain sum rules. Their deviation goes back to the work of Bethe, although Heisenberg[6] was the first to derive them in the form we shall present here. The extension to nuclear physics has been carried out by several authors[13]. Later, we shall attempt to derive their relativistic analogue which will hopefully be applicable to the nucleon. In any case, we shall show that these sum rules can be used to motivate the phenomenon of Bjorken scaling[14] for non-relativistic systems, i.e., we shall show that as $q^2 \to \infty$, the combination $vW(q^2, \nu)$ becomes a function of the dimensionless variable $x \equiv q^2/2M\nu$ only.

Returning to the representation (3) it is clear that integrating over ν at fixed q leads to

$$\begin{aligned} I(q^2) &\equiv \int_{-\infty}^{\infty} d\nu W(\nu, q^2) = \sum_{ij=1}^{Z} \langle \Psi_o | Q_i Q_j e^{iq.(r_i - r_j)} | \Psi_o \rangle \\ &= \sum_{i=1}^{Z} Q_i^2 + \sum_{ij=1}^{Z} Q_i Q_j \langle \Psi_o | e^{iq.(r_i - r_j)} | \Psi_0 \rangle \end{aligned} \tag{46}$$

Notice that by integrating over ν we now only require the coordinates r_i and r_j at the same time so that, as operators, they now commute. Effectively, this means that by forming the sum rule, the explicit dynamics is integrated out. It is convenient to separate the double sum over i and j into incoherent and coherent contributions; thus

$$I(q^2) = \sum_{i=1}^{Z} Q_i^2 + \sum_{ij=1}^{Z} Q_i Q_j \langle \Psi_o | e^{iq.(r_i - r_j)} | \Psi_0 \rangle \tag{47}$$

Notice that the second term (the "two-particle correlation function") is similar in structure to the elastic form factor in that it is a Fourier transform. As such, it can be expected to drop rapidly to zero when $q^2 \to \infty$. Thus, for identical particles with $Q_i = 1$,

$$I(q^2) \to \begin{cases} Z \text{ when } q^2 \to \infty \\ Z^2 \text{ when } q^2 = 0 \end{cases} \tag{48}$$

showing how the two extreme regimes pick out the incoherent from the coherent. In general, the *sum rule has integrated out the explicit dependence on dynamics so that the approach to scaling for $I(q^2)$ is completely governed by correlations alone.*

Now, below elastic threshold where the target stays intact and recoils (in the Lab. frame) with energy $q^2/2M$, W necessarily vanishes; thus, for $\nu < q^2/2M$, $W = 0$. The asymptotic form of the sum rule therefore reads

$$\lim_{q^2 \to \infty} \int_{q^2/2M}^{\infty} d\nu W(\nu, q^2) \approx \sum_{i=1}^{Z} Q_i^2 \tag{49}$$

It is obviously convenient to scale q^2 out of the limits on the integral by introducing the non-relativistic version of the Bjorken scaling variable [7]

$$x \equiv \frac{q^2}{2M\nu} \tag{50}$$

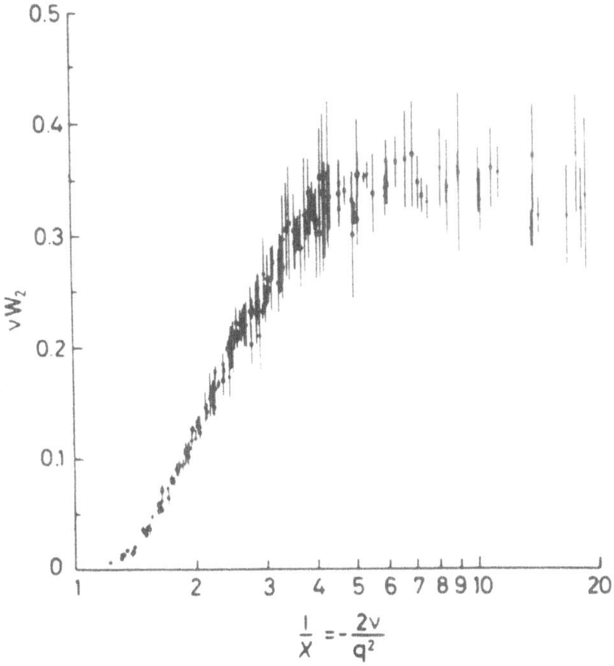

Figure 8. Plot of μW vs. 1/x for various values of q^2 taken from early SLAC data. The data lies on a universal scaling curve.

In that case, Eq. (14) becomes

$$\lim_{q^2 \to \infty} I(q^2) = \lim_{q^2 \to \infty} \int_o^1 \frac{dx}{x} \nu W(\nu, q^2) = \sum_{i=1}^{z} Q_i^2 \tag{51}$$

This is identical in structure to the sum rule derived above for the watershed problem, namely, that an integral which naively might have been expected to depend on q^2 is, in fact, a constant. As in the rainfall problem this result followed from a conservation law. The similarity can be carried further by recalling that (just as we had there $q > 0$) so here $W > 0$. $W > 0$, suggests (but certainly does not prove) that the integrand, namely

$$F(q^2, x) \equiv \nu W(q^2, \nu) \tag{52}$$

itself becomes independent of q^2 and a function of x alone. This is Bjorken x-scaling and is illustrated in Fig. 8. Note that the data shown there is taken in a relativistic domain with q^2 being the square of the 4-momentum transferred. As already discussed, the "derivation" of scaling from the sum rule is no more than heuristic since to prove that $F(q^2, x)$ scales would require showing that every moment sum rule of F exists and is independent of q^2. In fact, in relativistic quantum field theory based on the QCD Lagrangian, scaling is proven via a consideration of all such moments. We return to this later.

III Dynamics and Scaling

It would be nice to derive scaling directly for the structure function itself. To do so, let us examine the first-quantized expression, Eq. (29). It is worth remarking that although much formal and phenomenological work has been based upon the 2nd quantized representation, Eq. (32), (especially for liquids)[11,13] it turns out to be much more convenient for our purposes to stay with the first quantized version. We had

$$W(\nu,q^2) = \int_{-\infty}^{\infty} \frac{dt}{2\pi} e^{i\nu t} \langle \Psi_o | \sum_{i,j} Q_i Q_j e^{iq.\underline{r}_i(t)} e^{-iq.\underline{r}_j(o)} | \Psi_0 \rangle \tag{53}$$

The phase operator can be re-expressed as follows:

$$\begin{aligned} e^{-iq.\underline{r}_i(t)} e^{iq.\underline{r}_j(o)} &= \left[e^{iHt} e^{-iq.\underline{r}_i(o)} e^{iHt} \right] e^{iq.\underline{r}_j(o)} \\ &= e^{iHt} \left[e^{-iq.\underline{r}_i} e^{-iHt} e^{iq.\underline{r}_i} \right] \left[e^{-iq.\underline{r}_i} e^{iq.\underline{r}_j} \right] \end{aligned} \tag{54}$$

where, in the second line, we have inserted $1 \equiv e^{iq.\underline{r}_i} e^{-iq.\underline{r}_i}$. Notice that all operators are now to be evaluated at equal times. The terms in the second square bracket of the second line simply distinguish the coherent ($i \neq j$) from the incoherent ($i = j$) as in Eq. (47) of the sum rule. If we think of H as expressed in terms of conjugate coordinates $\underline{p}_i$ (momentum) and $\underline{r}_i$ then the first bracket can be expressed as

$$e^{-iq.\underline{r}_i} e^{iH(\underline{p}_i,\underline{r}_i)} e^{iq.\underline{r}_i} = e^{-iH(\underline{p}+q,\underline{r}_i)} \tag{55}$$

i.e., simply as a shift of the momentum of the 'ith particle by q. If we assume that H has the usual general structure represented in Eq. (31), then

$$H(\underline{p}_i + q, \underline{r}_i) = H(\underline{p}_i, \underline{r}_i) + \frac{q^2 + 2\underline{p}_i.q}{2\mu} \tag{56}$$

This allows us to write

$$e^{iq.\underline{r}_i(t)} e^{-iq.\underline{r}_j(o)} = e^{iHt} e^{-i[H+\underline{p}_i.q/\mu]t} e^{iq^2 t/2\mu} e^{iq.(\underline{r}_i-\underline{r}_j)} \tag{57}$$

We now make use of the operator identity:

$$e^{iHt} e^{-i[H+\underline{p}_i.q/\mu]t} = T e^{iq/\mu . \int_o^t \underline{p}_i(t')dt'} \tag{58}$$

where T is the usual time-ordering symbol[15]. This can be proven as a variant of the Baher-Hansdorf lemma. Putting all of this together we arrive at the following expression for W:

$$W(\nu,q^2) = \int_{-\infty}^{\infty} \frac{dt}{2\pi} e^{i[\nu - q^2/2\mu]t} \langle \Psi_o | \sum_{ij=1}^{z} Q_i Q_j e^{iq.(\underline{r}_j - \underline{r}_i)} T e^{iq/\mu . \int_o^t p_i(t')dt'} | \Psi_o \rangle \tag{59}$$

If we express this as a function of q^2 and x rather than q^2 and ν by using the definition (50), then the first phase-factor in (59) becomes

$$i\left(\nu - \frac{q^2}{2\mu}\right)t = -i\frac{q^2 t}{2\mu x}\left(x - \frac{\mu}{M}\right) \tag{60}$$

The second phase factor $e^{iq\cdot(\underline{r}_j-\underline{r}_i)}$ distinguishes between the incoherent ($i = j$, where it ceases to oscillate) and the coherent ($i \neq j$); this was discussed in the context of the sum rule following Eq. (47). For large q^2 we need only keep the incoherent piece where $\sum Q_i Q_j \to \sum Q_i^2$. The final phase factor (which involves the momentum operator p_i) remains $O(q)$ when $q^2 \to \infty$ at fixed x. In this limit the first factor, Eq. (60) therefore dominates since it is $O(q^2)$. *Thus, as with sum rule, all explicit dependence on dynamical operators eventually disappears in the Bjorken limit* and we are left with

$$\begin{aligned} F(q^2, x) &\equiv \nu W(q^2, \nu) \\ &\approx \left(\sum_i Q_1^2\right) \delta\left(x - \frac{\mu}{M}\right) \end{aligned} \tag{61}$$

In other words νW does indeed scale to a function of x only but the result is independent both of dynamics and the structure of the target! The sum rule (49) is thereby satisfied in an essentially trivial fashion: by choosing this set of variables, one is effectively making the scattering appear as if from completely static constituents. This is therefore not a particularly useful way of presenting the data for non-relativistic systems since one learns little directly about the dynamics or momentum distribution of the target. As already indicated above, such is not the case for the relativistic situation.

IV y-Scaling

We saw in the previous section that, although νW can be expected to scale to a function of x only, the result is relatively uninteresting as far as extracting useful information about the target is concerned. As already intimated above, the reason is that in the Bjorken limit the quasielastic piece in (59) grows like q^2 [as explicitly shown in (60)] whereas the dynamical piece only grows like q. To extract dynamics we need to make both of these pieces of comparable magnitude when $q \to \infty$. This is the rationale for y-scaling.

To further motivate y-scaling it is useful to use the equation of motion:

$$\frac{d\underline{p}_i}{dt} = i[H, \underline{p}_i] = -\nabla_i V(\underline{r}_1, \cdots \underline{r}_Z) \equiv F_i \tag{62}$$

where F_i is the force felt by the ith constituent due to the presence of all other constituents. This can be formally solved to read

$$p_i(t) = p_i(o) + \int_o^t dt' F_i(t'). \tag{63}$$

When substituted into (59) this leads to the following exact expression:

$$W(\nu, q^2) = \langle \Psi_0 | \sum_{i,j=1}^{Z} Q_i Q_j e^{iq\cdot(\underline{r}_i - \underline{r}_j)} T \int_{-\infty}^{\infty} \frac{dt}{2\pi} e^{i\frac{qt}{\mu}[\mu y - p_{iz} - \int_o^t (1-t'/t) F_{iz}(t') dt']} | \Psi_0 \rangle \tag{64}$$

Here we have defined the z-direction as that of q and introduced the dimensionless variable

$$y \equiv \frac{2\mu\nu - q^2}{2\mu q} \tag{65}$$

If we now think in terms of $q \to \infty$ at fixed y (rather than x) then the static quasielastic ($q^2 = 2\mu\nu$) and dynamical contributions have equal weight. To see how this leads to y-scaling introduce $\beta \equiv qt$ (and $\beta' \equiv qt'$) then the incoherent part of Eq. (64) can be re-expressed as

$$qW(\nu, q^2) = \langle \Psi_0 | \sum_{i=1}^{\mathcal{Z}} Q_i^2 T \int_{-\infty}^{\infty} \frac{d\beta}{2\pi} e^{i\beta[y - \frac{p_{iz}}{\mu} - \frac{1}{q}\int_0^{\beta} d\beta'(1-\frac{\beta'}{\beta})\frac{F_i(\beta'/q)}{\mu}]} | \Psi_0 \rangle \tag{66}$$

Apart from suppressing the coherent contribution which vanishes rapidly with q^2, this expression is exact. Now, if we take $q \to \infty$ at fixed y, it is clear that the term in the exponent containing F_i also eventually vanishes and we are left with

$$\mathcal{F}(y, q^2) \equiv qW(\nu, q^2) \to < \Psi_0 | \sum_{i=1}^{\mathcal{Z}} Q_i^2 \delta(y - \frac{p_{iz}}{\mu}) | \Psi_0 > \tag{67}$$

Thus F becomes a function of y only; its form clearly depends on the internal structure of the targets through the momentum operator p_i.

Like the result of x-scaling, y-scaling reflects incoherent quasi-elastic scattering from the constituents. However, whereas the former corresponds to a "static" snapshot of the target, the latter allows for a "dynamic" picture. To see this more explicitly let us express (67) in a momentum representation (in which k_i is the eigenvalue of p_i):

$$\mathcal{F}(y, q^2) \approx \sum_i Q_i^2 \int \frac{d^3 k_1}{(2\pi)^3} \cdots \frac{d^3 k_{\mathcal{Z}}}{(2\pi)^3} | < \Psi_0 | \underline{k}_1 \cdots \underline{k}_{\mathcal{Z}} > |^2 \delta(k_{iz} - \mu y). \tag{68}$$

If $|f(\underline{k}_i)|^2$ is a single-particle momentum distribution defined by

$$|f(k_i)|^2 \equiv \left[\int \frac{d^3 k}{(2\pi)^3} \right]_i | < \Psi_0 | \underline{k}_1 \cdots \underline{k}_i \cdots \underline{k}_{\mathcal{Z}} > |^2 \tag{69}$$

where the integration symbol means integrate over the momenta of <u>all</u> the constituents <u>except</u> the i'th, then (in the symmetric case), (68) reduces to

$$\mathcal{F}(y, q^2) \approx \mathcal{Z} \int \frac{d^2 k_\perp}{(2\pi)^3} \int_{-\infty}^{\infty} dk_z |f(k_\perp, k_z)|^2 \delta(k_z - \mu y) \tag{70}$$

Thus for large q^2 , $\mathcal{F}(y, q^2) \equiv qW(\nu, q^2)$ *scales to a function of* y *which measures the longitudinal momentum distribution of constituents inside the target.*

It is clear from this discussion that the approach to $y-$ scaling is governed by correlations as well as explicit dynamics. The expression given in Eq. (64) allows for a systematic expansion in powers of $1/q$. [Actually, with some reasonable approximations, one can translate this into an expansion in power of $e^{1/q}$][16]. Thus the scaling phenomenon simply reflects the fact that the target can be well described by $\mathcal{Z}$ scattering centers. In this sense, it is the correction and the approach to scaling that contain the really interesting physics. On the other hand, in the high energy case discussed above where it was <u>not</u> known that hadrons were definitely composed of quarks, the scaling phenomena itself was the clearest evidence for the ultimate establishment of the quark model. It should be pointed out that the relativistic analogue of y-scaling is, in fact, x-scaling (even though x-scaling is "trivial" non-relativistically!) Thus in the relativistic Bjorken limit $F(q^2, x) \equiv \nu W(q^2, \nu)$ "measures" the momentum distribution of quarks inside hadrons much like $\mathcal{F}(q^2, y) \equiv qW(q^2, \nu)$ measures that of nucleons inside nuclei or atoms inside liquids.

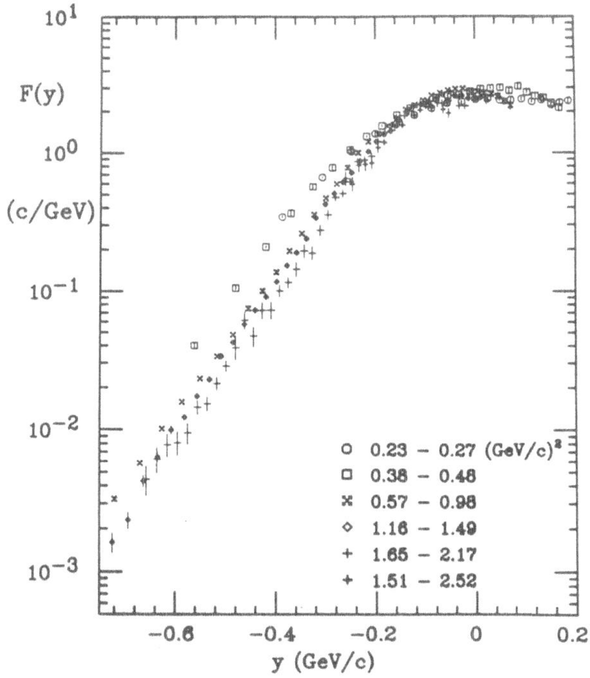

Figure 9. Y-scaling for quasi elastic electron nucleus scattering on ^{12}C.

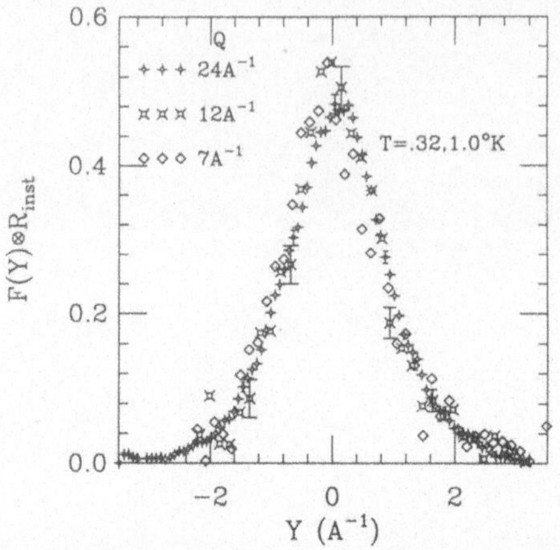

Figure 10. Y-scaling for deep inelastic neutron scattering on superfluid ^{4}He. Data from ref. [18].

Typical scaling curves for electron scattering from nuclear targets ($\lesssim GeV$range) and for neutron scattering from liquids (($\lesssim KeV$range) are shown in Figs. 9[17] and 10[18]. When developed, the theoretical discussion above leads to many interesting results which are in agreement with these data. Some of these are the following:

- Scaling results whether F_i is a confining force or not; this is clear from Eq. (26). Thus even for interparticle potentials $V(r) \sim r^n$ for $r \longrightarrow \infty$, the system behaves as if the constituents were essentially free.

- Corrections arising from dynamical effects (i.e. from finite F_i/q effects) dominate those due to correlations. An expansion in this parameter leads to the conclusion that, for (non-relativistic nuclei), scaling should be approached from above as $q^2 \longrightarrow \infty$; see Fig. 9. Furthermore, this correction should vanish at $y = 0$. These systematics are confirmed by the data - see Fig. 9.

- For a symmetric system one can derive the exact result that [3]

$$\mathcal{F}(0, q^2) \equiv \langle \frac{\mu}{2k} \rangle \tag{71}$$

  Taking $u(r) \sim e^{-\alpha r}/r$ as a single-particle wave function for a nucleus (where $\alpha \approx 170\, MeV$ is solely determined by the binding energy) leads to $\mathcal{F}(0) \sim 2$. This is again in reasonable agreement with the data showing how the overall normalization of the data can be understood.

- In terms of $\mathcal{F}$, the sum rule (49) reads

$$\int_{-\infty}^{\infty} dy \mathcal{F}(y, q^2) \approx \sum Q_i^2 \tag{72}$$

  which, because $|\Psi_0\rangle$ is normalized to unity, is in agreement with Eq. (49).

- It is straightforward to derive other sum rules; for example

$$\int_{-\infty}^{\infty} dy y^2 \mathcal{F}(y\ ,\ q^2) \approx (\sum Q_i^2)\frac{2}{3}\langle\frac{T}{\mu}\rangle \tag{73}$$

where $T \equiv \bar{p}^2/2\mu$ is the kinetic energy operator. Thus this second moment of $\mathcal{F}$ measures the mean kinetic energy of the constituents. More generally one can derive an infinite sequence of sum rules which relate moments of $\mathcal{F}$ to matrix elements of operators:

$$\int_{-\infty}^{\infty} dy y^{2n} \mathcal{F}(y\ ,\ q^2) \approx (\sum_i Q_i^2)\langle\Psi_0|\sum_{m=0}^{\infty} a_m p^{2(n-m)} \left(\frac{F}{\mu q}\right)^m |\Psi_0\rangle \tag{74}$$

Although this is not particularly useful in non-relativistic systems where one can work directly with the original expression Eq. (64), its analogue in relativistic field theory is the key to progress, as briefly discussed in Section IV.

- In liquids (and even possibly in nuclei) the interparticle potential contains a hard core which means that F_i cannot be smoothly defined over all space. This requires special treatment –indeed, as discussed elsewhere in these proceedings, Silver [19] has suggested that, although scaling is not spoiled by the presence of hard-core potentials, the naïve interpretation in terms of momentum distribution needs to be revised. He has suggested a convolution structure which incorporates the hard-core as a final-state effect.

- Perhaps one of the most peculiar aspects of the nuclear data is that, over a considerable range of y, $\mathcal{F}(y) \sim e^{-a|y|}$. There seems to be no straightforward reason why $\mathcal{F}(y)$ should exhibit such a simple structure.

- Finally we should emphasize that relativistic corrections (to y-scaling) have been completely ignored . These are important for the nuclear case because much of the data is in a kinematic range where $|q| \gtrsim |GeV$ i.e. where $q^2/\mu^2 \gtrsim 0(1)$. Estimating these corrections in the region below which relativistic Bjorken scaling relevant to a quark-gluon description is a difficult business. Kinematic attempts in which relativistic kinematics is substituted in the essentially non-relativistic formulae are clearly not entirely justifiable even though they probably account for some important effects.[20] Unfortunately this clouds the issue of how one extracts meaningful information from the data. It is important to note that an added complication in the relativistic regime is that mesons can be produced. Since these are new degrees of freedom beyond the nucleonic ones, scaling is thereby broken, as is clearly seen in Fig. 9. Meson production is the origin of the scale violations seen for $y > 0$. It is amusing that the same problem occurs in the ultra- relativistic case where gluons are ultimately produced. However, it is the magic of QCD and its attendant property of asymptotic freedom that limits such scaling violations to be only logarithmic in nature. Indeed, as emphasized in Section IV, the precise nature of the logarithms are an "exact" prediction of the theory and their brilliant experimental confirmation is one of the main reasons that QCD is accepted today as the theory of the strong interactions!

V Relativistic Treatment (QCD)

A Preliminaries

The relativistically covariant generalization of the structure function W, introduced in Eq. (26), is the tensor

$$W_{\mu\nu} = \sum_N \langle p|j_\mu(0)|N\rangle\langle N|j_\nu(0)|p\rangle(2\pi)^3\delta^{(4)}(p_N - p - q). \tag{75}$$

Here $j_\mu(x)$ is the electromagnetic current operator (in the Heisenberg representation) and N is supposed to indicate an arbitrary final state. An average over the polarization in the initial state is implied in $\sum_N$. Note that gauge invariance implies that

$$q^\mu t_{\mu\nu} = t_{\mu\nu}q^\nu = q^\mu W_{\mu\nu} = W_{\mu\nu}q^\nu = 0. \tag{76}$$

The tensorial character of $W_{\mu\nu}$ merely reflects the spin 1 nature of the photon and thus automatically incorporates both electric as well as magnetic interactions.

Now the most general form of $W_{\mu\nu}$ consistent with general invariance properties (e.g., Lorentz, gauge and parity) is [21]

$$W_{\mu\nu} = -W_1(q^2,\nu)\left[g_{\mu\nu} - \frac{q_\mu q_\nu}{q^2}\right] + W_2(q^2,\nu)\left[p_\mu - \frac{M\nu}{q^2}q_\mu\right]\left[p_\nu - \frac{M\nu}{q^2}q^\nu\right] \tag{77}$$

where the W_i are scalar functions of the two independent scalar variables q^2 and $\nu \equiv p.q/M$; note that in the laboratory system ν does indeed reduce to the energy loss of the electron, q^o leads to

$$\frac{d^2\sigma}{dE'd\Omega'} = \left(\frac{d\sigma}{d\Omega'}\right)_{\text{Mott}}[W_2 + 2W_1\tan^2\frac{1}{2}\theta] \tag{78}$$

which is the analog of Eq. (25). The Rutherford cross-section $(d\sigma/d\Omega)_{\text{Ruth}}$ has here been replaced by the Mott cross- section

$$\left(\frac{d\sigma}{d\Omega}\right)_{\text{Mott}} = \frac{\alpha^2\cos^2\frac{1}{2}}{4E^2\sin^4\frac{1}{2}\theta} \tag{79}$$

which is the differential cross-section for the scattering of relativistic electrons from point-like fermions. Note that there are now two structure functions reflecting the possibility of magnetic as well as electric scattering; alternatively they can be related to the possibility of inducing transitions either by transverse (T) or by longitudinal (L) photons. In fact, equivalent total cross-sections for the absorption of either transverse or longitudinal virtual photons are often introduced in place of the W_i. There is obviously some ambiguity as to how one normalizes the invariant flux for such virtual particles and it has become conventional to adopt the Hand[22] definition where the flux is evaluated as if the photons were massless. One thereby finds that

$$W_1(q^2,\nu) = \frac{W^2 - M^2}{2M}\frac{\sigma_T(q^2,\nu)}{4\pi^2 \propto}. \tag{80}$$

and

$$W_2(q^2,\nu) = \frac{-q^2}{\nu^2 - q^2}\frac{W^2 - M^2}{2M}\frac{[\sigma_T(q^2,\nu) + \sigma_L(q^2,\nu]}{4\pi^2 \propto} \tag{81}$$

where we have introduced $W^2 = (p+q)^2 = M^2 + 2M\nu + q^2$; note that W is the invariant mass of the final state.

W_1 is thus a purely transverse structure function whereas W_2 is a combination of longitudinal and transverse. It will prove convenient to introduce a purely longitudinal structure function

$$W_L = W_2\left(1 - \frac{\nu^2}{q^2}\right) - W_1 = \frac{W^2 - M^2}{2M}\frac{\sigma_L(q^2,\nu)}{4\pi^2 \propto}. \tag{82}$$

As before, a use of unitarity (i.e. completeness of the final set of states $|N>$) allows one to express $W_{\mu\nu}$ as a ground state expectation value, analogous to Eq. (29):

$$W_{\mu\nu}(p,q) = \int d^4x e^{iq.x} < p|[j_\mu(x), j_\nu(0)]|p > \tag{83}$$

With quarks as the fundamental degrees of freedom which carry charge, the electromagnetic current is $j_\mu = \sum_i \overline{q}_i Q_i \gamma_\mu q_i$ where the sum runs over all quark-types. Note also that $W_{\mu\nu} = Im\ T_{\mu\nu}$, where $T_{\mu\nu}$ is the corresponding Compton amplitude obtained from (83) by replacing the commutator by a time ordered product:

$$T_{\mu\nu} = \int d^4x e^{iq.x}\langle p|T[j_\mu(x), j_\nu(o)]|p\rangle \tag{84}$$

Below, we shall discuss an essentially free-field toy model for the time-ordered product derived from a scalar field theory. In the real world, of course, the currents are derived from the QCD Lagrangian. This is given by

$$\mathcal{L} = -\frac{1}{4}F^a_{\mu\nu}F^{\mu\nu}_a + \sum_i \overline{q}_i(i\gamma.D - M_i)q_i \tag{85}$$

where

$$F^a_{\mu\nu} \equiv \partial_\mu A^a_\nu - \partial_\nu A^a_\mu + igf^a_{bc}A^b_\mu A^c_\nu \tag{86}$$

and

$$D_\mu \equiv \partial_\mu - igA_\mu \tag{87}$$

The Latin indices (a, b..) refer to colour, f_{abc} are the structure coefficients of the colour group SU(3) and g is the coupling strength.

B The Role of the Light Cone

As already stressed we are interested in the behavior of the W_i when $q^2 \rightarrow \infty$. Relativistically, one might guess that this limit is sensitive to the behaviour of the T-product (or commutator) near $x^2 \approx 0$, i.e. near the lightcone. It is instructive to examine more closely how this comes about. To do so introduce light-cone variables

$$
\begin{aligned}
q_{\pm} &\equiv q_o \pm q_z &(88)\\
\text{and } x_{\pm} &\equiv x_0 \pm z &(89)
\end{aligned}
$$

with the z-direction defined along $\underline{q}$, $[i.e. \underline{q}_{\perp} = \underline{0}]$. Thus $q^2 = q_+q_-, x^2 = x_+x_- - x_{\perp}^2$ and the phase occurring in Eq. (84) is

$$
q.x = 1/2(q_+x_- + q_-x_+). \qquad (90)
$$

Now, in the large q^2 limit

$$
\begin{aligned}
q_+ \approx 2\nu[1 - q^2/4\nu^2 + \cdots] &= 2\nu[1 - x^2/q^2 + \cdots]\\
\text{and } q- \approx q^2/2\nu[1 - (3/4)q^2/\nu^2 + \cdots] &= -x[1 - 3x^2/q^2 + \cdots]\\
\text{where } x &\equiv -q^2/2\nu. \qquad (91)
\end{aligned}
$$

The limit $q^2 \rightarrow \infty$, with x fixed defines the Bjorken limit. In this limit $q^2 \approx 2\nu \rightarrow \infty$. By virtue of the properties of Fourier transforms this drives $x_- \sim 0(2/q_+) \sim 0(1/\nu)$ in the representation (83). Similarly the major contribution to the x_+ integration comes from the region $x_+ \sim 0(2/q_-) \sim 0(2/x)$. Clearly, then, the region that dominates the integrand in Eq. (83) in the Bjorken limit is given by $x^2 \approx -x_{\perp}^2 \leq 0$, i.e. whenever x_μ is **space-like or null**. On the other hand, causality requires that the commutator in (83) vanishes outside of the (forward) light-cone, i.e. the integrand can only be non-zero when x_μ is **time-like or null** ($x^2 \geq 0$). Thus, in the Bjorken limit, all of the contribution to the integral can only come from x_μ null, i.e. from the light- cone itself $x^2 \approx 0$. We therefore need to know the behaviour of products of currents near $x^2 \approx 0$. To get an idea of what this involves it is useful to consider a toy model.

C Toy Model

The toy model[4] consists of treating the fundamental fields $\phi(x)$ (the quarks) as scalars and defining a fictitious scalar current $j(x) = \phi^2(x)$ which is a bilinear in $\phi(x)$ – just as the real current $j_\mu(x)$ is bilinear in the quark fields $q(x)$. As is usual when dealing with singular products of fields, a normal ordering of operators is presumed; this is simply a ruse to remove the infinite zero point energy. We then manipulate the fields as if they were free. In that case the standard Wick expansion leads to

$$\begin{aligned} T[j(x)j(0)] &= T[\phi^2(x)\phi^2(0)] \\ &= -2\Delta_F^2(x,m^2) + 4i\Delta_F(x,m^2)\phi(x)\phi(0) + \phi^2(x)\phi^2(0) \end{aligned} \tag{92}$$

where

$$\Delta_F(x,m^2) \equiv \int \frac{d^4k}{(2\pi)^4}\frac{e^{-ik.x}}{k^2 - m^2 + i\epsilon} \tag{93}$$

is the Feynman propagator, m being the mass associated with $\phi(x)$. Diagramatically, the Compton amplitude, of which W is the imaginary part, is shown in Fig. 11. The first term contains no operator and gives rise to a disconnected graph which does not contribute to the physical deep inelastic scattering. The other two terms give contributions which are precisely analogous to the result of the non-relativistic analysis, and which break up into coherent and incoherent pieces as in Fig. 12. In fact, the analogy can be taken even further when we recall that when $x^2 \approx 0$

$$\Delta_F(x,m^2) \approx \frac{i}{4\pi^2}\frac{1}{x^2 - i\epsilon} + 0(m^2x^2) \tag{94}$$

so that the second term in (92) dominates the third when $x^2 \approx 0$. Thus the leading behaviour for W is given by

$$W(q^2,\nu) \approx Im\int d^4x e^{iq.x}\Delta_F(x,m^2)\langle p|\phi(x)\phi(0)|p\rangle. \tag{95}$$

Suppose now that we introduce a momentum distribution function

$$|f(k)|^2 \equiv \int d^4x e^{-ik.x}\langle p|\phi(x)\phi(0)|p\rangle \tag{96}$$

then Eq. (95) can be re-expressed as

$$W(q^2,\nu) \approx \int \frac{d^4k}{(2\pi)^4}|f(k)|^2\delta[(k+q)^2 - m^2]\theta(k_0+q_0). \tag{97}$$

Now,

$$\delta[(k+q)^2 - m^2] = \frac{1}{2\nu}\delta\left[k_- - x + \frac{k^2 - m^2 - xk_+}{2\nu}\right] \tag{98}$$

so, in the Bjorken limit, where q^2 and ν both $\to \infty$, we are lead to the scaling result:

$$\begin{aligned} \nu W(q^2,\nu) &\equiv F(x,q^2) \\ &\approx \int \frac{d^4k}{(2\pi)^4}|f(k)|^2\delta(k_- - x) \end{aligned} \tag{99}$$

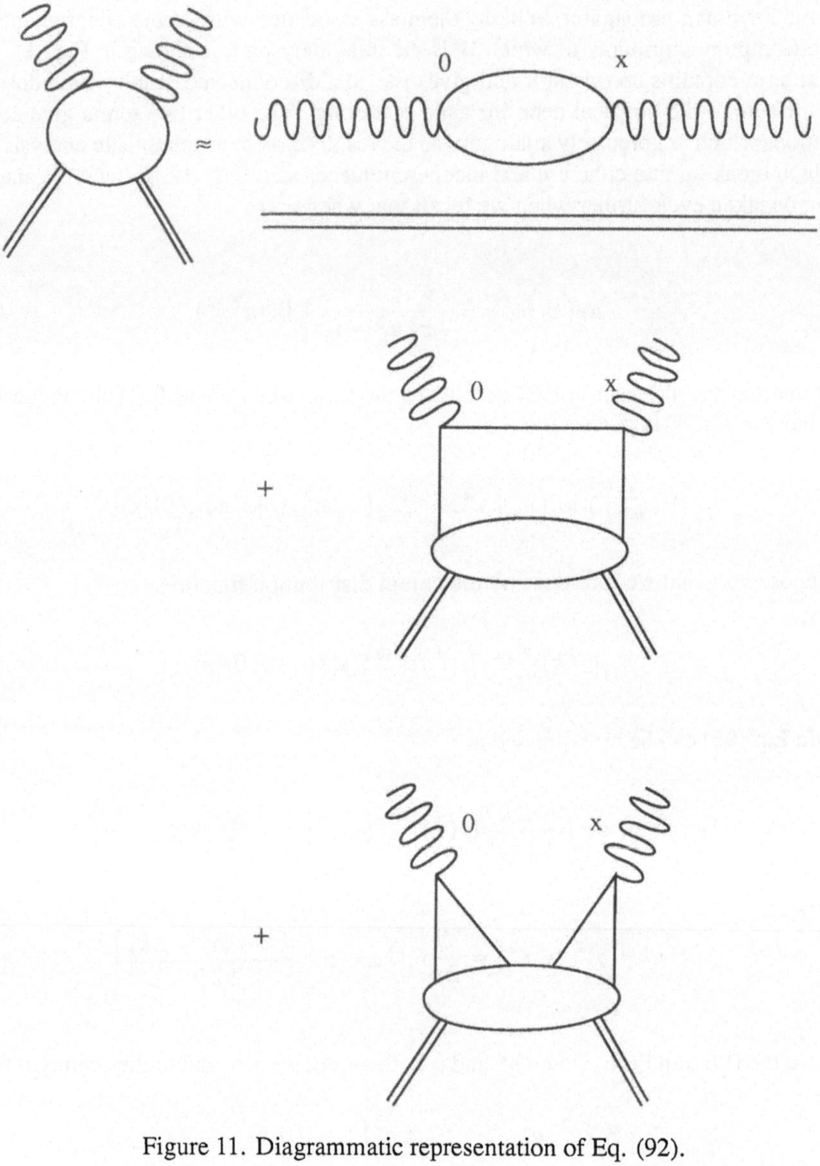

Figure 11. Diagrammatic representation of Eq. (92).

$$q \, W(q^2, v) \equiv F(q^2, y)$$

$$= \text{Im} \sum_i \qquad \text{INCOHERENT}$$

$$+ \text{Im} \sum_{i \neq j} \qquad \text{COHERENT}$$

$$+ \, ...$$

$$+ \text{Im} \sum_{i \neq j} \qquad \text{DYNAMICS}$$

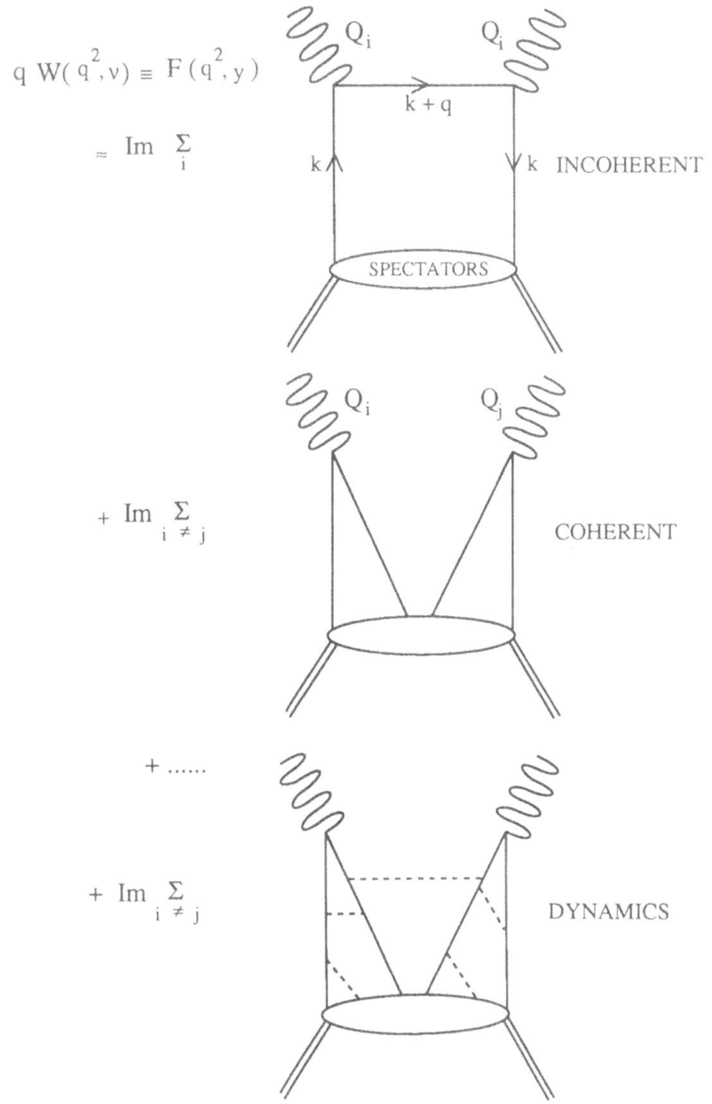

Figure 12. Expansion of the non-relativistic $F(y)$ into incoherent, coherent and dynamical corrections as follows from Eq. (66).

This is clearly the analogue of the non-relativistic many-body formula derived in Eq. (70) and justifies identifying $|f(k)|^2$ of Eq. (96) as a momentum distribution function. It shows that νW scales to a function of x which in the Lab frame measures the k_- ("the longitudinal light-cone momentum") distribution of constituents in the target. The situation in this toy model is therefore just like the non-relativistic case.

D Moments and the Operator Product Expansion

The situation in the real world is more complicated; fields cannot be treated as if they were free. However, the generalization from the free to interacting case is actually quite straightforward. The crucial characteristic of the expansion (92) which was based on treating ϕ as a free field is that it is in the form of $c-$ number singular functions of x^2 (such as Δ_F) multiplied by (composite) operators [e.g. $\phi(x)\phi(0)$]. Wilson[23] suggested (and it was later proven valid) that *this structure is maintained even in the fully-interacting theory*; so, for the scalar case, one would write:

$$T[j(x)j(0)] \approx \sum_m C_m(x^2)O_m(x) \tag{100}$$

where the $C_m(x^2)$ are functions like $\Delta_F(x^2)$ which are singular near the light cone and the $O_m(x)$ are the complete set of <u>all</u> possible composite operators occuring in the theory. Notice that the $O_m(x)$ are, like $\phi(x)\phi(0)$ of the toy model, <u>not</u> local operators (i.e. they depend on at least two different space-time points, x_μ and 0 in this case). Near the light-cone, however, the operators $O_m(x)$ can be expanded in a Taylor series whose coefficients <u>are</u> local operators:

$$O_m(x) = \sum_n x_{\mu_1}, \cdots x_{\mu_n} O_{mn}^{\mu_1 \cdots \mu_n}(0) \tag{101}$$

Inserting this in (100) we obtain the <u>operator product expansion:</u>

$$T[j(x)j(0)] \approx \sum_{m,n} C_{m(x^2)} x_{\mu_1}, \cdots x_{\mu_n} O_{mn}^{\mu_1 \cdots \mu_n}(0) \tag{102}$$

From the intuition gained in the toy model, where the operators $O_m(x)$ were interpreted as analogous to the wave-function of the non-relativistic theory the expansion (101) seems a little strange. For it is as if one were expanding a spatial wave-function around the origin ($x \sim 0$) in a Taylor series expansion. However, for the Bjorken limit this is a natural thing to do since knowledge of the most singular behaviour of the $C_m(x^2)$ is in principle sufficient to determine the large q^2 behaviour of W.

One can use dimensional analysis to deduce from (102) that the most singular $C_m(x^2)$ occur for operators $O_{mn}^{\mu_1 \cdots \mu_n}$ which are <u>bilinears</u> in the fundamental fields (i.e. quarks and gluons). For, suppose that when $x^2 \to 0, C_m(x^2) \sim (x^2)^{-dc/2}$ and that the dimension of the tensorial operator 0 is d_o, then, for the dimensions of (102) to match, requires

$$d_c = 2\,d_j - (d_o - n) \tag{103}$$

Thus d_c is maximized when the *twist* $\tau \equiv d_o - n$ is minimized. In other words the most singular behaviour of C_m (which dominates the large q^2 behaviour), *arises from operators of lowest twist.* These operators are, of course, constructed from the quark and gluon fields and it is a simple exercise in dimensional analysis to check that the lowest possible twist ($\tau = 2$) does indeed arise from bilinear forms. Typical examples might be[7,8]

$$\begin{aligned} &\bar{q}[\gamma_{\mu_1} D_{\mu_2} \;\cdots\; D_{\mu_n}]q \\ \text{or}\;\; &F_{\mu_1\nu}[D_{\mu_2} \;\cdots\; D_{\mu_{n-1}}]F^{\nu}{}_{\mu_n} \end{aligned} \tag{104}$$

Higher twist operators are multilinear in the quark and gluon fields and give rise to less singular $C_m(x^2)$ and therefore to corrections to the leading large q^2-behaviour.

We clearly need the matrix elements of these operators, these have the general structure

$$\langle p_{\mu_1} \cdots \mu_n | p \rangle = A_n p_{\mu_1} \cdots p_{\mu_n} + B_n g_{\mu_1\mu_2} p_{\mu_3} \cdots p_{\mu_n} + \cdots \tag{105}$$

Upon substitution of this in Eq. (84) for $T_{\mu\nu}$, we can derive the following asymptotic series in the Bjorken limit:

$$T_2(q^2, x) \approx \sum_n A_n \frac{C_n(q^2)}{q^2} x^{-n} \tag{106}$$

Here the $C_n(q^2)$ are <u>dimensionless</u> coefficients given by

$$q^2 \left(i \frac{\partial}{\partial \ln q^2} \right)^n \int d^4x e^{iq.x} C_n(x^2) \tag{107}$$

We have already remarked that $W_2(q^2, x) = \operatorname{Im} T_2(q^2, x)$ [see Eqs. (83) and (84) as well as fig. 2]. When combined with Eq. (106) this leads to an infinite sequence of asymptotic sum rules or moment relations:

$$\begin{aligned} M_n(q^2) &\equiv \int_0^1 dx\; x^{n-2} F_2(x, q^2) \\ &\approx A_n C_n(q^2) \end{aligned} \tag{108}$$

It is worth emphasizing that the $C_n(q^2)$ are independent of the target but probe (and therefore q^2) dependent whereas the A_n are, of course, target dependent, though independent of the probe (and therefore q^2). It is clear that the operator product expansion has therefore allowed one to separate the infrared features of the problem from the ultra-violet; this is referred to as <u>factorization.</u>

By this ruse the determination of q^2-dependence is disentangled from the knotty problems of dealing with the structure of the target - which, of course, is a non-perturbative infrared problem. The leading q^2 behaviour of the moments is thereby tied to the behaviour of the $C_n(q^2)$ and therefore the twist-2 quark and gluon bilinear operators. One of the great theoretical triumphs of recent years is the calculation of the $C_n(q^2)$ which can be effected by the special property of QCD, namely that it is <u>asymptotically free.</u>

E Calculating $C_n(q^2)$ - Asymptotic Freedom

Let us for simplicity consider massless QCD; this would seem to imply that the only scale available is associated with an external momentum such as q. This, however, is not correct by virtue of the phenomenon of renormalization. Any quantity calculated in the theory involves Feynman graph loops and the implied momentum integrations typically diverge logarithmically when the internal momentum becomes large. It turns out that these divergences can be consistently controlled by introducing some cut-off scale (Λ) and by rescaling the various physical quantities in the theory. For example, the finite coupling (g) is related to the "bare" coupling occurring in the original Lagrangian (g_o) by

$$g = Z_g g_o \tag{109}$$

Similarly, a *finite* C_n that does not depend on Λ, can be derived by rescaling if, at the same time, one rescales g similarly:

$$C_n = Z_n C_n^o \tag{110}$$

The crucial property of these scaling factors is that they are independent of the physical momenta (such as q) but depend on Λ in such a way that when the cutoff is removed, C_n and g remain finite. In other words, when $\Lambda \to \infty$, Z_n and Z_g must develop infinities of their own that precisely compensate for the infinities of C_n^o and g_o. The original so-called *bare* parameters in the theory calculated from the Lagrangian therefore have no physical meaning – only the renormalized parameters do.

Now let us apply some ordinary dimensional analysis to these remarks. Because they are simply scale factors, the Z's must be dimensionless. However, the Z's are functions of Λ but not of q. But that is very peculiar: a dimensionless function cannot depend on a *single* mass parameter! Thus, in order to express the Z's in dimensionless form, *a new finite mass scale μ must be introduced* so that one can write $Z = Z(\Lambda^2/\mu^2, g_o)$. *An immediate consequence of renormalization is therefore to induce a mass scale not manifest in the Lagrangian.* This is extremely interesting because it provides a possible mechanism for generating mass even though no mass parameter appears in the Lagrangian. We therefore have the exciting possibility of being able to calculate the masses of *all* the elementary particles in terms of just *one* of them. Similar considerations for the dimensionless C_n clearly require that they be expressible as $C_n = C_n(q^2/\mu^2, g)$.

To recapitulate, the physical finite renormalized propagator C_n is related to its bare and divergent counterpart (calculated from the Lagrangian using a cutoff mass) by an infinite rescaling:

$$C_n\left(\frac{q^2}{\mu^2}, g\right) = \lim_{\Lambda \to \infty} Z_n\left(\frac{\mu^2}{\Lambda^2}, g_o\right) C_n^o\left(\frac{q^2}{\Lambda^2}, g_o\right). \tag{111}$$

Notice that the physical coupling g now depends implicitly on the renormalization scale parameter μ. Thus, in QED, for example, it is not strictly sufficient to state that the fine structure constant $\alpha \approx 1/137$; rather, one must also specify the corresponding scale. From this point of view there is nothing magic about the particular number 137 since a change of scale would produce a different value.

As already mentioned, renormalization makes the bare parameters occurring in the Lagrangian effectively irrelevant; the theory has been transformed into one that is now specified by the value of its physical coupling constants at some mass scale μ. In this sense μ plays the role of the hidden scale parameter M in ordinary dimensional analysis by setting the scale of units by which all quantities are measured.

This analogy can be made almost exact by considering a scale change for the arbitrary parameter μ in which $\mu \rightarrow \lambda^{1/2}\mu$. This change allows us to rewrite Eq. (110) in a form that expresses the response of C_n to a scale change:

$$C_n\left(\frac{q^2}{\lambda\mu^2}, g(\lambda\mu^2)\right) = Z(\lambda)C_n\left(\frac{q^2}{\mu^2}, g(\mu^2)\right). \tag{112}$$

The scale factor $Z(\lambda)$, which is independent of q^2 and g, must, unlike the Z's of Eqs. (109) and (110), be *finite* since it relates two finite quantities. Notice that all explicit reference to the bare quantities has now been eliminated. The structure of this equation is *identical* to Eq.(21), the scaling equation derived for the classical case; *the crucial difference is that $Z(\lambda)$ no longer has the simple power law behaviour expressed in Eq.(13).* In fact, the general structure of $Z(\lambda)$ and $g(\mu)$ are not known in field theories of interest. Nevertheless we can still learn much by converting this equation to the differential form analogous to Eq.(24) that expresses scale invariance. As before we simply take $\partial/\partial\lambda$ and set $\lambda = 1$, thereby deriving the so-called *renormalization group equation*:

$$-q^2\frac{\partial C_n}{\partial q^2} + \beta(g)\frac{\partial C_n}{\partial g} = \gamma(g)C_n, \tag{113}$$

where

$$\beta(g) = \mu^2\frac{\partial g}{\partial \mu^2} \tag{114}$$

and

$$\gamma(g) = \frac{\partial \ln Z(\lambda)}{\partial \lambda}\Big|_{\lambda=1}. \tag{115}$$

Comparing Eq.(113) with the scaling equation of classical dimensional analysis Eq. (4), we see that the role of the dimension is played by γ. For this reason, and to distinguish it from ordinary dimensions, γ is usually called the *anomalous dimension* of C_n, a phrase orginally coined by Wilson[23]. (We say anomalous because, in terms of ordinary dimensions and again by analogy with Eq. (24), C_n is actually dimensionless!). It would similarly have been natural to call $\beta(g)/g$ the anomalous dimension of g; however, conventionally, one simply refers to $\beta(g)$ as the β-function. Notice that $\beta(g)$ characterizes the theory as a whole (as does g itself since it represents the coupling) whereas $\gamma(g)$ is a property of the particular object or field one is examining.

The general solution of the renormalization group equation Eq.(113) is given by[24]

$$C_n\left(\frac{q^2}{\mu^2}, g\right) = e^{A(g)} f\left(\frac{q^2}{\mu^2} e^{K(g)}\right), \tag{116}$$

where

$$A(g) = \int^g dg \frac{\gamma(g)}{\beta(g)} \tag{117}$$

and

$$K(g) = \int^g \frac{dg}{\beta(g)}. \tag{118}$$

The arbitrary function f is, in principle, fixed by imposing suitable boundary conditions. (Equation (24) can be viewed as a special and rather simple case of Eq. (113). If this is done, the analogues of $\gamma(g)$ and $\beta(g)/g$ are constants, resulting in trivial integrals for A and K. One can then straightforwardly use this general solution Eq. (116) to verify the claim that the scaling equation Eq. (21) is indeed exactly equivalent to using ordinary dimensional analysis.) The general solution reveals what is perhaps the most profound consequence of the renormalization group, namely, that in quantum field theory the momentum variables and the coupling constant are inextricably linked. C_n for instance, appears at first sight to depend separately on the momentum q^2 and the coupling constant g. Actually, however, the renormalizability of the theory constrains it to depend effectively, as shown in Eq.(116), on only *one* variable $(q^2 e^{K(g)}/\mu^2)$. This, of course, is exactly what happens in ordinary dimensional analysis.

In essence, we use the same modeling-theory scaling technique used by ship designers. Going back to Eq. (116), one can see immediately that the high-energy or short-distance limit ($q^2 \to \infty$ with g fixed) is identical to keeping q^2 fixed while taking $K \to \infty$. However, from its definition Eq. (118), K diverges whenever $\beta(g)$ has a zero. Similarly, the low-energy or long-distance limit ($q^2 \to 0$ while g is fixed) is equivalent to $K \to -\infty$, which also occurs when $\beta \to 0$. Thus *knowledge of the zeros of β, the so-called fixed points of the equation, determines the high- and low-energy behaviours of the theory.*

If one assumes that for small coupling quantum field theory is governed by ordinary perturbation theory, then the β-function has a zero at zero coupling $(g \to 0)$. In this limit one typically finds $\beta(g) \approx -bg^3$ where b is a calculable coefficient. Of course, β might have other zeroes, but, in general, this is unknown. In any case, for small g we find (using Eq. (118)) that $K(g) \approx (2bg^2)^{-1}$, which diverges to either $+\infty$ or $-\infty$ depending on the sign of b. In QED, the case originally studied by Gell-Mann and Low[25], $b < 0$ so that $K \to -\infty$, which is equivalent to the low-energy limit. One can think of this as an explanation of why perturbation theory works so well in the low-energy regime of QED: the smaller the energy, the smaller the effective coupling constant. With $b > 0$ the high-energy limit is related to perturbation theory and is therefore calculable and understandable. I shall now give an explicit example of how this comes about, using the propagator, which also satisfies Eq. (116).

First we note that no boundary conditions have yet been imposed on the general solution Eq. (116). The one boundary condition that *must* be imposed is the known free field theory limit ($g = 0$). For the photon in QED, or the gluon in QCD, the propagator $G\,(= D/q^2)$ in this limit is just $1/q^2$. Thus $D(q^2/\mu^2, 0) = 1$. Imposing this on Eq. (116) gives

$$D\left(\frac{q^2}{\mu^2}, 0\right) = \lim_{g \to 0} e^{A(g)} f\left(\frac{q^2}{\mu^2} e^{K(g)}\right) = 1. \tag{119}$$

Now when $g \to 0, \lambda(g) \approx -ag^2$, where a is a calculable coefficient. Combining this with the fact that $\beta(g) \approx -bg^3$ leads, by way of Eq.(117), to $A(g) \approx (a/b)\, lng$. Since $K(g) \approx (2bg^2)^{-1}$, the boundary condition (Eq. 119) gives

$$\lim_{g \to 0} f\left(\frac{q^2}{\mu^2} e^{1/(2bg^2)}\right) = g^{-a/b}. \tag{120}$$

Defining the dimensionless variable in the function *f* as

$$x \equiv \left(\frac{q^2}{\mu^2}\right) e^{1/(2bg^2)}, \tag{121}$$

it can be shown that with $b > 0$ Eq. (120) is equivalent to

$$\lim_{x \to \infty} f(x) = (2b\ln x)^{a/2b}. \tag{122}$$

An important point here is that the $x \to \infty$ limit can be reached either by letting $g \to 0$ or by taking $q^2 \to \infty$. Since the $g \to 0$ limit is calculable, so is the $q^2 \to \infty$ limit. The free field ($g \to 0$) boundary condition therefore determines the large x behaviour of $f(x)$, and, once again, the "modeling technique" can be used – here to determine the large q^2 behaviour of the propagator G.

In fact, combining Eq. (116) with Eq. (122) leads to the conclusion that

$$\lim_{q^2 \to \infty} D\left(\frac{q^2}{\mu^2}, g\right) = e^{A(g)} \left(2b\ln\frac{q^2}{\mu^2}\right)^{a/2b}. \tag{123}$$

This is the generic structure that finally emerges: the high-energy or large $-q^2$ behaviour of the propagator $G = D/q^2$ is given by free field theory ($1/q^2$) modulated by calculable powers of logarithms. The wonderful miracle that has happened is that all the powers of $\ln(\Lambda^2/q^2)$ originally generated from the divergences in the "bare" theory have been summed by the renormalization group to give the simple expression of Eq. (123). The amazing thing about this "exact" result is that it is far easier to calculate than having to sum an infinite number of individual terms in a series. Not only does the methodology do the summing, but, more important, it justifies it!

We have therefore shown that all the moments of F deviate from constants by small, but calculable, powers of $\ln\, q^2$: thus

$$M_n(q^2) \approx \frac{C_n}{(\ln q^2)^{\gamma_n}} \tag{124}$$

where the γ_n are known. Thus exact Bjorken scaling is actually violated logarithmically although in a predicted pattern. Fig. 13 shows a plot of M_n^{1/γ_n} vs. $\ln q^2$ for n=3, 4, 5 and 6, together with the theoretical predictions which are (unambiguously) calculated from QCD. The agreement is remarkably good and is one of the main reasons why QCD is believed as the theory of the strong interactions.

The target dependent piece, $\langle p|O_n|p\rangle$, remains in general undetermined since it requires a solution of the bound state problem. Thus the light-cone only determines the q^2-evolution of the structure functions - their shape and normalization are infrared properties. Remarkably, however, the normalization can in fact be, in some sense, determined. The reason for this is that the lowest moment (n = 2) corresponds in Eq. (102) to the 2-tensor $O^{\mu_1\mu_2}$ which must contain the energy-momentum tensor. This is not only a conserved quantity (so that its anomalous dimension $\gamma_2 = O$) but, furthermore, its matrix elements at rest are known, being given by the mass of the target. Thus the complete right-hand-side is known. One finds

$$\begin{aligned} M(q^2, 2) &\equiv \int_0^1 F_2(x, q^2)\, dx \\ &= \left(\frac{\sum_f Q_f^2}{N_f}\right)\left(\frac{N_q}{N_q + N_g}\right) \end{aligned} \tag{125}$$

where f means flavour. This sum rule can be thought of as measuring the fraction of momentum carried by the quarks. For $SU(3)$ this reduces to

$$\int_0^1 F_2(q^2, x)\, dx \approx \frac{5N}{6(3N+8)} \tag{126}$$

where N is the number of quark generations. Thus, for $N = 4$, this gives 5/42 whereas for $N = 3$, 5/34. The data are shown in Fig. 14.

These indicate that $M(q^2, 2)$ is approaching a constant which appears to be consistent with 3 generations. Note, incidentally, that the operator $O^{\mu_1\mu_2}$ contains another operator beyond the energy-momentum tensor and that this is not conserved and so has a non-vanishing value for its γ_2. This means that there are corrections to the sum rule, Eq. (102), which are of the form $a(\ln q^2)^{-\gamma_2}$. Remarkably, a can be shown to be positive so that the approach to scaling must be from above which is in agreement with the data. Further corrections are given by the higher twist operators containing more than just two quark and gluon fields. These are down by $O(1/q^2)$ and so are presumably not of importance for high values of q^2.

An Aside - Application to the EMC Effect

A remarkable property of the sum rule, Eq.(126) beyond the fact that its right-hand-side is independent of q^2 (i.e. of the probe) is that it is also independent of the target!

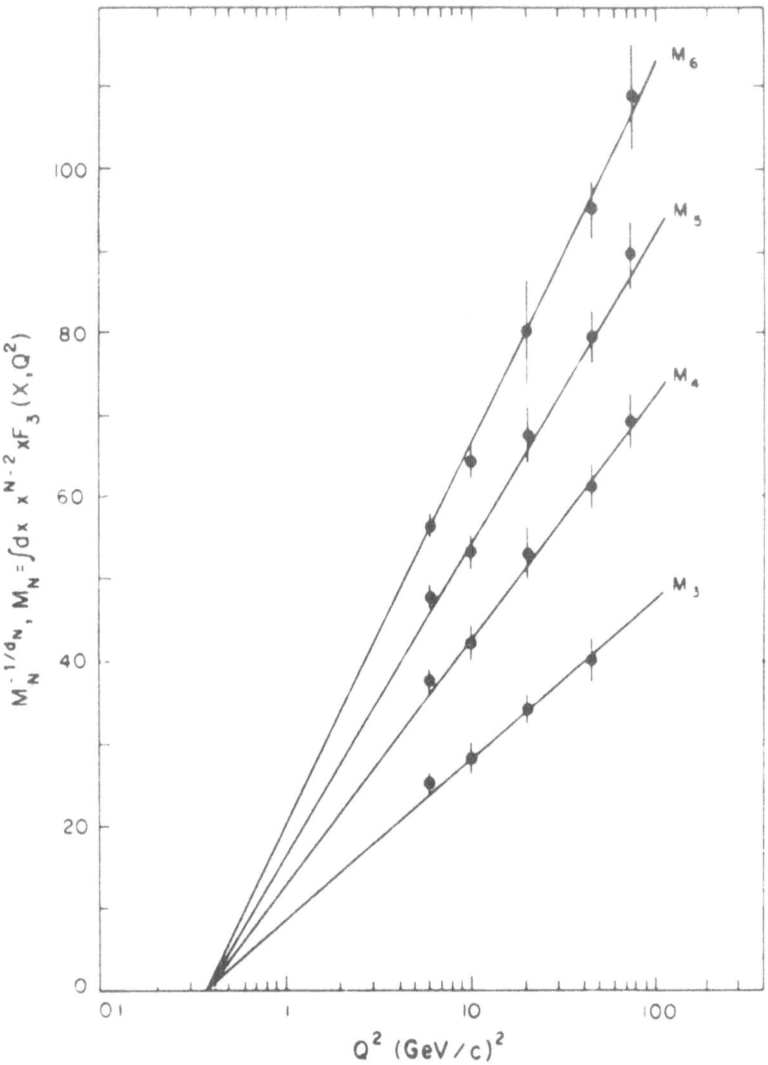

Figure 13. Graph showing agreement of QCD predictions for $M_n(q^2)$ with the experimental data [see Eq. (124)].

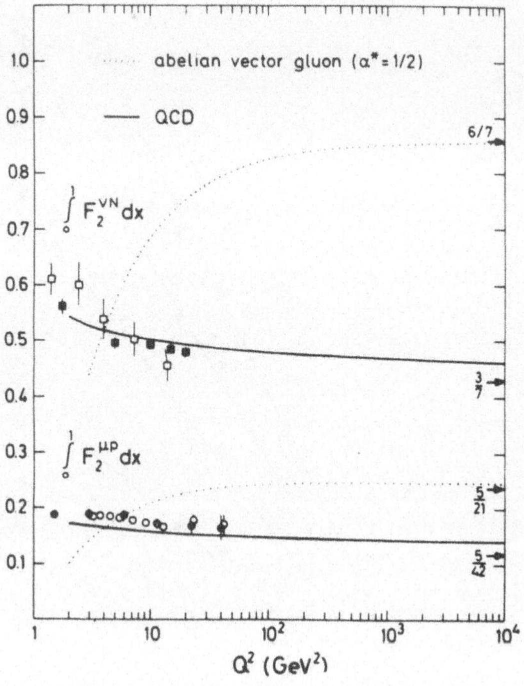

Figure 14. The behaviour of the n=2 moment vs. q^2 for neutrino and muon scattering showing approach to a constant from above, see Eq. (126).

Thus, if one introduces the difference

$$\Delta(q^2, x) \equiv \frac{F_A(q^2, x)}{A} - F_N(q^2, x) \tag{127}$$

[A denoting a nucleus and N the nucleon], then

$$\Delta M(q^2, 2) \equiv \int_0^A \Delta(q^2, x)\, dx \approx \frac{(C_A - C_N)}{(ln\, q^2)^{\gamma_2}} \tag{128}$$

In fact <u>all</u> moments of Δ vanish asymptotically so ultimately Δ itself must vanish, with increasing q^2, albeit very slowly. Thus at very large q^2, the EMC effect must eventually disappear. Notice also, incidentally, that $|\Delta M(q^2, 2)|$ must decrease monotically with q^2 which is, in fact, violated when the original EMC data is compared to the later SLAC data! [26] Since that time the EMC points near $x \approx O$ which were the largest deviations of Δ from zero $x \approx O$ have been amended so that the data is now consistent with this requirement on $|\Delta M(q^2, 2)|$.

Correlations, Higher Twist and Shadowing

We have seen that the operator product expansion on the light cone leads to sum rules with the structure:

$$\begin{aligned} M(q^2, 2) &\equiv \int_0^1 F_2(q^2, x)\, dx \\ &\approx \frac{< Q^2 >}{(1 + 16/3N_f)} + \frac{C}{(ln\, q^2)^{\gamma_2}} + O\left(\frac{1}{q^2}\right) + \cdots\cdots \end{aligned} \tag{129}$$

The first two terms represent the lowest twist contribution arising from quark and gluon bilinears. These can be represented by graphs of the kind shown generically in Fig. 12. These incorporate the naive parton model, modulated with leading logarithmic gluon radiative corrections which give rise to the second term in Eq. (129). The leading corrections to these asymptotic estimates come from higher twist terms; the four-quark operator, as illustrated in Fig. 12, gives rise to $O(1/q^2)$ corrections. Notice that these leading graphs are identical in structure to those that arose in the $1/q^2$ expansion for the structure function in non-relativistic many-body theory.

Let us take this connection with the many-body result seriously - after all, the basic physics is clearly the same. In that case, as one comes down to modest values of q^2 (below a few GeV^2) correlations in the system begin to dominate. Let us therefore write

$$M(q^2, 2) = M_{RAD}(q^2, 2)[1 - f(q^2)] \tag{130}$$

where $M_{RAD}(q^2, 2)$ just includes the "soft-gluon" radiative corrections that we typically calculated from asymptotic freedom, i.e. the first two terms in Eq. (129). This is, of course, a slowly ranging function of q^2. Writing Eq.(130) in this form simply factors out the QCD radiative corrections in much the same way one removes radiative corrections in QED. What remains, i.e. $f(q^2)$, contains "dynamics". Now, suppose we mimic the non-relativistic sum rule, Eq. (46), and identify f with correlations in the target (i.e. loosely with $\langle e^{i\mathbf{q}\cdot(\mathbf{r}_1-\mathbf{r}_2)}\rangle$), then below the "correlation length" (a few GeV), it becomes very rapidly varying. Of course for large q^2, it rapidly vanishes. A crude approximation for f is simply the square of the elastic form factor of the target, $G_{el}^2(q^2)$:

$$i.e.\ f(q^2) \approx G_{el}^2(q^2) \tag{131}$$

This can be "justified" by noting that diagramatically (Fig. 5) f is the overlap of two triangles, each one approximately the elastic form factor. Thus, a crude approximation would have

$$M(q^2,2) \approx M_{\mathrm{RAD}}(q^2,2)[1 - G_{el}^2(q^2)] \tag{132}$$

For the nucleon $G_{el}(q^2)$ is a remarkably smooth function, well approximated by a dipole form:

$$G_{el}(q^2) \approx \frac{1}{(1 - q^2/M_0^2)^2} \tag{133}$$

where $M_0 \sim 0.7\,\mathrm{GeV}$. Thus the approach to the asymptotic regime governed by the light cone should, for the nucleon, be smooth - as indeed it is, as can readily be seen in Fig. 15. Indeed this approach is remarkably well fit by Eq. (132). On the other hand for

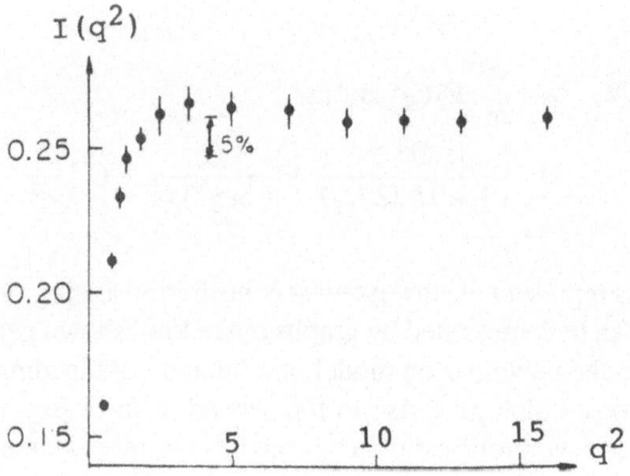

Figure 15. Smooth approach to scaling for the sum rule, Eq. (126), in agreement with Eq. (132).

systems such as nuclei and liquids which have spatial "edges" $G_{el}(q^2)$ is oscillatory, reflecting diffraction. In that case the approach to asymptopia should be oscillatory. For liquids this is indeed the case. Relevant data on nuclei are not yet available.
We can take this argument one step further, if we are willing to be bold: we can suppose that $f(q^2)$ dominates the approach to scaling not just for the sum rule but for the structure function itself: this suggests writing:

$$F_2(q^2,x) \approx F_2^{\mathrm{RAD}}(q^2,x)[1 - f(q^2)] \tag{134}$$

where again $F_2^{\mathrm{RAD}}(q^2,x)$ contains only the "soft-gluon radiative corrections". In that

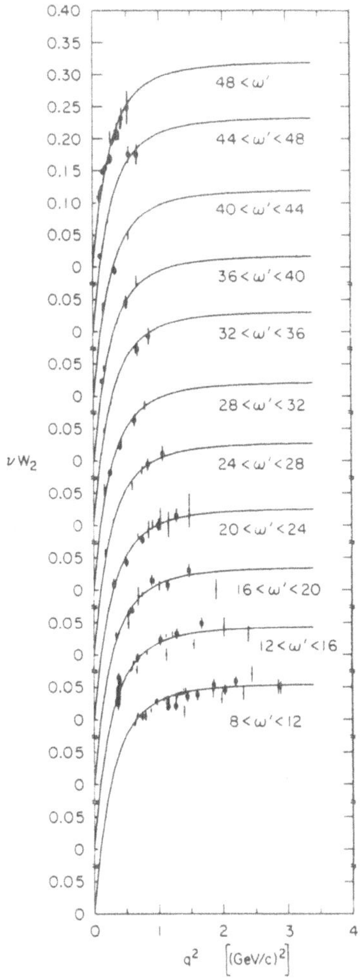

Figure 16. $F_2(x, q^2)$ vs. q^2 for fixed $x(\equiv 1/w^1$ showing smoothness as reflected in Fig. 6). The solid lines are $[1 - G_{el}^2(q^2)]$; see Eq. (135).

case, it follows that

$$\widetilde{F}_2\,(x) \equiv \frac{F_2(q^2,x)}{1-G_{el}^2(q^2)} \tag{135}$$

should (up to logarithms) scale down to very small values of q^2 (i.e. well below a few GeV^2 and possibly even down to $q^2 = 0$!!). A fit with this formula was performed many years ago[27] on early data and is reproduced in Fig. 16. It does indeed show a remarkably good agreement.

Suppose we go even further and try to continue this formula down to $q^2 = 0$ (with ν fixed). On the left- hand-side $x \rightarrow 0$ when $q^2 \rightarrow 0$. On the right-hand-side we have

$$F_2(x,q^2) \rightarrow \frac{q^2\sigma_\tau(\nu)}{4\pi^2\,\alpha} \tag{136}$$

where $\sigma_\tau(\nu)$ is the total photo-absorption cross-section. If we therefore set $q^2 = 0$ and $\nu = \infty$ in Eq. (135) we obtain

$$\begin{aligned}\widetilde{F}_2\,(0) &\approx \frac{m_0^2\sigma_\gamma(\infty)}{8\pi^2\,\alpha} \\ &\approx 0.38\end{aligned} \tag{137}$$

which is in remarkably good agreement with experiment!

References

[1] For early reviews of the phenomenology see, e.g., F. Gilman, Phys. Rep. *4c*, 94 (1972) or R. P. Feynman "Photon-Hadron Interactions," (W.A. Benjamin, Reading, MA 1972). See also refs. [3] and [4].

[2] This is generally the attitude expressed in "The Eightfold Way," by M. Gell-Mann and Y. Ne'eman. (W.A. Benjamin, NY 1964).

[3] G. B. West, Phys. Rep. *18c*, 264 (1975).

[4] T-P. Cheng and L-F. Li, "Gauge Theory of Elementary Particle Physics Particle Physics," (Oxford Univ. Press, NY 1984).

[5] J. J. J. Kokkedee "The Quark Model," (W.A. Benjamin, NY 1969).

[6] H. Bethe Ann. der Phys. *5*, 325 (1930); W. Heisenberg, Physik Z *32*, 737 (1932).

[7] A. Gross and F. Wilczek, Phys. Rev. Letters *26*, 1343 (1973); H. D. Politzer, idem. *26*, 1346 (1973).

[8] See, e.g., H. D. Politzer, Phys. Rep. *14c*, 129 (1974).

[9] G. B. West, "Particle Physics, A Los Alamos Primer", (Eds. N. G. Cooper and G. B. West, Cambridge, 1988) p. 2.

[10] T. A. McMahon, Science, *173*, 349 (1971).

[11] See, e.g., A. D. B. Woods and R. A. Cowley, Rep. Prog. Phys., *36*, 1135 (1973).

[12] R. Hofstadter, "Nuclear and Nucleon Structure" (Benjamin, N.Y. 1963).

[13] K. W. McVoy and L. van Hove, Phys. Rev. *125*, 1034 (1962); W. Czyz, Phys. Rev. *131*, 2141 (1963); T. de Forest and J. D. Walecka, Adv. in Physics *15*, 1 (1966).

[14] J. D. Bjorken, Phys. Rev. *179*, 1547 (1969).

[15] See any standard text on quantum mechanics.

[16] H. A. Gersch and L. J. Rodriguez, Phys. Rev. *8A*, 905 (1973); the work of this paper implies the existence of y-scaling. I thank S. A. Gurvitz and R. Silver for recently bringing this paper to my attention.

[17] D. B. Day et al., Phys. Rev. Letts. *59*, 427 (1987).

[18] T. R. Sosnick et al. Los Alamos preprint LA-UR-88-505 and W. G. Stirling et al. J. Low Temp. Phys. (to be published).

[19] R.N. Silver, Phys. Rev. *B37*, 3794 (1988).

[20] I. Sick, Phys. Lett. *110B*, 411 (1982).

[21] S. D. Drell and J. D. Walecka, Ann. Phys. (N.Y.) *28*, 18 (1964)

[22] L. Hand, Phys. Rev. *129*, 1834 (1963).

[23] K. G. Wilson, Phys. Rev. *179*, 1499 (1969).

[24] G. B. West, Phys. Rev. *D27*, 1402 (1983).

[25] M. Gell-Mann and F. E. Low, Phys. Rev. *95*, 1300 (1954).

[26] G. B. West, Phys. Rev. Letts. *54*, 2576 (1985).

[27] S. Stein et al., Phys. Rev. *D12*, 1884 (1984).

CHIRAL QUARK/PARTON MODELS: THE WAY QCD IS REALIZED?

Anthony W. Thomas

Department of Physics and Mathematical Physics, Adelaide University
SA 5001, Australia

INTRODUCTION

Quantum chromodynamics (QCD) is almost certainly the correct theory of the strong interaction. In the perturbative regime, involving high momentum transfer, it is well understood and phenomenologically successful. However, the matter of which we are made contains protons and neutrons. Their stucture is critically dependent on the long-distance behaviour of QCD, where the theory is not under control. It is believed that as a consequence of its non-Abelian structure QCD is singular at large distances, and that this singular behaviour means that only color singlet quark clusters have finite mass – the phenomenon of confinement.

Given that QCD cannot be solved exactly to yield the structure of hadronic matter there are three attitudes which may be taken. First one could dismiss strong interaction physics as "chemistry" and move on to grander things. Second one could try to use a combination of powerful computers and clever numerical techniques to solve for hadronic ground-states on a space-time lattice. This approach does appear to be yielding convergent results for the pure-glue sector[1], however, it is not clear (to me at least) that this method has yet led to any insight into the structure of the nucleon. A third approach is to build models of hadron structure which incorporate as much of our knowledge of QCD as possible. These models should then be refined or rejected on the basis of how well they describe experimental data (including lattice "measurements", when those become reliable).

These lectures follow the third philosophy. In particular we shall concentrate on one class of models known as chiral bags, and especially the cloudy bag model (CBM). This conforms with my own beliefs and the wishes of the organisers. Nevertheless the reader should be aware that there are a number of very different models of hadron structure, and that the field is not without controversy. During the discussion of various types of experimental data we shall point out where the predictions of one model differ in a significant way from others. Unfortunately there are not many such examples amongst low energy phenomena, and for this reason we turn eventually to deep-inelastic scattering (DIS) as a potentially unambiguous tool for choosing between models.

Of course much of physics is involved with modelling physical systems. A lot of the skill in such work lies in knowing where the model should not be used. Thus the proposal that DIS could be used to distinguish between models[2,3] is often countered by claims that one model or another was only meant to describe low-energy phenomena. This argument may be logically correct in some cases. On the other hand, as we shall see, there are explicit quark models which not only allow one to calculate low energy hadronic properties in a simple, transparent way, but which also give a surprisingly good description of data in the deep-inelastic regime. This strongly suggests that such models are closer to the truth.

The purpose of these notes is to explain the key ideas behind, and some important applications of, the cloudy bag model. As we move from low energy properties like masses, charge radii, magnetic moments and axial form-factors to meson-baryon scattering, the short-distance N-N force and ultimately DIS we shall highlight the open questions and problems as well as the sucesses. Throughout the emphasis will be on conceptual development rather than algebraic details. For earlier reviews of bags and chiral bags we recommend particularly those by De Tar and Donoghue[4], Miller[5], Myhrer[6] and Thomas[7].

BARYON STRUCTURE IN THE CLOUDY BAG MODEL

Given that any model should as far as possible reflect what is known about QCD, we should first summarise some general ideas on which (almost) everyone can agree. For very heavy quarks (Q = c or b) one finds an effective potential which is Coulomb-like at short-distances but rises linearly at large distances. The latter feature is responsible for "confining" the heavy quarks, in the sense that it would require infinite energy to separate them by an infinite amount. The mechanism for generating the linearly rising potential is the self-interaction of the gluons, which means that lines of chromo-electric flux tend to be concentrated in tubes of constant energy density (~1 GeV/fm). From the study of the spin-dependence of the long-distance force on a lattice it is believed to be a Lorentz scalar.

Once we introduce the light quarks (q = u or d), which make up most of the matter in the universe, the situation changes rather dramatically. It will always be energetically favourable for heavy $Q - \bar{Q}$ systems to decay to two color neutral mesons ($Q\bar{q}$ and $\bar{Q}q$) at large distance. The natural theoretical framework for studying sysyems of heavy quarks is the adiabatic, or Born-Oppenheimer approximation. This has been supplemented by models of light-quark pair creation (or "string breaking") to handle the break-up process which we just described. Unfortunately these phenomenological models are not well constrained at the present time because of the difficulty of the experiments above the break-up threshold.

If we move at last to systems made purely of light quarks and gluons the situation is far more complicated. At the Lagrangian level the u and d are approximately massless. Thus the adiabatic approximation can not be expected to yield any insight into their dynamics. Of course, if $\bar{q}$-q pair creation could be suppressed one would still expect the long-range inter-quark force to lead to confinement. In reality one must deal simultaneously with the highly relativistic motion of the quarks, long-range confining forces and pair creation. Given the evident complexity of the problem it is not surprising that there are so many models of nucleon structure which are apparently so different.

As explained in the introduction we shall consider just one class of models which have developed from the MIT bag model. The key features of QCD which are retained by such models are the relativistic motion of the quarks, the long-range confinement and finally a feature we have not mentioned before, namely asymptotic freedom. That is, at short distances (or high momenta) the quarks should almost behave as free particles. These ideas are incorporated by suggesting that the QCD Lagrangian allows two different vacuum states. Inside the "bag" quarks move as free, relativistic particles which interact only perturbatively through gluon exchanges. Outside the bag the quarks feel an infinitely repulsive scalar potential which stops them at the boundary. The stability of the system is ensured by postulating a higher energy density (B) for the vacuum inside the bag. Once B is chosen to fit one hadronic mass the rest of the baryon spectrum may be calculated.

Although the model was formulated in a completely Lorentz invariant way[8], in practice it has usually been solved in the approximation where the bag is fixed at some point in space and assumed spherically symmetric. Crude though this approximation may seem, the model has enjoyed impressive phenomenological success. Most important from our point of view is the fact that it allows analytic investigation of all the properties of the hadrons – including their symmetries.

At this point the astute reader might object that while the model has accounted for relativity, asymptotic freedom and confinement, $\bar{q}$–q pair creation has been ignored. Our discussion of heavy $\bar{Q}$–Q systems suggested that this should not be ignored. We have deliberately waited to raise this matter until after the mention of the key word "symmetry". In particular, QCD for massless u and d quarks has an exact SU(2) x SU(2) chiral symmetry. Any model, like the MIT bag, which confines quarks through an effective scalar potential breaks this symmetry. The only way that the symmetry can be recovered is to include massless, pseudo-scalar mesons (Goldstone bosons) coupled to the quarks. Models which incorporate this feature are known as chiral quark models, and the one on which we concentrate is the cloudy bag model (CBM) of Miller, Théberge and myself[9]. From the point of view of advocates of such models it is actually an advantage that the u and d quarks are very light, for this guarantees that pion creation and absorption is the dominant effect of allowing for $\bar{q}$–q creation and annihilation, and furthermore gives us a model independent way to calculate it.

After this somewhat lengthy introduction we are almost ready to give the details of the MIT bag and the cloudy bag models, and their applications. However we would first make some remarks concerning the philosophy we have adopted. This may be helpful to students whose concerns must include the question, "where next?". The MIT and cloudy bag models are certainly incorrect in detail. Hadrons are not static, the bag surface (even if that has a meaning) would not be spherical or without thickness. A sharp transition between two different vacua is at best an idealisation. Neither confinement nor asymptotic freedom are as simple as the model suggests. Nevertheless the CBM probably does contain elements of truth which will be found in any more sophisticated treatment. Experience with this simple model may guide the more sophisticated work. We think for example of the importance of relativity in understanding the nucleon axial current and magnetic moment, the role of pion coupling (particularly open channels) in spectroscopy, etc. From this point of view chiral soliton models, at least those in which the quarks are confined by a scalar field which is <u>not</u> the chiral partner of the pion, are natural extensions of the CBM – as are the less sophisticated relativistic potential models which include pion coupling.

The MIT Bag Model

For the details of the covariant formulation of the bag we refer to the original papers.[8,11] In the approximation of a static, spherical cavity of radius R the Lagrangian has the form:

$$L = \left[\frac{i}{2} \bar{q} \overleftrightarrow{\partial\!\!\!/} q - B \right] \theta\ (R-r)$$

$$- \tfrac{1}{2}\, \bar{q}\, q\ \delta\ (r-R). \qquad (1)$$

We have specialised to the case of massless quarks (inside the cavity), and for simplicity we have dropped the gluon fields which are to be treated in low-order perturbation theory so as not to overcount. (As usual $\overleftrightarrow{\partial\!\!\!/}$ is $\gamma^\mu\ (\overrightarrow{\partial}_\mu - \overleftarrow{\partial}_\mu)$, and θ is one for r $\leqslant$ R and zero otherwise). The equations of motion are obtained by requiring that the corresponding action (S) should be stationary under variation of q, $\bar{q}$ and R. If we define n^μ as a unit vector normal to the bag surface (n^μ = (O,$\hat{r}$)), under the change R $\rightarrow$ R + δR we have

$$\theta\ (R-r) \rightarrow \theta\ (R-r) + \delta R\ \delta(r-R),$$
$$\delta\ (r-R) \rightarrow \delta\ (r-R) - \delta R\ n.\partial\ \delta(r-R) \qquad (2)$$

Using these results, and equating the coefficients of δq, $\delta q\ \delta\ (r-R)$ and δR in δS to zero we find the equations:

$$i \not\partial q = 0 \qquad r < R, \tag{3}$$

$$i\ \gamma .\ n\ q = q \qquad r = R, \tag{4}$$

$$B = -\tfrac{1}{2}\ n.\partial\ [\bar{q}q] \qquad r = R. \tag{5}$$

Thus the quarks obey the free Dirac equation inside the bag, but are subject to a linear boundary condition, equ. (4), at the surface. This boundary condition has the simple interpretation that there should be no flow of (color) current through the surface. To improve it we note that equ. (4) implies that $\bar{q}$ equals $-\ i\bar{q}\ \gamma.n$ (at $r = R$), and hence at $r = R$:

$$i\ n^{\mu}\ j_{\mu} = i\bar{q}\ \gamma.n\ q = \bar{q}\ (q) = (-\bar{q})\ q = 0. \tag{6}$$

This is the meaning of confinement in the bag model and it is a consequence of the surface δ-function in equ.(1). If we look for solutions of the free Dirac equation with angular momentum zero we find

$$\psi_s\ (\underline{r}) = N \begin{bmatrix} j_0\left[\omega\ r/R\right] \\ i\underline{\sigma}.\hat{r}\ j_1\left[\frac{\omega r}{R}\right] \end{bmatrix} \chi, \tag{7}$$

with χ a Pauli spinor and N the normalisation constant. The linear boundary condition implies that ω must satisfy

$$j_0\ (\omega) = j_1\ (\omega), \tag{8}$$

for which the lowest solutions are $\omega = 2.04\ (1s_{\frac{1}{2}})$ and $5.40\ (2s_{\frac{1}{2}})$.

For three quarks in the 1s state the energy is

$$E = 3\ \frac{\omega}{R} + \frac{4\pi}{3}\ B\ R^3 \tag{9}$$

where the quark kinetic energies and the volume energy and obvious. The final boundary condition equ.(5) is equivalent to the statement that B and R are related by the condition

$$\frac{\partial E}{\partial R} = 0, \tag{10}$$

which ensures stability. Using equs.(9) and (10) once easily finds that $E = 4\omega/R$, so that each quark carries one quarter of the nucleon energy. In this crude version of the bag we could set E to be the average of nucleon and delta masses, in which case R is 1.46 fm and B is 21 MeV/fm^3. Once B is fixed the masses and sizes of all excited states are determined.

Of course hadron spectroscopy is a little more complicated than equ.(9). As in any mean field theory the bound quarks will have some spurious c.m. kinetic energy which should be removed. In the simplest phenomenology this is just parameterised as an additional term, of the form $-\ Z_0/R$, on the right of equ.(9) $-$ where Z_0 is a constant to be determined by fitting data. This has the advantage that other corrections, like the zero-point energy of the cavity which also goes like $^1/R$, may be included in the best-fit value of Z_0.

One can also include finite mass terms for the quarks in the Lagrangian. In the case of the u and d one would expect these masses to be of order 10 MeV with the d a few MeV higher to explain the n-p mass difference. Unless one is interested in small charge-symmetry breaking effects these are unimportant corrections. On the other hand, a strange quark mass of order 200 MeV is essential to explain the SU(3) - flavour breaking of the masses in the nucleon octet.

Finally, within the original bag model, one needs to consider the spin-dependent mass corrections arising from the gluon exchange. To do so one introduces the gluon fields ($\vec{E}^{\alpha}$, $\vec{B}^{\alpha}$) which to lowest order in α_s obey Maxwell's equations inside the cavity, plus the boundary conditions (at r = R):

$$\hat{r}\,.\,\vec{E}^{\alpha} = 0\;, \qquad \vec{r} \times \vec{B}^{\alpha} = 0\;. \tag{11}$$

The sources for $\vec{E}^{\alpha}$ and $\vec{B}^{\alpha}$ are the color currents of the quarks, $\bar{\psi}\,\gamma^{\mu}\,\lambda_{\alpha}\,\psi$, with λ_{α} the usual SU(3) matrices. It is usual to argue away the colour-electric contribution (at least for all quarks in s-wave) as small and spin-independent, leaving the chromomagnetic interaction. After some hard work this can be shown to give a mass correction of the form

$$\Delta\, M_g = -\frac{\lambda \alpha_c}{R} \sum_{i<j} M_{ij}\; \underline{\sigma}_i \cdot \underline{\sigma}_j\;. \tag{12}$$

Here λ is a color factor equal to $-8/3$ for baryons and $-16/3$ for mesons, α_c is the strong coupling constant (equal to 2.2 in the original fits) and M_{ij} is a slowly varying function of the bag radius and the masses of quarks i and j. We note that for a pair of quarks in a spin-triplet state equ.(12) is repulsive, while for spin-singlet it is attractive. This immediately tells us that the delta(Δ) will be heavier than the nucleon (N) and the rho (ρ) heavier than the pion (π).

For the ground-state mesons and baryons the mass formula works extremely well. Furthermore, since one has analytic wavefunctions, the low-energy properties like magnetic moments, charge radii and axial charges can all be obtained analytically. For example the magnetic moment is:

$$\underline{\mu} = \tfrac{1}{2} \int_{\text{Bag}} d^3r \quad (\underline{r} \times \underline{j}^{em})\,, \tag{13}$$

with j^{em} the electromagnetic current of the bound quarks (charges e_i):

$$\underline{j}^{em} = \sum_i e_i\, \bar{q}_i\, \underline{\gamma}\, q_i\,, \tag{14}$$

and q given (for massless quarks) by equ.(7). Substituting for q and doing the integral in equ. (13) one finds a result that looks like the usual non-relativistic one:

$$\underline{\mu} = \mu_0 \sum_i e_i\, \underline{\sigma}_i\,, \tag{15}$$

which is to be evaluated between non-relativistic spin-flavor wavefunctions. The dynamics of the bag model is hidden in the scale parameter μ_0, which dimensionally must be proportional to the bag radius R. For massless quarks one actually finds:

$$\mu_0 = \frac{4\,\omega - 3}{12\omega\,(\omega-1)}\, R. \tag{16}$$

The connection with the constituent quark model, where μ_0 would be $(2m_q)^{-1}$, is evident if ω/R, the quark eigen-energy in the bag, is identified with m_q.

As a second example, of importance for the next section, we consider the axial current:

$$A_k^{\mu}\,(\underline{r}) = \bar{q}\,(\underline{r})\,\gamma^{\mu}\,\gamma_5\,\tau_k/2\;\; q\,(\underline{r})\;\theta\,(R-r)\,. \tag{17}$$

(Here τ_k is the k'th component (in isospace) of the quark isospin operator). In particular the axial charge, g_A, is defined by the relationship

$$\int d^3r \quad \langle p|\, \underline{A}_k\,(\underline{r})\, |n\rangle = g_A \quad \langle p\,|\, \underline{\sigma}\, \frac{\tau_k}{2}\, |\, n\rangle_{s-f} \tag{18}$$

where the subscript s–f denotes a spin–flavor matrix element only, $|p\rangle$ and $|n\rangle$ on the left are composite states built of quarks and $|p\rangle$ and $|n\rangle$ on the right are treated as elementary. Using the explicit quark wave function of equ.(7) we can again write the left hand side of equ.(18) in a form resembling the non-relativistic result. That is:

$$\int d^3r < p \,|\, \underset{\sim}{A}_k (\underset{\sim}{r}) \,|\, n> \propto \sum_{i=1}^{3} <p \,|\, \underset{\sim}{\sigma}^i \frac{\tau_k^i}{2} \,|\, n>_{s-f} \tag{19}$$

and using SU(6) wavefunctions the right hand side is 5/3 $<p|\,\underset{\sim}{\sigma}\,\tau_k/2\,|n>_{s-f}$, which is the origin of the non-relativistic quark model result of 5/3 for g_A. The key difference, and one of the major successes of the bag model, is that the constant of proportionality in equ. (19) is not unity but

$$\frac{\int_0^R dr\, r^2 \left[j_0^2 \left[\omega r/_R\right] - \frac{1}{3} j_1^2 \left[\frac{\omega r}{R}\right] \right]}{\int_0^R dr\, r^2 \left[j_0^2 \left[\omega r/_R\right] + j_1^2 \left[\frac{\omega r}{R}\right] \right]} = 0.65 \tag{20}$$

The lower component of the quark wave-function plays a key role, reducing g_A to 1.09 which is in much better agreement with the experimental value of 1.258.

We must end the discussion of the MIT bag model at this point in order to discuss chiral symmetry and the CBM. However, it would be misleading to move on without a mention of the situation for spectroscopy of excited states. The removal of spurious c.m. energy is much more complicated for excited states. In addition spin-orbit corrections are not under control in any quark model, including the bag. The numerical results for excited state masses obtained by De Grand[11] were not very impressive. One major problem was that the lowest $\Lambda(\frac{1}{2}^-)$ and $\Lambda(^3/_2{}^-)$ states were predicted in the opposite order from experiment. In view of our results[12] with the SU(3) x SU(3) version of the CBM (as discussed below), this now seems desirable and when viewed with progress on the Roper resonance[13] perhaps it is time for renewed effort on the spectrum of excited states of the bag. In any case the reader should not be left with the impression that this is a solved problem, nor that the phenomenology is as satisfactory as for the ground states.

Chiral Symmetry

The Lagrangian for massless QCD is invariant under the global chiral transformation

$$q \to q - i\, \underset{\sim}{\tau} \cdot \underset{\sim}{\epsilon}\, \gamma_5\, q. \tag{21}$$

(where $\underset{\sim}{\epsilon}$ is infinitesimal). Associated with this invariance or symmetry property is a conserved Noether current (the axial current)

$$\underset{\sim}{A}^\mu = \bar{q}\, \gamma^\mu \gamma_5 (\underset{\sim}{\tau}/2) q. \tag{22}$$

That is, $\partial_\mu \underset{\sim}{A}^\mu$ is zero throughout all space.

If the MIT bag, or any other model for that matter, is supposed to model QCD one would expect it to preserve the symmetries of QCD. In particular one would expect the axial current to be conserved. That this is not the case can be seen very easily. Consider the expression for the axial current in the MIT bag model given in equ.(17). The divergence of $\underset{\sim}{A}^\mu{}_{bag}$ is in fact proportional to a δ-function at the bag surface – the δ-function arising from ∂_μ acting on $\theta(R-r)$. It is not hard to find the source of the problem. Under the chiral transformation (21), $\bar{q}$ behaves as:

$$\bar{q} \to \bar{q} - i\, \bar{q}\, \gamma_5\, \underset{\sim}{\tau} \cdot \underset{\sim}{\epsilon}\ . \tag{23}$$

As a consequence any mass term, like the surface δ-function in equ. (1), will not be invariant under a chiral transformation and will break chiral symmetry. That is, under the transformation (21) and (23):

$$L_{MIT} \rightarrow L_{MIT} - i\, \bar{q}\, \gamma_5\, \underset{\sim}{\tau} \cdot \underset{\sim}{\epsilon}\, q\, \delta(r-R). \tag{24}$$

The very term responsible for confining the quarks is also responsible for breaking chiral symmetry.

A somewhat more picturesque way of stating the problem is the following. In massless, perturbative QCD a quark's helicity (or chirality) does not change when it emits or absorbs a gluon. On the other hand a positive helicity quark striking the bag surface will be reflected (confinement) but will not have its spin flipped because the surface interaction is a Lorentz scalar. Thus the helicity of the quark is altered at the bag surface - in contradiction with perturbative QCD.

We cannot stress too much that this is not a pathology of the MIT bag model, but is a much more general problem. Any theory in which quarks are confined by interacting with a Lorentz scalar potential will also break chiral symmetry. Since we suggested earlier that the long-distance force between quarks calculated in lattice QCD seems to be scalar, we might conclude that <u>any</u> QCD-based model will have the same problem.

From general considerations there appears to be only one way out of this impasse. The Goldstone theorem allows an alternative realization of chiral symmetry in which the vacuum structure is altered to contain massless, pseudoscalar Goldstone bosons. That is, if we define the axial charge $\underset{\sim}{Q}_5$ in the usual way:

$$\underset{\sim}{Q}_5 = \int d^3r\, \underset{\sim}{A}^0\, (\underline{r}) \tag{25}$$

then $\underset{\sim}{Q}_5 |0\rangle$ is non-zero. The particular symmetry which concerns us is the one given in equ.(21), that is a chiral transformation with an isospin rotation. In this case the massless pseudoscalar bosons are isovector and clearly the pion, with its mass which is extremely low by hadronic standards, is a prime candidate. Indeed the conventional understanding of chiral symmetry is that in an idealised world with massless quarks the pion would also be massless and exact chiral symmetry would be realized in the Goldstone mode ($Q_5 |0\rangle \neq 0$). Since the quark masses are small one can work with low-order perturbation theory and the physical pion mass is related to the u and d quark masses by

$$f_\pi^2\, m_\pi^2 = (m_u + m_d)\, \langle\bar{\psi}\psi\rangle. \tag{26}$$

Here f_π is the pion decay constant (93 MeV) and $\langle\bar{\psi}\psi\rangle$ is the vacuum expectation value of $\bar{u}u$ or $\bar{d}d$ (assumed equal). The non-zero value of $\langle\bar{\psi}\psi\rangle$ indicates that the vacuum contains a quark condensate. To lowest order $\langle\bar{\psi}\psi\rangle$ is taken to be independent of (m_u+m_d).

To summarise, the chiral symmetry of QCD and the fact that the long-distance confining force is a Lorentz scalar implies that any consistent quark model of hadron structure must include pions as well. The cloudy bag model was based on this realization plus the fact that the MIT bag model had achieved considerable phenomenological success. Our philosophy was to build on that success by making the minimal changes necessary to restore its broken chiral symmetry.

Since it was the surface that broke chiral symmetry the initial idea was to introduce a pion field coupled to the quarks at the bag surface and transforming in exactly the right way under a chiral rotation such that chiral symmetry was restored.[9,14-16] Simple though this sounds there is still an ambiguity. We recall that the stability of the bag relied on the fact that the interior had a higher energy density than the exterior. This two phase picture suggests that one might identify the exterior of the bag as a region with a non-zero quark condensate, and the interior as a region where $\langle\bar{\psi}\psi\rangle$ is zero. In that case chiral symmetry would be realized in the Wigner mode (no pions and $Q_5|0\rangle=0$) inside the bag, and in the Goldstone mode outside. In other words pions would be strictly excluded from the bag. This is the working hypothesis adopted by the Stony Brook group with their little bag model.

On the other hand we have already expressed caution about some features of the MIT bag – especially its sharp, static surface. The bag radius could be thought of as that distance which a quark can escape on average before the confining forces of the other quarks pull it back. For light quarks we noted that an alternative would be for a q-$\bar{q}$ pair to be created and the lines of force broken. This would tend to give a reflected quark plus a meson emitted. Since the pion is by far the lightest meson it could be expected to dominate such processes, and restore chiral symmetry too! From this point of view it is clear that pions could be created anywhere in the baryon. It is just that the probability would be greatest at the surface, and the pion would spend most of its time outside the bag because of its long wavelength. The initial version of the CBM concentrated the production and absorption of pions at the bag surface, but allowed for a more continuous transition by allowing them to propagate inside the bag too.

At this point we must emphasise that it does matter whether the pion field is excluded from the bag or not. To see this we note that once pions are included the conserved axial current has two pieces, the usual quark term given in equ.(17) and a pionic piece proportional to $f_\pi \partial_\mu \underset{\sim}{\varphi}$ (with $\underset{\sim}{\varphi}$ the pion field). Suppose we estimate g_A (as above) in terms of the integral of the space piece of the axial current. If $\underset{\sim}{\varphi}$ is smooth the integral vanishes, as the integral of a total divergence must. However, if $\underset{\sim}{\varphi}$ is excluded from the bag we get a surface contribution to g_A which undoes the good work of the MIT model – i.e. g_A goes back up to 5/3!

One important objection raised against all chiral bag models is that the pion is known to be made of quarks and anti-quarks and has a charge radius of order o.6 fm – not much smaller than the nucleon. What right do we have to introduce it into the Lagrangian as an elementary field? The only answer I can give is that we are at best developing an effective theory applicable for some region of relatively low momentum transfer. Certainly if one hits the nucleon with a deep-inelastic probe it will find q-$\bar{q}$ pairs not elementary pions. The reason for treating the pion as "elementary" at all is that it alone among the mesons is a collective state – see e.g. the model of Weise and collaborators[17]. That is why its mass is small. Just as a Cooper pair need not be physically small to be treated as a unit neither must the pion. Of course it would be reassuring to derive the pion wavefunction, its mass and its coupling to baryons from QCD. (One would expect equ.(26) to also come out of such a calculation.) Some interesting work on this problem has recently been carried out by the Seattle group[18], but there is a long way to go. In the meantime the limits of validity are probably best established phenomenologically. On the practical side the high-momentum cut-off is imposed by truncating the baryon space – e.g. to N and Δ bags in calculating nucleon properties. (Such a procedure is already familiar from the non-relativistic quark model where the one-gluon-exchange interaction is usually diagonalised in a limited space, 1 or 2 $\hbar\omega$).

This introductory section has been rather long. However, there are some very important considerations which underly the form of the Lagrangian chosen for the cloudy bag model. Having been through these arguments we can present the details of the model rather concisely.

The Cloudy Bag Model

As for MIT bag we shall exclude explicit mention of gluons for the sake of clarity. The associated corrections can be added later in perturbation theory. In order to restore chiral symmetry we add an "elementary" pion field $\underset{\sim}{\varphi}$ to obtain

$$L = \left[\frac{i}{2} \bar{\psi} \overleftrightarrow{\not{\partial}} \psi - B \right] \theta(R-r) - \frac{1}{2} \bar{\psi} e^{i \underset{\sim}{\tau} \cdot \underset{\sim}{\varphi} \gamma_5 / f} \psi \; \delta(r-R)$$

$$+ \tfrac{1}{2} (D_\mu \underset{\sim}{\varphi})^2 \tag{27}$$

In equ.(27) we have called f_π simply f, and $D_\mu \underset{\sim}{\varphi}$ is a covariant derivative

$$D_\mu \underset{\sim}{\varphi} = (\partial_\mu \varphi)\, \hat{\varphi} + f \sin(\varphi/f)\, \partial_\mu \hat{\varphi}, \tag{28}$$

where $\hat{\varphi} = \underset{\sim}{\varphi} / |\underset{\sim}{\varphi}|$. This Lagrangian is invariant under the chiral transformation

$$\psi \longrightarrow \psi - i \frac{\underset{\sim}{\tau} \cdot \underset{\sim}{\epsilon}}{2} \gamma_5 \psi ,$$

$$\underset{\sim}{\varphi} \longrightarrow \underset{\sim}{\varphi} + \underset{\sim}{\epsilon} f + f (\underset{\sim}{\epsilon} \times \hat{\varphi}) \times \hat{\varphi} \left[1 - \left[\frac{\varphi}{f}\right] \cot\left[\frac{\varphi}{f}\right] \right], \tag{29}$$

Clearly equs. (27)-(29) give a non-linear realization of chiral symmetry. This realization is unique only up to first-order in $\underset{\sim}{\varphi}$, which is all that was required in many of the early applications. For processes in which higher order terms matter one should keep an open mind. Indeed it has been claimed[19] that the Weinberg representation[20] gives a better description of the $0(\varphi^3)$ terms. For none of the applications considered here shall we need to wory about such terms.

The historical approach for calculating hadron properties was to linearise equ.(27) (in $\underset{\sim}{\varphi}$), and then remove explicit mention of quarks by projecting the result onto the space of colorless, non-exotic baryons.[9,21,22] This yielded a theory of bare (bag model) hadrons coupled to the pion field in a unique way - that is all coupling constants and form-factors were determined. Rather than follow this approach we would like to first consider the result of an apparently simple unitary transformation

$$q = S \psi$$

$$S = \exp \left[i \underset{\sim}{\tau} \cdot \underset{\sim}{\varphi} \gamma_5 /2f \right]. \tag{30}$$

After some algebra this yields the Lagrangian

$$L' = (i \bar{q} \not{D} q - B)\, \theta\, (R-r)$$

$$- \tfrac{1}{2} \bar{q} q\, \delta(r-R) + \tfrac{1}{2} (D_\mu \underset{\sim}{\varphi})^2 + \frac{\theta(R-r)}{2f} \bar{q} \gamma^\mu \gamma_5 \underset{\sim}{\tau} q \cdot D_\mu \underset{\sim}{\varphi} , \tag{31}$$

where the covariant derivative on the new (dressed) quark field is

$$D_\mu q = \partial_\mu q - \frac{i}{2} \left[\cos \left[\varphi/f\right] - 1 \right] \underset{\sim}{\tau} \cdot \left[\hat{\varphi} \times \partial_\mu \hat{\varphi} \right] q. \tag{32}$$

While the transformed and untransformed theories should be equivalent if calculated to all orders we wish to work to low order in $\underset{\sim}{\varphi}$. In that case one version may be more rapidly convergent. Because of the well-known result that soft-pion theory leads to pseudo-vector coupling, we suspect that eqn. (31) could be the better starting point. This has been confirmed by explicit calculation for s-wave pion nucleon scattering[24], where to order φ^2 the covariant quark derivative guarantees the Weinberg-Tomozawa relationship[23]. To order $\underset{\sim}{\varphi}^2$ the new version of the CBM Lagrangian becomes:

$$\begin{aligned} L'_{CBM} &= (i\, \bar{q} \not{\partial} q - \bar{q} m q - B)\, \theta(R-r) - \tfrac{1}{2} \bar{q} q\, \delta(r-R) \\ &- \frac{\theta(R-r)}{4f^2} \bar{q} \gamma^\mu \underset{\sim}{\tau} q \cdot (\underset{\sim}{\varphi} \times \partial_\mu \underset{\sim}{\varphi}) \\ &+ \frac{\theta(R-r)}{2f} \bar{q} \gamma^\mu \gamma_5 \underset{\sim}{\tau} q \cdot \partial_\mu \underset{\sim}{\varphi} \\ &+ \tfrac{1}{2} (\partial_\mu \varphi)^2 - \tfrac{1}{2} m_\pi^2 \varphi^2 . \end{aligned} \tag{33}$$

Note that through the explicit quark and pion mass terms we have allowed for the fact that the axial current is only partially conserved in the real world. As noted in our discussion of chiral symmetry the CBM in this form does not provide a microscopic link between m and m_π.

The remarkable feature of L'_{CBM} is that pions now couple to quarks throughout the bag volume. In fact, in this representation the chiral transformation on q is $q \to q - (i/2f)\tau.(\epsilon \times \varphi)q$, from which it is easily seen that the surface δ-function is chiral invariant! A chiral transformation here turns a quark into a quark plus or minus a pion. On the other hand it turns out that when one computes the coupling constant and form-factor for the $NN\pi$ and $BN\pi$ vertices eqns. (27) and (31) give the same result (up to a small correction which vanishes with quark mass m). The lesson is clearly that one should be careful of reading too much physics into mathematics. The second version of the CBM, known as the volume-coupling version, clearly corresponds much more closely to the physical picture described in our discussion of chiral symmetry. Nevertheless its predictions for all physical processes involving single pion emission and absorption are essentially identical to those of the surface coupled version!

The Structure of the Nucleon

Equation (33) naturally breaks into three pieces: one describing free MIT bags, the second describing free pions and the third giving their interaction. In order to exploit this structure one can project the Lagrangian onto the space P of non-exotic bags $|\alpha>$ (like N, Δ, etc.) and the Q-space of everything else (e.g. $4q$-$\bar{q}$ states). We shall quote an example of the exchange current corrections associated with the Q-space later on. For the present we drop it. With this approximation the Hamiltonian corresponding to eqn. (33) becomes (to order $\underset{\sim}{\varphi}$ only):

$$H = \sum_\alpha |\alpha> m_\alpha^{(0)} <\alpha| + \sum_\alpha \omega_k a_k^+ a_k$$
$$+ \sum_{k,\alpha,\beta} (v_k^{\beta\alpha} |\beta><\alpha| a_k + \text{h.c.}). \tag{34}$$

Here $m_\alpha^{(0)}$ is the mass of the bare bag state $|\alpha>$, $\omega_k = (\underline{k}^2 + m_\pi^2)^{\frac{1}{2}}$ as usual, a_k is a destruction operator for a meson of momentum and isospin formally labelled k. Finally, $v_k^{\beta\alpha}$ is the essential prediction of the model namely the form-factor for the vertex at which a pion of momentum and isospin k is absorbed by the (bare) bag state $|\alpha>$ leaving the bag state $|\beta>$. It is calculated by evaluating the matrix element of the pseudo-vector volume-coupling term in eqn. (33) between the appropriate states. For example, for the $NN\pi$ and $\Delta N\pi$ vertices we find:

$$v_k^{NN} = i(4\pi/2\omega_k)^{\frac{1}{2}} (f_{NN\pi}^{(0)}/m_\pi)\, v(\underline{k})\, \tau_k\, \underline{\sigma}.\underline{k},$$
$$v_k^{\Delta N} = i(4\pi/2\omega_k)^{\frac{1}{2}} (f_{\Delta N\pi}^{(0)}/m_\pi)\, v(\underline{k})\, T_k\, \underline{S}.\underline{k}. \tag{35}$$

where $\underline{S}$ and $\underset{\sim}{T}$ are transition spins and isospins and the coupling constants are:

$$(f_{NN\pi}^{(0)}/m_\pi) = (25/72)^{\frac{1}{2}} (f_{\Delta N\pi}^{(0)}/m_\pi) = g_A/(4\pi)^{\frac{1}{2}} f. \tag{36}$$

The appearance of g_A (actually g_A predicted by the bag model) and f in eqn. (36) is obvious given the fact that the coupling involves A^μ/f explicitly. Equation (36) is the Goldberger-Treiman relationship for the bare parameters of the theory. The form-factor (for massless quarks) is determined just by the bag radius (R), that is:

$$v(k) = 3\, j_1(kR)/kR. \tag{37}$$

Details of the couplings for all members of the nucleon octet are given in the paper of Theberge and Thomas[25].

To find the nucleon wavefunction for the CBM, which we call $|\tilde{N}>$, we can use low-order perturbation theory about the bare bag state $|N>$. This remarkable statement can be rigorously justified[26] for bag radii greater than (0.7–0.8)fm, provided we restrict the space of bare baryons allowed to $|N>$ and $|\Delta>$ as discussed earlier. (Expanding the space to include one or two $\hbar w$ excitations would not alter this conclusion. The condition is necessary only to avoid a formal but unphysical divergence which arises if one sums over infinitely many excited bag states in a bag of the same radius. This of course is nonsense for an effective theory). Indeed the solution to the Schrödinger equation

$$H\ |\tilde{N}> = m_N\ |\tilde{N}> \tag{38}$$

can be accurately written as

$$|\tilde{N}> = Z^{\frac{1}{2}}\ |N> + \sum_k c_k\ |N\pi_k> + \sum_k c_k'\ |\Delta\pi_k> \tag{39}$$

for the radii quoted above. The formal summation over spin and isospin labels means that the correct Clebsch–Gordon coefficients are included to ensure that $|\tilde{N}>$ is an eigenstate of total angular momentum and isospin. The probability amplitudes c_k and c_k' can be calculated directly from eqns. (34) and (38). Clearly the constant Z is the probability that a dressed nucleon will be found to contain a bare bag. It is typically 70% or greater for R in the range quoted – another indication of the rapid convergence of the theory.

There are many fascinating aspects of nucleon structure which we could discuss at this stage. We shall concentrate on just four: the neutron charge distribution; the renormalisation of g_A and particularly the role of the Δ–bag; the role of the pion in breaking the N–Δ degeneracy; the pionic corrections to the baryon magnetic moments.

For the neutron charge distribution the $\Delta\pi$ component of the wave function (39) is not qualitatively important. If we drop it the neutron wavefunction becomes:

$$|\tilde{n}> \cong Z^{\frac{1}{2}}|n> + c[(^2/_3)^{\frac{1}{2}}|p\pi^-> - (^1/_3)^{\frac{1}{2}}|n\ \pi^0>]. \tag{40}$$

To first order the charge distribution arises from a proton bag with a negative pion; that is, a <u>well understood</u> positive core and a negative tail. There can be little doubt that this picture is qualitatively correct. The key advance over earlier meson theory is the rapid convergence and the fact that the core is simple! A good measurement of $G_{En}(q^2)$ would be extremely valuable for comparison with the theory[22]. At the moment only the mean-square charge radius is accurately known – it is negative and $|<r^2>_{ch}^n|^{\frac{1}{2}} = 0.342$ fm. The CBM gives a value between 0.33 and 0.39 fm for R between 1.1 and 0.8 fm, which is quite impressive.

Equation (36) related the bare πNN coupling constant to the bag value of g_A. The effect of the pion coupling is to renormalise both sides of this equation in the same way so that it also holds for the renormalised values. In an old-fashioned meson-nucleon field theory like that of Chew and Wick the main effect of renormalisation is to reduce the bare pion coupling. This happens because the wave function renormalisation constant Z is very small in such models (typically $\frac{1}{4}$ or less), and this is not compensated by the corresponding vertex connection. To be specific, in the CBM the renormalised value of g_A (or $f_{\pi NN}$) is related to the bare (bag) value by:

$$g_A = ZZ_1^{-1}\ g_A^{Bag}\ , \tag{41}$$

where

$$Z_1^{-1} = 1 + \Lambda_{NN} + \Lambda_{N\Delta} + \Lambda_{\Delta\Delta}. \tag{42}$$

In the Chew–Wick theory only Λ_{NN} would appear. It corresponds to a nucleon bag emitting a pion but staying as a nucleon which interacts with the axial current and then reabsorbs the pion. (Clearly $\Lambda_{\Delta N}$ and $\Lambda_{\Delta\Delta}$ involve excitation of a Δ in at least one intermediate state). Obviously, Λ_{NN} involves the calculation

$$\Lambda_{NN} \propto \sum_k \underline{\sigma}.\hat{k}\tau_k\underline{\sigma}\ \underset{\sim}{\tau}\ \underline{\sigma}.\hat{k}\tau_k = {}^1/_9 \underline{\sigma}\ \underset{\sim}{\tau} \sum_k (\sigma.\hat{k})^2 \tau_k^2 . \tag{43}$$

The factor of $^1/_9$ is responsible for Z_1 giving negligible compensation for Z.

For the CBM the explicit inclusion of the intermediate Δ completely alters matters:

$$\Lambda_{NN} : \Lambda_{\Delta N} : \Lambda_{\Delta\Delta} = 1:32:20, \tag{44}$$

and now the product ZZ_1^{-1} is near unity – decreasing by about 15% as R goes from 1.1 to 0.7 fm[22]. *We cannot stress too much the importance of the explicit appearance of the bare Δ in improving the convergence of the theory.* It is only at this stage that the small value of g_A given by the bag model becomes a clear problem. Initial work on c.m. corrections suggested that they might give an 18% increase in g_A, but later work does not support this conclusion[27].

Two solutions to this problem have been proposed. With the surface coupling version of the CBM, Høgaasen and Myhrer[28] have shown that the modified boundary condition (c.f. equ. (4)):

$$i\ \gamma.n\ \psi = e^{i\underset{\sim}{\tau}.\underset{\sim}{\varphi}\ \gamma_5/f}\ \psi, \quad r=R. \tag{45}$$

leads to an increase in g_A of 16% or greater. In the volume coupling version, which we favour, the boundary condition on the quark field is not altered, although there is some coupling throughout the bag volume. In this case the biggest correction is an extra piece in the axial current (proportional to the quark vector current cross φ). Morgan and collaborators showed that this can also improve the calculated value of $\tilde{g}_A$ significantly. They found g_A between 1.4 at R = 0.7 fm and 1.22 at R = 1.1 fm.[70]

The pion coupling required by chiral symmetry also has important consequences for spectroscopy. In our brief summary of the MIT bag model we mentioned that the breaking of the N–Δ degeneracy is usually attributed to the chromomagnetic interaction. However, the pion self–energies can also contribute. In the work of Thomas, Théberge and Miller[21] the virtual $\Delta\pi$ contribution to the mass of the nucleon was about 80 MeV more attractive than the (real part of the) $N\pi$ contribution to the Δ. This has the attractive feature that a smaller colour coupling constant is required to fit the observed mass difference. Incidentally our reference to the real part of the delta mass shift hints at a much deeper issue, namely the role of open channels in the calculation of hadron structure. The major motivation of the initial work in the CBM was in fact to obtain a consistent description of the Δ-resonance <u>as a resonance</u> in πN scattering. We shall return to this issue in a later section.

The CBM has also been used to investigate the magnetic moments of the whole nucleon octet[25]. (For the corresponding work on axial charges see ref. (29)). As this has been adequately reviewed elsewhere, and the overall agreement with data is quite satisfactory, we wish to make just two points of general interest. First the major uncertainty in the work is in the estimation of c.m. corrections where more work is needed. Secondly it is an essential feature of the CBM that pion coupling mixes other octet and decuplet states into the physical hadron. For example the Λ includes small admixtures of Σ and Σ^* bags (with a pion) which contribute in a vital way. Thus it is not true (as often stated) that the pionic corrections are purely isovector.

SYSTEMS OF MORE THAN ONE NUCLEON

An enormous amount of effort has been put into calculating the N–N force. Most of this effort has concentrated on the boson exchange picture[30] where essentially point-like nucleons exchange observed mesons like π, ρ and ω. With very few parameters this approach has provided a successful description of a vast amount of data on nuclear binding energies and reactions. One naturally hesitates to suggest that we could learn anything new from the quark model. Nevertheless nucleons have radii of order $^{8}/_{10}$ fm which means that they overlap at nucleon separations of just under 2 fm. This is a characteristic nearest neighbour separation at nuclear matter densities. It would be astonishing if we learnt nothing significant from the quest to understand how such composite systems can conspire to produce the boson exchange model.

From our discussion of the CBM it should be clear that long distances present no problem. Indeed with the CBM form-factors the one pion exchange N–N force is identical to that between point-like nucleons until the bag surfaces touch (r=2R). Only inside 2R is there a reduction because of the finite size of the nucleon. Of course, the asymptotic d/s ratio of the deuteron places severe constraints on the one pion exchange N–N force. Ericson and Rosa-Clot[31] have shown that in the simple model where the pion exchange is given by the CBM alone when the nucleons overlap the parameter R should not be greater than 0.6 fm. However, when the extra physics which can arise at short distances is accounted for (e.g. quark exchange and gluon exchange), this limit is much less restrictive. Indeed it could be as large as 0.8 or 0.9 fm [32] which is more in the CBM range.

Since Δ excitation is a natural feature of the pion coupling in the CBM the intermediate range attraction is in principle accounted for by the model. However, no quantitative calculation of this piece of the force has yet been made using the CBM.

A major issue for any explicit quark model description of the N–N force is whether explicit vector meson exchange need be added. Within the CBM they are <u>certainly not needed</u> to explain the nucleon electromagnetic properties <u>in the space-like region</u>. Of course, viewed from the t-channel photon coupling to a bound valence quark looks exactly like the photon becoming a quark-anti-quark pair with mass twice the quark eigen-energy – about 800 MeV. This is so close to m_ρ and m_ω that the <u>duality</u> of the two descriptions <u>is obvious</u>.

A number of explicit quark models of the short distance N–N force including quark and gluon exchange have demonstrated that the well known N–N repulsion, usually attributed to ω-exchange, can be understood this way [33, 34]. The key question is whether any significant contribution from additional anti-quark-quark pairs is required. It is a remarkable feature of meson and baryon spectroscopy that such admixtures are very small up to excitations of more than 1 GeV. Since the reason for this suppression is not well understood for a single baryon we would like experimental guidance on the baryon-number two system if that is feasible. We should like to present one possible test.

<u>Charge Symmetry as a Probe of the Short-Distance N–N Force</u>

There has been quite some interest recently in the study of the charge symmetry breaking N–N force of class-IV [35], which mixes spin triplet and spin singlet states in the n–p system. A TRIUMF experiment confirmed the existence of such a force at 477 MeV (E_n^{lab}), at a single angle [36] – that is where $A_n(\theta)$ vanishes. The theoretical analysis of this experiment, based on conventional boson exchange, suggests that the nucleon mass difference in single pion exchange accounts for the observed effect [37, 38]. Amongst other possible mechanisms the photon exchange is small, so is ρ exchange and all other mesons are negligible.

The mechanism of interest to us is ρ–ω mixing (η–π mixing vanishes in this case). Near the energy and angle where the class-IV signal ($A_n(\theta)\neq A_p(\theta)$) was seen at TRIUMF, it can be shown in a model independent way that the ρ–ω contribution goes through zero [37]. On the other hand, just 20^0 either side of this point it becomes the dominant term. Now the essential point is that ρ–ω mixing is dominated by the up–down mass difference in the QCD Lagrangian $(\bar{u}u-\bar{d}d)(m_u-m_d)$. If one adopts the alternate view of the short-distance force that one needs no $\bar{q}$–q pairs this mass-difference term cannot give a class-IV transition.

Thus in principle one has a very clear test. If the experiments can be performed away from cross-over ($A_n(\theta)=0$) and do not show the characteristic ρ–ω signature we shall have a very firm indication that the valence quark description of the short-distance N–N force is correct. If on the other hand such a signal is seen it will be clear that $\bar{q}$–q admixtures are required and ultimately the boson exchange approximation may be most effective. Our proposal represents quite a challenge to the experimenters, but it is worth the effort!

Nuclear Matter

At the other end of the scale from the N–N problem, and yet intimately linked to it, we have the problem of the saturation of nuclear matter. The conventional approach is perhaps typified by the Walecka model[39], in which point-like nucleons move in a mean-field generated by the exchange of isoscalar (σ) and vector (ω) mesons. Since the strength of the mean scalar and vector fields is typically found to be 300 or 400 MeV one has to question the consistency of neglecting the internal structure of the nucleon. We shall briefly review some recent work by Guichon[40] in which this internal structure instead plays a key role.

Suppose we consider isoscalar nuclear matter of uniform density ρ in which quarks confined in nucleon bags interact through the exchange of σ and ω mesons (for the present purposes we do not ask whether these are real mesons or merely a simple way of accounting for two pion exchange and quark interchange). The source of vector mean-field ($\bar{\omega}$) is the quark current $\bar{q}\,\gamma^0\,q$, or q^+q, which just measures the number of nucleons present. On the other hand the source of the scalar mean-field ($\bar{\sigma}$) is $\bar{q}q$ which depends on the spatial distribution of the quarks. Since the scalar field coupling is attractive it acts as a negative mass, and makes the quark wave function more and more relativistic as $\bar{\sigma}$ increases. This in turn decreases $\bar{q}q$ and hence $\bar{\sigma}$. Thus we have a very simple saturation mechanism. The vector field gives a repulsion proportional to ρ while the scalar field attraction initially grows as ρ but then saturates.

For a series of bag radii between 0.6 and 1.0 fm Guichon adjusted g_σ and g_ω to fit the saturation energy and density of infinite nuclear matter[40]. It is remarkable that for each of these solutions the incompressibility ($K=9\,\rho^2\,\partial^2W/\partial\rho^2$ at $\rho=\rho_0$) of nuclear matter was within the experimental limits. This may be compared with the point-nucleon approach which badly overestimates this parameter. Another attractive feature of this approach is the fact that the mean scalar and vector potentials required were considerably smaller than one finds in the literature – typically −140 MeV and +50 MeV respectively at nuclear matter density. Finally the predicted changes in the properties of the bound nucleon were quite small – typically a 1% decrease in R and only a few per cent change in the magnetic moment and charge radius.

In conclusion, we stress that this is at present a very crude model of nuclear matter in which the usual ingredients of Fermi motion and the Pauli Exclusion Principle play no role. Clearly the model needs to be made much more sophisticated. Nevertheless the beauty of this new way of viewing nuclear matter is undeniable.

MESON BARYON SCATTERING

One of the outstanding defects of much quark model spectroscopy is that highly unstable resonances are treated as stable. It is ridiculous to believe that a state with a πN decay width of several hundred MeV will not have its position altered significantly by the channel coupling. The CBM was constructed to deal with this problem from the very beginning[8,15]. In particular the treatment of the Δ involved a calculation of the P_{33} phase shifts in πN elastic scattering.

We do not intend to repeat that discussion, here, but simply to draw attention to it. (We note also the recent extraction of the Δ magnetic moment from πp bremmstrahlung[41]). The reason such effects are usually ignored is simply that to include them correctly involves a lot of work. One should strictly make a full scattering calculation, including channel coupling, for each resonance. Realistically this is not on, of course, and one will probably need to adopt some simple approximation scheme for all but a few special cases.

One such special case was mentioned in the section on bag model spectroscopy, that is the $\Lambda(\frac{1}{2}^-)$ at 1405 MeV. This state is badly fit even in the Isgur-Karl work,[42] and for the MIT bag seemed like a disaster. The bag predicted[11] that the $\Lambda(\frac{1}{2}^-)$ should be 100 MeV heavier than the $\Lambda(^3/_2{}^-)$, while experimentally it is the $\Lambda(^3/_2{}^-)$ that is over 100 MeV heavier. Only recently has this problem been re-examined in a version of the volume-coupled CBM based on SU(3) x SU(3) chiral symmetry.[43,44]. Our conclusion was that the $\Lambda(\frac{1}{2}^-)$ observed at 1405 MeV is not a 3-quark state but a $\bar{K}N$ state bound by the strong channel coupling to $\Sigma\pi$. These effects are so strong because the $\Lambda(\frac{1}{2}^-)$ couples to both of these channels in s-wave. The $\Lambda(^3/_2{}^-)$ couples to these decay channels in d-wave, and there is no comparable effect. In order to fit the existing $\bar{K}N$ and $\bar{K}N \to \Sigma\pi$ scattering data, Veit et al. found that the three-quark state with $\Lambda(\frac{1}{2}^-)$ quantum numbers had to be over 1600 MeV[43]. Thus the original bag model result may be right after all.

With respect to this problem we note that the $\Lambda(1405)$ is below $\bar{K}p$ threshold and hence difficult to study. Nevertheless a current experiment at Brookhaven[45] may shed some light on the problem. Most naive quark model calculations up to now have had the decays $\bar{K}p \to \Lambda\,\gamma$ and $\bar{K}p \to \Sigma^0\gamma$ proceed through a three-quark $\Lambda^*(1405)$. The physics is much more complicated in the CBM and one might hope that the measurements of absolute branching ratios would help to choose between models. From the theoretical point of view it seems impossible to justify any calculation which does not include the channel coupling effects. For example in the CBM work of Zhong et al.[46] the $\bar{K}p \to \Lambda\gamma$ amplitude is essentially real while the $\bar{K}p \to \Sigma^0\gamma$ amplitude is mostly imaginary. In the naive quark model both are real.

With the appearance of CEBAF and possibly a kaon factory in the next decade, we can expect this area to become very topical. In particular there is a desperate need to check the existence and properties of a large number of so-called "missing states", which are predicted by the quark model but have not yet been seen.

DEEP INELASTIC SCATTERING

We have hitherto considered the low energy properties of hadrons such as masses and form - factors, as well as their interactions. The cloudy bag model clearly gives an acceptable, quantitive description of such data. In this final section we should like to briefly review recent work which shows that it also leads to a reasonable understanding of deep inelastic scattering (DIS) data. We have argued elsewhere [2,3] that DIS may be the only way to unambiguously distinguish between the multitude of models of hadron structure which exist in the literature. The challenge is therefore out to the proponents of other models to compute the consequences of them for DIS.

Before we turn to the computation of structure functions themselves, we would like to make some comments on the sum-rule for the spin-dependent structure function $g_1(x)$ of the proton. There has been considerable fuss over the EMC result[47] that quarks appear to carry very little of the proton spin. Some authors have gone so far as to suggest abandonning the conventional quark models because of this result[48]. We shall suggest that the data may actually provide important confirmation of the physics involved in the cloudy bag model[49,50].

The Quark-Parton Model

There are many reviews of the quark-parton model which can be consulted for details[51,52]. We shall simply collect a few key results here. Inclusive lepton scattering (e.g. (e,e'), (ν_μ,μ^-) etc.) involves the measurement of a cross-section as a function of energy loss (ν) and scattering angle (θ). Conventionally these are converted to two Lorentz invariant variables, Q^2 which is minus the 4-momentum transfer squared, and Bjorken x which is $Q^2/2m\nu$ (with m the target mass - here assumed to be a nucleon).

If one chooses to look only at events with ν greater than 1 or 2 GeV, and Q^2 greater than 1 or 2 GeV^2, all DIS data can be characterised by a small number of distribution functions $u(x,Q^2)$, $\bar{u}(x,Q^2)$, $d(x,Q^2)$ etc. The observation that these distributions are only weakly dependent on Q^2 (logarithmically) is known as scaling. It confirms the existence of point-like quarks in the nucleon. The interpretation of the distributions is simplest in a frame where the proton has extremely high momentum $\underline{P}$. Then u(x) x dx is the fraction of the momentum of the proton carried by up-quarks with momentum between x $\underline{P}$ and (x+dx) $\underline{P}$. A similar definition applies to anti-up quarks ($\bar{u}$), strange quarks (s), and so on. We have also acknowledged the slow Q^2 dependence by dropping Q^2 as an argument of u.

Any experimental cross-section can be parameterised as a few structure functions, which in turn can be expressed in terms of the distribution functions described above. Electromagnetic DIS from an unpolarised target (T) is essentially given by one structure function, $F_2^{eT}(x)$:

$$F_2^{eT}(x) = x \sum_i e_i^2 \; f_i^T(x) \tag{46}$$

where e_i is the charge of quark i and f_i^T labels the u,d,s.... distributions in target T. If the target is polarized there is another measureable structure function;

$$g_1^T(x) = \tfrac{1}{2} \sum_i e_i^2 \; (f_i^{T\uparrow} - f_i^{T\downarrow}) \quad . \tag{47}$$

The arrow up indicates a quark polarised parallel to the target and the arrow down a quark anti-parallel. (Clearly $f_i^T = f_i^{T\uparrow} + f_i^{T\downarrow}$).

For the weak interaction we shall again be interested in just two structure functions for an isoscalar target. The so-called singlet structure function is

$$F_2^T(x) = x\,(u^T(x) + \bar{u}^T(x) + d^T(x) + \bar{d}^T(x) + s^T(x) + \bar{s}^T(x)), \tag{48}$$

while the non-singlet (or valence) structure function is

$$x\,F_3^T(x) = x\,(u^T(x) + \bar{u}^T(x) + d^T(x) \,\bar{d}^T(x)). \tag{49}$$

(In writing equ. (49) we follow the common assumption that $s(x) = \bar{s}(x)$, however this is at best a good approximation[53]). We note that equs. (46) - (49) are only correct in leading order QCD. In next-to-leading order there are logarithmic corrections to the relations between the structure functions and the quark distributions[54]. As a consequence, whereas we might expect the excess of quarks over anti-quarks in a nucleon to be three, and therefore the integral of $F_3(x)$ to be three, in next-to-leading order QCD the integral is actually $3\,(1 - \alpha(Q^2)/\pi)$.

The Sum Rule For $g_1(x)$

For a given nucleon target (N = p or n) one can use the usual commutation relations to prove the following remarkable sum-rule[51,52]:

$$S_N \equiv \int_0^1 g_1^N (x)\, dx = \tfrac{1}{2} < N \uparrow | \bar{\psi}(0)\, \gamma_z \gamma_5 Q^2 \psi(0) | N \uparrow > \tag{50}$$

Note that here $|N\uparrow>$ is a translationally invariant state of definite polarisation and Q^2 is a quark charge operator. Using the usual quark model to relate Q^2 to I_3, B and Y one can then establish the well-known Bjorken sum-rule

$$S_p - S_n = g_A/6 \tag{51}$$

The beauty of equs. (50) and (51) is that it relates very high energy measurements to a low energy matrix element which can be calculated for any model. If the neutron wavefunction is a $\underset{\sim}{56}$ of SU(6), S_n is easily seen to be zero and hence S_p should be $g_A/6$. The shock of the recent EMC measurement of S_p is that they found only about half of this expected result!

For simplicity we shall discuss the neutron sum rule (S_n) and rely on equ. (51) to infer the corresponding effect on the proton. We consider first the CBM expansion of the neutron wavefunction given in equ. (40). Of the possible $N\pi$ configurations the Clebsch-Gordon coefficients favour a proton core with spin anti-parallel to that of the original neutron, together with a p-wave $\pi-$ (with $m_\ell = +1$). Since the pion does not contribute to S_n clearly the spin-down proton gives a negative result. While one must also include the delta, the dominant contribution found by Schreiber and Thomas[49] was the $p\pi-$ term just described. Overall S_n varied from −0.010 with R = 1.1 fm to −0.017 at R = 0.8 fm.

The second correction to the sum rule implicit in the usual bag model arises from gluon exchange. We already saw that the chromomagnetic interaction helps break the N-Δ degeneracy. It can also mix other configurations than $(1s)^3$ into the ground-state wavefunction. Høgaasen and Myhrer[55] recently calculated such corrections to low energy hadronic properties in the MIT bag model. In particular they found important effects for the ratio $\Sigma^- \to ne\nu/\Lambda \to pe\nu$ and for the Ξ^- magnetic moment. For the nucleon axial current, however, this effect gave only a 2% correction. From equ.(50) it should be clear that the calculation of the correction to the sum rule, S_n, due to these non - SU(6) admixtures in the bag wavefunction is essentially identical to that for δg_A. Myhrer and Thomas[50] found a contribution to S_n of −0.019 (for α_s = 2.2), which was dominated by configurations with 4 quarks in the 1s state and one anti-quark in the $1p_{\frac{1}{2}}$ or $1p_{3/2}$ state.

Together the pionic and gluonic corrections give a maximum contribution to S_n of −0.036. In next-to-leading order there is a correction factor of $(1-\alpha/\pi)$ (also on the r.h.s. of the Bjorken sum rule (51)) which would lower this to −0.033. Of course one cannot simply add the pion and gluon corrections together without re-adjusting α_s. Nevertheless a neutron sum-rule of −0.030 seems quite reasonable for the CBM. This is barely compatible with the EMC result[47] (assuming the Bjorken sum-rule to be satisfied) namely −0.078 ± 0.012 ± 0.026. However it does agree very nicely with the re-analysis of the data of Close and Roberts[56], namely −0.043 ± 0.012 ± 0.026.

It is too early to draw firm conclusions, and much more accurate proton and neutron data are urgently needed. Nevertheless it seems quite clear that the EMC result provides no reason whatsoever to discard quark models like the CBM. On the positive side, this experience confirms the utility of polarisation phenomena in probing details of the theory which are otherwise difficult to isolate.

The Quark Distribution Functions

Using the operator product expansion one can show that the structure functions $F_2(x)$ and $F_3(x)$ are given in terms of two functions $H(x)$ and $\bar{H}(x)$, such that for $x>0$:

$$F_2(x) = x\,(H(x) + \bar{H}(x))$$

$$F_3(x) = x\,(H(x) - \bar{H}(x)) \tag{52}$$

(This is strictly a "leading-twist" result. That is, there are corrections of $0(1/Q^2)$ which we neglect. The work of Jaffe[57] and of Ellis, Furmanski and Petronzio[58] shows how the $1/Q^2$ terms could also be calculated – at least in principle.) These functions are the Fourier transform of the following connected matrix elements (for $x > 0$):

$$H(x) = \frac{m}{2\pi}\int_{-\infty}^{\infty} dz \quad e^{-imxz} \quad \langle N|\, \psi_+^+(\xi^-)\, \psi_+(0)\,|N\rangle_c\ , \tag{53}$$

and

$$\bar{H}(x) = \frac{m}{2\pi}\int_{-\infty}^{\infty} dz \quad e^{-imxz} \quad \langle N|\, \psi_+(\xi^-)\, \psi_+^+(0)\,|N\rangle_c\ , \tag{54}$$

where ξ^- is (z; 00 −z) and ψ_+ is $(1 + \alpha_3)\,\psi/2$. We have specifically chosen to write equs. (53) and (54) in the rest frame of the target N.

Let us start with the simplest model for the state $|N\rangle$, say three quarks in the 1s-state of the bag. Then it is tempting to write the time – dependence of the operator $\psi_+^\dagger(\xi^-)$ as $\exp(-i\ \omega z/R)$ with ω/R the 1s eigenergy. This has been the approach adopted almost universally up to now[59–63]. Unfortunately once such an approximation is made, translational invariance in time and hence energy conservation is lost. As a result the nucleon structure function is no longer zero in the unphysical region $x > 1$.

One can easily solve this problem at the formal level by introducing a complete set of states $|n;p\rangle$ such that

$$H(x) = \frac{m}{2\pi}\int dz \sum_n \int \frac{d\underline{p}}{(2\pi)}\ e^{-imxz}\ \langle N|\psi_+^+(\xi^-)|n;\underline{p}\rangle$$

$$\langle n;\underline{p}|\ \psi\ (0)\,|N\rangle. \tag{55}$$

Then using the translational invariance of $\psi_+(\xi^-)$ to write

$$\langle N|\ \psi_+^+\ (\xi^-)\ |\ n;\ \underline{p}\rangle = e^{imz-ip_n^+z}\ \langle N|\psi_+^+(0)|\ n;\underline{p}\rangle \tag{56}$$

with

$$p_n^+ = (m_n^2 + \underline{p}^2)^{\frac{1}{2}} + p_z \tag{57}$$

and m_n the rest mass of the state $|n;\underline{p}\rangle$, we find:

$$H(x) = \frac{m}{(2\pi)^3}\sum_n \int d\underline{p}\,\delta[m(1-x)-p_n^+]\ |\langle n;\underline{p}|\psi_+(0)|N\rangle|^2 \tag{58}$$

As $p_n^+ > 0$ the δ-function can only be satisfied for $x < 1$ and H(x) is zero for $x \geqslant 1$. In a similar way one finds that $\bar{H}$ is given by

$$\bar{H}(x) = \frac{m}{(2\pi)^3}\sum_n \int d\underline{p}\ \delta[m(1-x)-p_n^+]\ |\langle N;\underline{p}|\psi_+^+\ (0)\,|N\rangle|^2 \tag{59}$$

Only recently has it been realized that these expressions constitute a practical starting point for the calculation of quark-parton distributions for a given model.[64,65] Our proposal is to use whatever model is of interest for the states $|N\rangle$ and $|n;\underline{p}\rangle$ in equations (58) and (59) – not before. The key assumption is that one should use the mass m_n of the model, ignoring the fact that these intermediate states are necessarily colored. This is clearly in the spirit of the parton model and the MIT bag model . The physical idea is that the intermediate, colored, spectator state only exists while the struck quark travels a fermi or so at the velocity of light. Therefore it does not have time to develop the infinite flux tube necessary for it to have infinite energy. (In fact the true intermediate state is $|n;\underline{p}>$ plus a fast quark which is overall color neutral.)

For the harmonic oscillator (naive non-relativistic) quark model it is straightforward to write down translationally invariant states. In the case of the bag model we use the Peierls-Yoccoz approximation[66]:

$$|n;p> = \varphi_n^{-1}(\underline{p}) \int d\,\underline{x}\; e^{i\underline{p}.\underline{x}}\, |n;\,\underline{x}>, \tag{60}$$

where $|n;\underline{x}>$ is a bag centered at $\underline{x}$ with internal state n. The wave-packet $\varphi_n(p)$ is fixed by requiring δ-function normalisation for $|n;p>$. This method is essentially a non-relativistic one which is best for matrix elements between states of similar momenta. It should not be taken too seriously for large values of p in equs. (58) and (59). Solving the δ-function for p_z at fixed $p_T{}^2$ we find:

$$p_z = \frac{m^2\,(1-x)^2 - m_{nT}{}^2}{2m\,(1-x)}\quad, \tag{61}$$

where $m_{nT}{}^2$ is $m_n{}^2 + p_T{}^2$. Clearly large, negative p_z corresponds to $x \to 1$, while large positive p_z corresponds to negative x where we do not need it. The p_z integral can be performed leaving a Jacobian:

$$J = \frac{m_{nT}{}^2 + m^2\,(1-x)^2}{2m^2\,(1-x)}\quad, \tag{62}$$

and an integral over transverse momentum. This integral converges rapidly because of the behaviour of the bound-state wave functions.

We now turn to the question of which intermediate states contribute to H(x). Supposing that $|N>$ contains just three quarks in the 1s level the obvious term, n=2, is that where the intermediate state has two quarks in the 1s state. This would be expected to have a mass order $^3/_4$ m, or 700 MeV, in the bag model. (For the present, subtle effects like gluon exchange are ignored). There is an additional (n=4) term corresponding to the insertion of an anti-quark into any bag energy level. In fact, the term where the $\bar{q}$ is put into the 1s state will dominate in the physical region. (Note that for wavefunctions peaked at small $|p|$ the δ-function implies that H(x) will be maximum at $x \simeq (m-m_n)/m$. This is negative for n=4 and rapidly becomes more negative as the excitation energy of the state into which the $\bar{q}$ is inserted rises).

Turning next to $\bar{H}(x)$ the same line of argument suggests that the dominant term will be that where a fourth quark is inserted into the 1s-state in the bag (n=4 again). Clearly there are three contributions to H(x) for n=2 and twelve (three colors, two flavours, two spins) for n=4. For $\bar{H}(x)$ we find nine n=4 terms because three quarks are already in the 1s-state. These nine go with nine of the twelve n=4 terms in H(x) to give a finite, intrinsic "sea". The remaining three n=4 terms in H(x) go with the naive n=2 terms to give the valence distribution (recall equ.(52) for $F_3(x)$).

For the bag in 1-space and 1-time dimensions Signal and Thomas[64] found the integral of $F_3(x)$ to be 96% of the naive parton result of three. Of this 91% was from n=2 and 5% from n=4. Past work has invariably calculated the n=2 term only, and fixed the normalisation to 100% by hand. In three space dimensions the normalisation varies between 75% and 90% depending on the bag radius. We also find that each valence quark carries about 27% of the momentum of the nucleon (in both 1D and 3D). This is consistent with a scale of somewhat less than 1 GeV^2.

In order to compare with data we must evolve high-Q^2 data, where ($^1/Q^2$ or) higher twist effects are negligible, down to low Q^2 – using perturbative QCD[51,52]. Bickerstaff and Thomas[63] have done this for a variety of fits to the valence distributions at high Q^2. Before we actually show any comparison with this data, we shall discuss a subtle but nevertheless important correction.

Consider the n=2 term which dominates at large x. If we remove a d-quark two u-quarks remain. They necessarily have spin-1. If we hit a u-quark the spectator u-d pair will be equally likely to be found with spin-0 or spin-1. However we know that the chromomagnetic interaction (c.f. equ(12)) is repulsive for spin-1 and attractive for spin-0. With α_s chosen to fit the N-Δ mass difference this mass splitting would be 200 MeV. This is something of an overestimate because of the neglect of pionic corrections, nevertheless we shall use it for our first estimates.

Figure 1 shows that the calculated valence distributions[67] when the n=2 term uses a spin-0 pair of mass 650 MeV and a spin-1 pair of mass 850 MeV with equal weight. The results are shown for three bag radii in comparison with the "data" obtained in the manner described above[63]. Clearly the overall agreement is rather good up to $x \approx 0.7$. This corresponds to a struck quark of momentum about 1 GeV. It is not surprising that the bag, which is essentially a mean field theory, does not fit the data a higher momenta. This would be improved by including configuration mixing. Until this is done we would not like to draw conclusions about the best value of R.

Our discussion of the peak position for H(x) should make it clear that u(x) will dominate over d(x) at large x once the chromomagnetic splitting is included. Indeed we find that $d(x)/u(x) \to 0$ as $x \to 1$. It is well known[68] that this implies $F_2^{en}/F_2^{ep} \to 1/4$ as $x \to 1$. Our calculations of this ratio do agree rather well with recent data[69].

Finally we note that if the proton and neutron are in the $\underset{\sim}{56}$ of SU(6) there are distinct correlations between the spin and flavour of a quark and the spin of the spectator pair[51,67]. For example only a u-quark with spin parallel to that of the proton is found opposite a spin-0 pair. From this information we can calculate the spin polarisation asymmetry A^p and A^n ($A^T = 2xg^T{}_1(x)/F_2{}^{eT}(x)$), measured in the scattering of polarised electrons from a polarised target. The agreement between our calculations[67] and the EMC data on the proton[47] is quite impressive. This leads us to take seriously the predictions for the neutron, shown in Fig.2. It would be very nice to have data with which to compare. In particular the rapid rise between x of 0.3 and 0.7 is directly related to the chromomagnetic interaction so familiar from spectroscopy.

Summary

The calculations of structure functions from models like the CBM are just beginning to be understood. Much theoretical work remains to be done. For example we need to include configuration mixing, improve on the Peierls-Yoccoz procedure, include the effect of meson coupling and understand the treatment of spectator masses better. Nevertheless the agreement with experimental data, including some rather subtle spin-flavour effects, is already rather impressive.

CONCLUDING REMARKS

In such a brief review as this we have been able to paint only a broad picture of one particular model of hadron structure. We have seen that the MIT bag model, modified in the minimal way to restore chiral symmetry (as in the cloudy bag model), yields an impressive framework within which one can understand an enormous amount of data. As our discussion ranged from static properties to deep-inelastic scattering we tried to distinquish between those features which one can trust and those which need more work; those which will survive in more refined models and those which probably will not.

If we have stimulated students to read further, or perhaps to tackle one of the problems mentioned here, then the effort has been worthwhile.

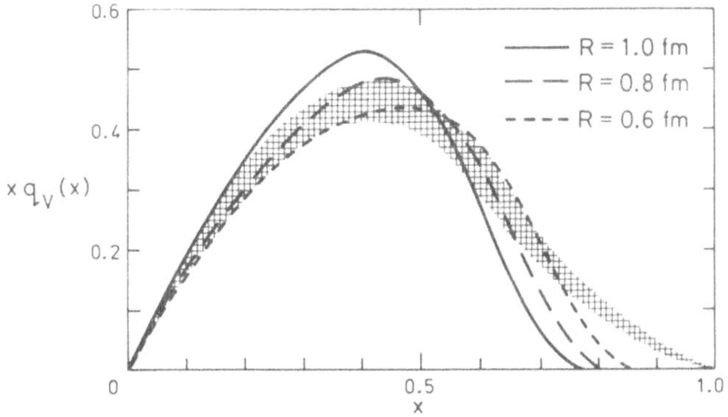

Figure 1. The total valence quark distribution, including the chromomagnetic correction in the diquark mass, compared with a selection of fits (hatched area) at 5 –10 GeV^2 evolved[63] to a Q^2-scale where each valence quark carries 1/4 of the momentum of the nucleon – from ref. (67).

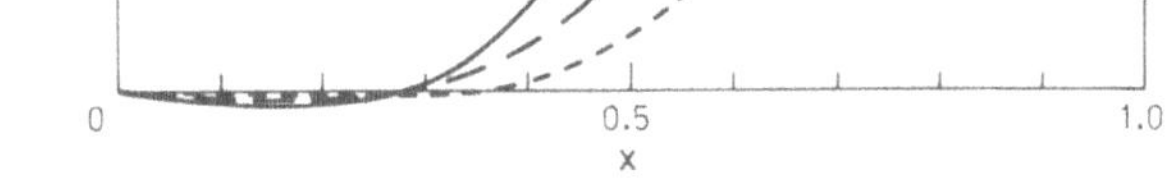

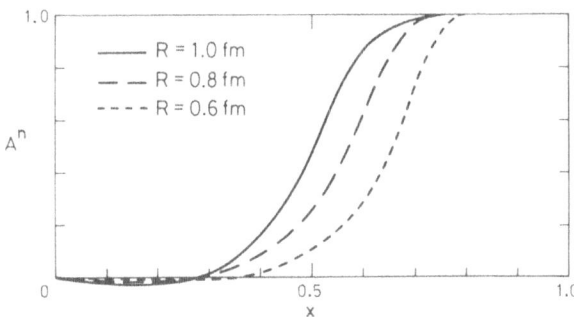

Figure 2. Predictions for the neutron polarisation asymmetry obtained after inclusion of chromomagnetic mass corrections – from Close and Thomas[67].

ACKNOWLEDGEMENTS

I would like first to acknowledge the efforts of all those who have collaborated with me on the work described here, particularly the present members of the Adelaide group, R.P. Bickerstaff, A.I. Signal, A.W. Schreiber and M. Weyrauch. These notes were prepared during a period of study leave at Oxford University and I would like to thank C.H. Llewellyn Smith for both his hospitality and a number of stimulating discussions. It is also a pleasure to thank C. Moody for her efforts in preparing the manuscipt.

This work was supported by the University of Adelaide, the Australian Research Council and the Science and Engineering Research Council.

REFERENCES

1. M.Teper, Phys. Lett. 185 B: 121 (1987)
2. A.W.Thomas, Prog. Part. Nucl. Phys. 11: 325 (1983)
3. A.W.Thomas, Prog. Part. Nucl. Phys. 20: 21 (1988)
4. C.E.De Tar and J.F.Donoghue, Ann. Rev. Nucl. Part. Sci. 33: 235 (1983)
5. G.A.Miller, Int. Rev. Nucl. Phys. 1:189 (1984)
6. F.Myhrer, in "Quarks in Nuclei", W.Weise, ed., World Scientific, Singapore,1: 325 (1984)
7. A.W.Thomas, Adv. Nucl. Phys. 13: 1 (1984)
8. A. Chodos et al., Phys. Rev. D9: 3471 (1974)
9. S. Théberge, A.W. Thomas and G.A. Miller, Phys. Rev. D22: 2838 (1980); D23: 2106 (E) (1981)
10. A. Chodos et al., Phys. Rev. D10: 2599 (1974)
11. T.A. De Grand, Ann. Phys. 101 496 (1976); in "Proceedings of Baryon 80", N. Isgur ed., Univ. of Toronto (1980)
12. E.A. Veit et al. Phys. Lett. 137 B:415 (1984)
13. P.A.M. Guichon, Phys. Lett. 164B: 361 (1985)
14. T. Inoue and T. Maskawa, Prog. Theor. Phys. 54: 253 (1975); A. Chodos and C.B. Thorn, Phys. Rev. D12: 2733 (1975)
15. G.E. Brown and M. Rho, Phys. Lett. 82B: 177 (1979); G.A. Miller, A.W. Thomas and S. Théberge, Phys. Lett. 91B: 192 (1980)
16. R.L. Jaffe, in Proc. 1979 Summer School, Ettore Majorana, ed. A. Zichichi, Vol. 17, Plenum Press, New York (1982)
17. W. Weise, Nucl. Phys. A434: 685 (1985)
18. G. Krein et al., University of Washington preprint 40427-11-N8 (1988)
19. G. Kalbermann and J.M. Eisenberg, Phys. Rev. D28: 71 (1983)
20. S. Weinberg, Phys. Rev. Lett. 18: 188 (1967)
21. A.W. Thomas, S. Théberge and G.A. Miller, Phys. Rev. D24: 216 (1981)
22. S. Théberge, G.A. Miller and A.W. Thomas, Can. J. Phys. 60: 59 (1982)
23. A.W. Thomas, J. Phys. G7: L283 (1981)
24. E.D. Cooper and B.K. Jennings, Nucl. Phys. A 458: 717 (1986)
25. S. Théberge and A.W. Thomas, Nucl. Phys. A393: 252 (1983)
26. L.R. Dodd, R.F. Alvarez-Estrada and A.W. Thomas, Phys. Rev. D24: 1961 (1981)
27. P.A.M. Guichon, Phys. Lett. B129: 108 (1983)
28. H. Høgaasen and F. Myhrer, Zeit. Phys. C21: 73 (1983)
29. Y. Kohyama et al., Phys. Lett. B186: 255 (1987)
30. R. Machleidt, K. Holinde and Ch. Elster, Phys. Rep. 149: 1 (1987)
31. T.E.O. Ericson and M. Rosa-Clot, Phys. Lett. 110B: 193 (1982)
32. P.A.M. Guichon and G.A. Miller, Phys. Lett. 134B: 15 (1984)
33. M. Oka and K. Yazaki, Phys. Lett. 90B: 41 (1980)
34. A. Faessler et al., Phys. Lett. 112B: 201 (1982)
35. E.M. Henley and G.A. Miller, in "Mesons and Nuclei", M.Rho and D. Wilkinson eds., North Holland, Amsterdam 1: 416 (1980)
36. R. Abegg et al., Phys. Rev. Lett. 56: 2571 (1986)
37. G.A. Miller, A.W. Thomas and A.G. Williams, Phys. Rev. Lett. 56: 2567 (1986); A.G. Williams et al., Phys. Rev. C36: 1956 (1987)

38. B.H. Holzenkamp, K. Holinde and A.W. Thomas, Phys. Lett. B195:121 (1987)
39. B.D. Serot and J.D. Walecka, Adv. Nucl. Phys. 16: 1 (1986)
40. P.A.M. Guichon, Phys. Lett. B200: 235 (1988)
41. L. Heller et al. Phys. Rev. C35 : 718 (1987)
42. N. Isgur and G. Karl, Phys. Lett. B74: 353 (1978); Phys. Rev. D18: 418 (1978)
43. E.A. Veit et al., Phys. Rev. D31: 1033 (1985)
44. E.A. Veit et al., Phys. Rev. D31: 2242 (1985)
45. B.L. Roberts et al., "Radiative Kaon Capture and Hyperon Decay", BNL proposal (1987)
46. Y.S. Zhong et al., Adelaide preprint ADP-87-72/T52, to appear in Phys Rev. D: (1988)
47. J. Ashman et al., Phys. Lett. B206: 364 (1988); P.B. Renton, Oxford Report 88/87 (1987)
48. S.J. Brodsky, J. Ellis and M. Karliner, Phys. Lett. B206: 309 (1988)
49. A.W. Schreiber and A.W. Thomas, Adelaide preprint. ADP-88-83/T54 (1988)
50. F. Myhrer and A.W. Thomas, Oxford Report 51/88 (1988)
51. F.E. Close, "An Introduction to Quarks and Partons", Academic, New York (1979)
52. E. Leader and E. Predazzi, "An Introduction to Gauge Theories and the New Physics", Cambridge (1982)
53. A.I. Signal and A.W. Thomas, Phys. Lett. B193: 205 (1987)
54. A.J. Buras, Rev. Mod. Phys. 52: 199 (1980)
55. H. Høgaasen and F. Myhrer, Phys. Rev. D37: 1950 (1988)
56. F.E. Close and R.G. Roberts, Phys. Rev. Lett. 60: 1471 (1988)
57. R.L. Jaffe, Nucl. Phys. B229: 205 (1983)
58. R.K. Ellis, W. Furmanski and R. Petronzio, Nucl. Phys. B212: 29 (1983)
59. A. Le Yaouanc et al., Phys. Rev. D11: 2636 (1975)
60. R.L. Jaffe, Phys. Rev. D11 : 1953 (1975)
61. R.L. Jaffe and G.G. Ross, Phys. Lett. 93B: 313 (1980)
62. C.J. Benesh and G.A. Miller, Phys. Rev. D36:1344 (1987)
63. R.P. Bickerstaff and A.W. Thomas, Adelaide preprint ADP-87-1/T29 (1987)
64. A.I. Signal and A.W. Thomas, Adelaide preprint ADP-88-88/T56, to appear in Phys. Lett. (1988)
65. A.W. Thomas, Adelaide preprint. ADP-88-89/T57. To appear in Proc. Argonne Conference on Nuclear Chomodynamics (May 1988)
66. R.E. Peierls and J. Yoccoz, Proc. Phys. Soc. (London) A70: 381 (1957)
67. F.E. Close and A.W. Thomas, Phys. Lett. (1988), to appear
68. F.E. Close, Phys. Lett. 43B: 422 (1973)
69. EMC Collaboration, Nucl. Phys. B293: 740 (1987); BCDMS, A. Milsztajn, priv. comm. to A. Martin (1988)
70. M.A. Morgan et al. Phys. Rev. D33: 817 (1986)

PERTURBATIVE QCD, BARYONS, AND BARYON RESONANCES

C.E. Carlson

Physics Department
College of William and Mary
Williamsburg, VA 23185, U.S.A.

I. INTRODUCTION

We will discuss applications of QCD using perturbation theory to baryons[1,2] and to the baryon resonances. The subjects that nuclear physicists study are changing and Quantum Chromodynamics (QCD) is presumably the correct theory for the strong interactions, so that this is a suitable subject for this institute. At the same time, we should remember that many of the consequences of QCD, and all the ones to be mentioned in these lectures, are derived using perturbation theory and so are valid only at higher momentum transfers, perhaps at the upper reaches of what will be got at CEBAF. There are many motivations for pursuing these studies. The predictions are testable and this is always an encouragement to the experimenter. We can see what limits traditional nuclear physics must approach as the kinematics becomes more extreme. We may get some idea where the boundary lies between the "strong interaction region of QCD" (i.e., traditional nuclear modeling) and the "asymptotically free" region of QCD.

Also, as we probe the nucleus more and more carefully, it behooves us to better understand the simplest nucleus and its excited states. There have been many pleas for better calculations in the context of traditional nuclear physics so that we can be sure that unexpected observations signal new phenomena and not incomplete calculations. There is also a need for work from the other direction, where we elucidate the consequences of the quark-gluon picture of the nucleons and nuclei starting with the simplest results that follow from using perturbation theory and subsequently improving on them and extending their validity to lower momentum transfers as well as estimating their range of validity. These lectures represent a report on the simple beginning part of this project.

The results can be presented in the categories of results that require thinking but no detailed calculation and those that require significant calculations. The first category includes results that follow because the helicity of the hadrons must be conserved[3]. Relevant examples are the dominance of the magnetic over the electric form factor in electron-nucleon elastic scattering cross sections, the tendency of the tensor polarization in electron deuteron elastic scattering to move to its kinematic lower limit[4], and the dominance of one particular helicity amplitude over the others in baryon resonance electroproduction[5]. Again, these results follow if QCD is correct and if we are at high enough momentum transfers. Section II will be devoted to showing how these results can be demonstrated.

Other results in the first category are the scaling rules that tell how quickly a given helicity amplitude falls with increasing momentum transfer. Examples are the $1/Q^4$ falloff expected for the nucleon magnetic form factor or the $1/Q^{10}$ falloff for the deuteron elastic charge form factor[6]. See section III to see how these results are derived. (The baryon resonance transition form factors are not given as examples in the introduction only because the notation for these is not standardized. Section III will give the definitions we will use and then the results.)

Then we will discuss items requiring some serious calculation. It is possible to calculate, completely and almost *ab initio*, the leading helicity amplitude for a given process. In practical terms, the amount of labor increases greatly with the number of quarks involved, so that we have results only for three quark systems. Relevant to these lectures are the calculations of the nucleon magnetic form factor[1,2] and the leading nucleon-resonance transition amplitude[7], which we can also call a form factor. The presentation is divided into two parts. The first, in Section IV, shows how the form factor can be calculated if we know what the quarkic wave function of the hadrons is.

Then, in Section V, we show how that wave function, or at least the relevant piece for doing a complete high momentum transfer form factor calculation, can be got. Two steps are used. One is to get some constraints on moments of the wave function by the technique of QCD sum rules (what they are will be explained in Section V). This work was pioneered in the nucleon wave function context by Chernyak and Zhitnitsky[1]. Then we rely on an expansion of the wave function in orthogonal polynomials proposed by Brodsky and Lepage[2]. The rational behind this expansion is that one can derive an "evolution equation" that shows how the nucleon wave function evolves from some base point with increasing momentum transfer of the probe one examines the wave function with. The "evolution equation" can be solved to show that the higher the term in the polynomial expansion, the faster it disappears with increasing momentum transfer. This justifies, at high enough momentum transfers, keeping only the first so many terms in the polynomial expansion. The coefficients of these terms can then be determined from the QCD sum rule constraints.

We will from time to time compare the results we are able to obtain for the nucleon magnetic form factors and the leading nucleon-resonance transition form factors to the available data and make some comments about what we can expect in the future. There are great possibilities and opportunities for either verifying or falsifying the applications of perturbative QCD at experimentally accessible momentum transfers. The former would lead to much pleasure over our ability to understand nature and, more importantly, further work trying to augment the calculations to apply at lower momentum transfers. The latter, well....

II. HADRON HELICITY CONSERVATION

Helicity is the component of a particle's spin along its direction of motion. That the total helicity of the hadrons is conserved in a reaction at high momentum transfers follows because hadrons -- at least the ones we talk about here -- are made from quarks and the helicity of the quarks is conserved.

To start with the quark, we have a theorem that if a spin 1/2 particle is massless and on shell, then its interactions with vector particles such as the photon, the gluon, or the intermediate vector bosons, will not change its helicity.

The proof is easy and we give it in this here. Consider a quark or other spin 1/2 particle as depicted in Fig. 1 interacting with photons or gluons.

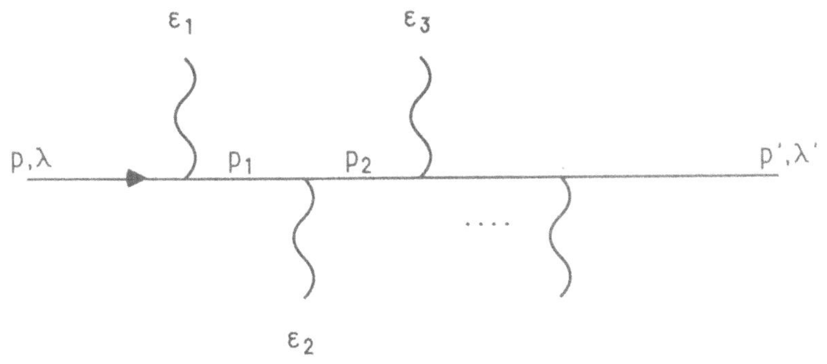

Fig.1. A quark line interacting with gluons and photons.

Algebraically this is proportional to

$$u_{\lambda'}^{\dagger}\gamma_0 \not{\varepsilon}_1 \not{p}_1 \not{\varepsilon}_2 \not{p}_2 \cdots \not{\varepsilon}_n u_\lambda$$

where p_i represent momenta of the internal lines, ε_i represent polarizations of the vector particles, and $\lambda = \pm 1/2$ and λ' represent the helicities of the initial and final quark. Insert $(\gamma_5)^2 = 1$ before the initial spinor. Use $\gamma_5 u_\lambda = (2\lambda) u_\lambda$ and after commuting the other γ_5 through the even number of gamma matrices use $u_{\lambda'}^{\dagger} \gamma_5 = (2\lambda') u_{\lambda'}^{\dagger}$ and obtain that the above expression is equal to

$$(2\lambda)(2\lambda') \text{ x itself.}$$

Hence $\lambda = \lambda'$.

To turn the statement of quark helicity conservation into hadron helicity conservation requires use of the high momentum transfer condition twice. The quarks are not quite massless nor are they on shell when bound inside a hadron. We must neglect these quantities and so need something like a momentum transfer to compare them to. Further, we want to say that the hadron helicity is the sum of the quark helicities, and this is true in general only if the quarks and the parent hadron are moving in the same direction. So we find a reference frame where the hadron is moving fast enough to carry the quarks in the same direction despite their fermi momentum. We can use the Breit frame, for example: the hadron comes in, absorbs whatever momentum transfer there is, and exits rapidly in the opposite direction. (We could boost so that one of the hadrons is at rest, and leave the reader to determine what to say then.)

Hence at high enough momentum transfers, we have[3]

$$\sum_{i=\text{incoming hadrons}} \lambda_i = \sum_{j=\text{outgoing hadrons}} \lambda_j \quad .$$

To see what consequences this has for nucleon elastic scattering or resonance electroproduction, it is useful to draw some pictures of the reactions as seen in the Breit frame, as in Fig. 2. The electron is not shown. A nucleon enters along the z-direction, absorbs the virtual photon, and a nucleon or resonance exits along the -z direction with the same three-momentum magnitude. We give the incoming nucleon helicity +1/2, obtaining helicity -1/2 by space inversion (parity) when necessary. There are three possibilities, distinguished by the helicity of the virtual photon.

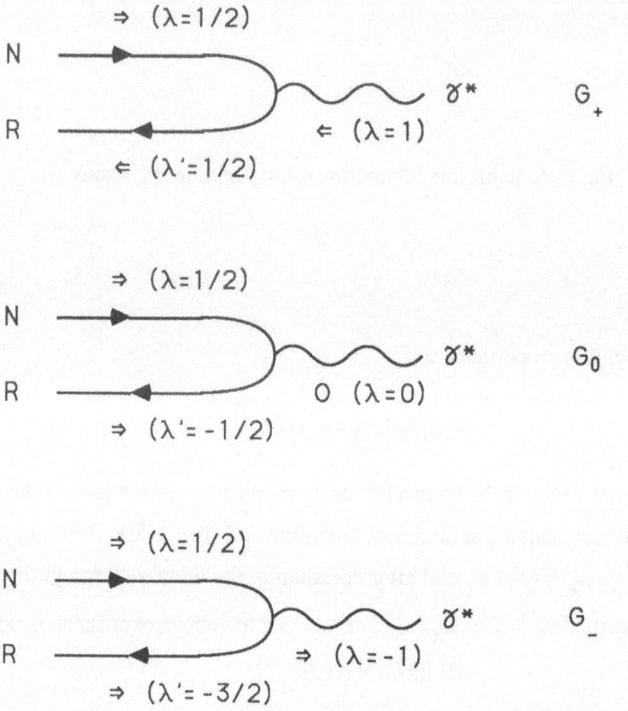

Fig. 2. Virtual photon plus nucleon gives baryon resonance. The diagrams are drawn in the Breit frame, and are distinguished by the photon's helicity.

Algebraically, the three amplitudes are

$$G_m = \left\langle R(p', \lambda') \right| \varepsilon_m^{\mu} \cdot J_{\mu} \left| N\,(p, \lambda = 1/2) \right\rangle / 2m_N$$

where R stands for the outgoing baryon, J_μ is the electromagnetic current operator and the factor $1/2m_N$ makes G_m dimensionless. The ε_m is a polarization vector for a photon of helicity m, and for photons moving in the -z direction,

$$\varepsilon_{\pm} = \frac{1}{\sqrt{2}}(0, \pm 1, -\,i, 0) \quad ,$$

and ε_0 satisfies $\varepsilon_0 \cdot q = 0$ and $\varepsilon_0 \cdot \varepsilon_0 = 1$. Angular momentum conservation tells us that

$$\lambda' = m - \lambda \quad ,$$

and the outgoing baryon's helicity in Fig. 2 is labelled accordingly.

Of the three helicity amplitudes, only one satisfies the requirement of hadron helicity conservation. That is G_+. The amplitudes G_0 and G_- require one or two units of helicity change, respectively, and which requires flipping one or two quark helicities. Hence G_+ is the dominant amplitude[5].

A reconsideration of the quark helicity conservation argument with masses included will show that helicity flip "costs" a factor m/Q, where m is some mass scale and Q is some momentum transfer. Hence

$$\frac{G_0}{G_+} = O(m/Q) \qquad \text{and} \qquad \frac{G_-}{G_+} = O(m^2/Q^2) \quad .$$

Of course, many people do not think in terms of helicity amplitudes and so for orientation we can consider nucleon elastic scattering and should rewrite the above results in terms of more conventional form factors. For the matrix element of the electromagnetic current between two nucleon states, we have

$$\langle N(p',\lambda')|J^\mu|N(p,\lambda)\rangle = \bar{u}(p',\lambda')[F_1(Q^2)\gamma^\mu + F_2(Q^2)\frac{i}{2m_N}\sigma^{\mu\nu}q_\nu]u(p,\lambda)$$

where F_1 and F_2 are the Dirac and Pauli form factors. The helicity amplitudes (or helicity form factors) were given algebraically above. Note that

$$\varepsilon_0 = (1,0,0,0)$$

for elastic scattering. A little bit of algebra now shows that

$$G_+ = \frac{Q}{m_N\sqrt{2}}G_M = \frac{Q}{m_N\sqrt{2}}(F_1 + F_2)$$

$$G_0 = G_E = F_1 - \frac{Q^2}{4m_N^2}F_2$$

so that the helicity amplitudes are simply related to the Sachs form factors G_M and G_E. (G_- of course doesn't exist for this case since the outgoing nucleon cannot have helicity ±3/2.)

Because of the extra kinematic factor Q in the relation between G_+ and G_M, we find that

$$\frac{G_E}{G_M} = \frac{Q}{m_N\sqrt{2}}\frac{G_0}{G_+} = const\,.$$

the constancy being valid at high Q^2. The available data for the proton runs from momentum transfers of zero to a few GeV^2 rather than from a few GeV^2 and up. However, we show it in Fig. 3 for the readers amusement. It would be interesting to see if there is any drift in the ratio G_{Ep}/G_{Mp} in the next few GeV^2. Many phenomenological fits to the existing data anticipate such a shift.

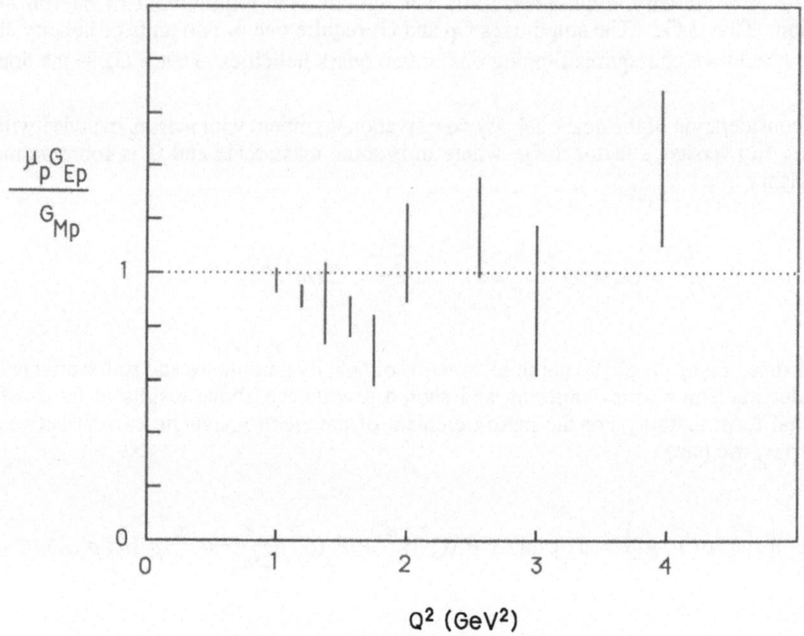

Fig. 3. Experimental values for the ratio of proton form factors. This graph is based on one in Ref. 8. (Data below 1 GeV^2 is not shown.)

The available relevant data for the baryon resonance electroproduction, eN→e'R, is shown in Fig. 4. The vertical axis is the ratio

$$R = \frac{G_+^2 - G_-^2}{G_+^2 + G_-^2}$$

which should approach unity with increasing Q^2. "Relevant data" means here data with Q^2 above 1 GeV^2 separated into helicity amplitudes and published in a referred journal. The two states shown, the $D_{13}(1535)$ and the $F_{15}(1688)$, are apparently the only two states where there is such data. The data is clearly sparse, but indeed seems to be behaving properly[9].

Those who wish to check the data themselves may wish to know that it is more often quoted in terms of helicity amplitudes $A_{1/2}$ and $A_{3/2}$ related to ours by

$$A_{1/2,3/2} = e\sqrt{\frac{m_N}{m_R^2 - m_N^2}}\,G_{+,-}$$

Persons who work only with QCD at high Q^2 prefer to work with helicity amplitudes because of the hadron helicity conservation rule. One or a few amplitudes will dominate and the others will be small. Of course, persons who are used to working at lower Q^2 are more familiar with multipole amplitudes. There is in principle no difficulty in translating between the two languages, and the perturbative QCD results are often more dramatic in the multipole language. For example, consider Δ(1232) electroproduction. There are three multipole amplitudes for this process, and two

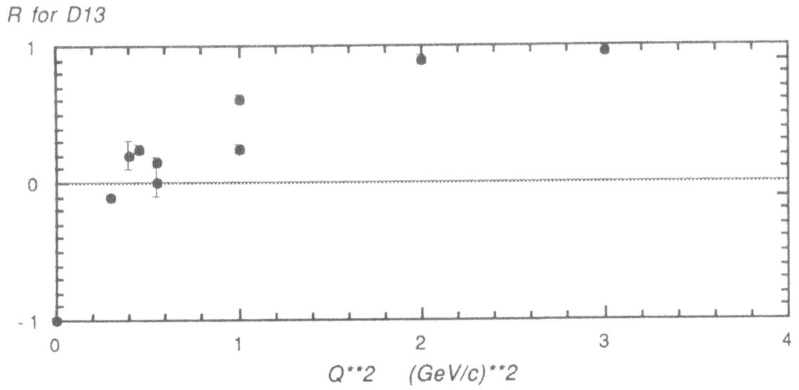

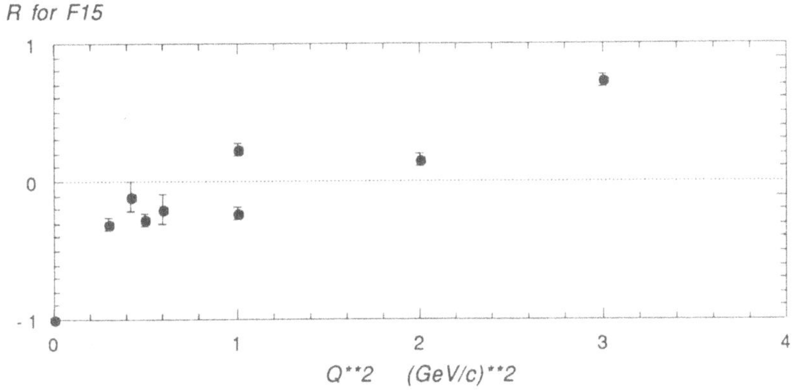

Fig. 4. Check of hadron helicity conservation for baryon resonance electroproduction. The ratio should approach one at high momentum transfers if the outgoing baryon has the same helicity as the target nucleon.

of them enter into the helicity amplitudes $G_\pm$:

$$G_+ \propto F_{M1} + \sqrt{3} F_{E2}$$
$$G_- \propto -\sqrt{3} F_{M1} + F_{E2}$$

The requirement that G_-/G_+ be small asymptotically dictates a cancellation and[5]

$$\frac{F_{E2}}{F_{M1}} \xrightarrow[Q^2 >> m^2]{} \sqrt{3}$$

(There are a number of different notations in this business. The above notation follows Donnelly. We could also quote the result as $E_{1+}/M_{1+} = 1$, or $G_E^*/G_M^* = -1$, or $E2/M1 = -\sqrt{5}$. All these would be the same if the actual result were quoted as ratios of experimental cross sections.)

As a side remark (for these lectures), there is a prediction for the high momentum transfer tensor polarization in electron-deuteron elastic scattering that is easy to obtain just from the hadron helicity conservation rule and the definition of tensor polarization. Again, there are three possible helicity amplitudes and they are diagrammed in the Breit frame in Fig. 5. It looks rather similar to a preceding diagram except that the helicities of the incoming and outgoing hadrons are ±1 and 0. Any other helicity amplitudes for this process can be gotten by parity inversion or time reversal from the ones shown.

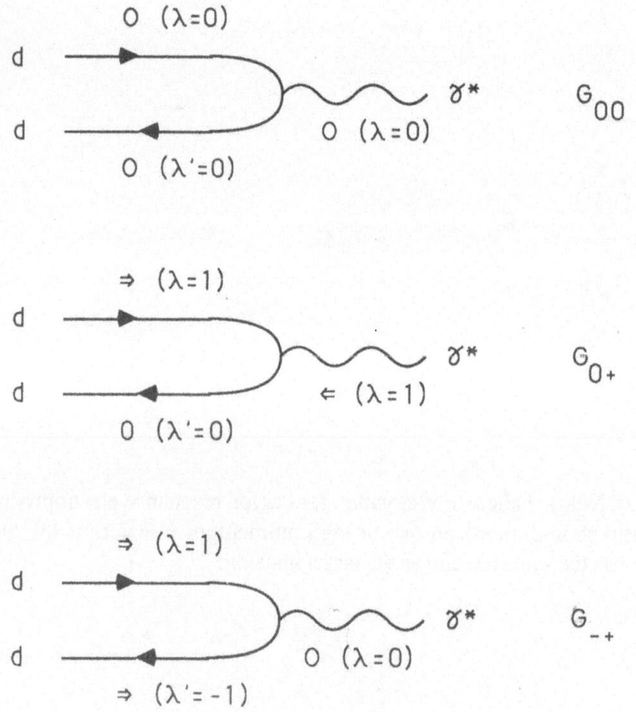

Fig. 5. Breit frame diagrams for electron-deuteron elastic scattering.

The three helicity amplitudes can be denoted G_{00} , G_{-+} , and G_{0+} , where the indices represent the helicities of the outgoing and incoming deuteron, respectively. Only G_{00} conserves hadron helicity, so it is the dominant amplitude at high Q^2. The tensor polarization is

$$t_{20} = \frac{1}{\sqrt{2}} \frac{\sigma_+ + \sigma_- - 2\sigma_0}{\sigma_+ + \sigma_- + \sigma_0}$$

where σ_λ represents the cross section for elastic e-d scattering on an unpolarized target and outgoing deuteron polarization λ. Notice that t_{20} is kinematically bounded by $-\sqrt{2}$ and $1/\sqrt{2}$. Cross sections $\sigma_\pm$ can only come from amplitudes that are subdominant at high momentum transfers. Hence σ_0 dominates and the prediction[4] is that t_{20} approaches its lower bound at high Q^2.

III. SCALING RULES

The scaling rules are easy to obtain using not much more than dimensional analysis[6]. A relevant diagram is shown in Fig. 6.

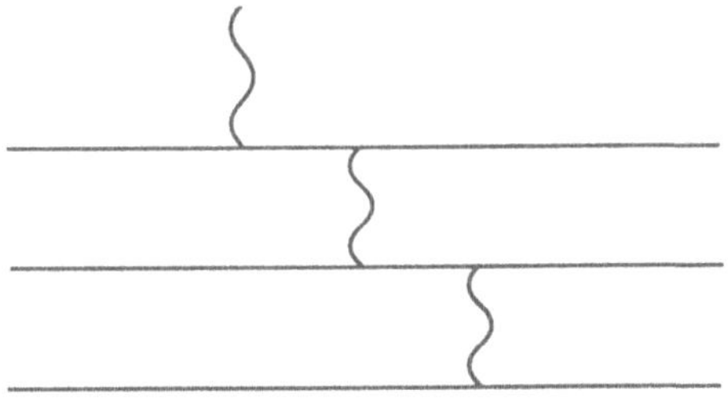

Fig. 6. A lowest order diagram for G_+.

We will be calculating G_+ so that there are no helicity flips, and shall neglect all masses and binding energies so that Q is the only scale. Each quark line in the evaluation of this diagram has dirac spinors u and $u^\dagger$ at its beginning and end respectively, with various dirac matrices (which are dimensionless) and propagators in between. The u and $u^\dagger$ themselves give a factor proportional to Q for each quark line,

$$u^\dagger \ldots u \propto Q \quad .$$

Also we have factors which are dimensionally 1/Q for each quark propagator and $1/Q^2$ for each gluon propagator so that

$$G_+ \propto Q^3 \cdot \frac{1}{Q^2} \cdot \left(\frac{1}{Q^2}\right)^2 = \frac{1}{Q^3} \quad .$$

Hence at high Q^2, we get[10] $A_{1/2} \propto 1/Q^3$ and G_M or $F_1 \propto 1/Q^4$. These can be checked out. We start checking by showing, in Fig. 7, $Q^4 F_{1p}$ vs. Q^2.

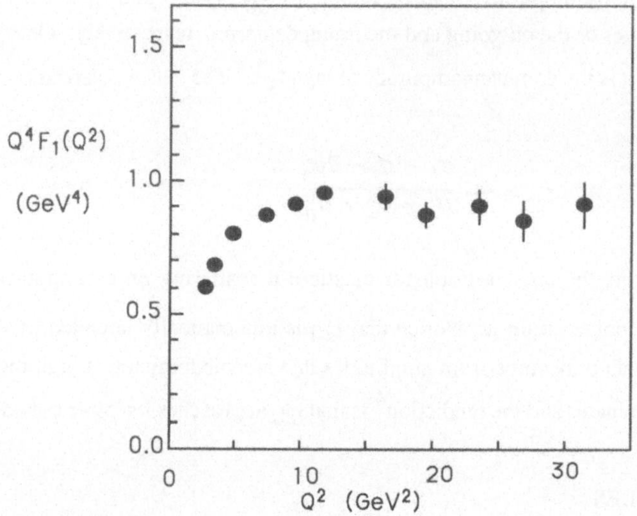

Fig. 7. Q^4 $F_1(Q^2)$ plotted vs. Q^2. This plot is based on one in Ref. 11, but only data from Ref. 12 is included.

If the PQCD expectation applies, the data for Q^4F_{1p} should be constant in Q^2 and this appears to work starting at 5 or so GeV^2 of Q^2.

Similarly we show in Figs. 8a, b, and c the results for $Q^3A_{1/2}$ for three resonances or bumps seen in baryon electroproduction. There is no separated data above 3 GeV^2 so these plots are based on total cross section data. With some optimism we can say that the scaling is o.k. for the 1535 and 1688 regions. These regions also satisfy another QCD based expectation, namely that the resonance/background ratio is roughly constant in Q^2. The Δ is less satisfying. If we look at the original data[13], we would see the Δ peak disappearing into the background with increasing Q^2; perhaps the falloff seen in the present plot may be more significant than the error bars indicate. There will be more comments about the delta below, including some explanation of why the delta can sink into the background when other resonances do not. (To anticipate: there may -- or may not -- be an accidental cancellation that makes the nominal leading helicity amplitude for the Δ smaller than is typical for other resonances.)

IV. NORMALIZED CALCULATIONS

A more stringent test of the theory is to calculate not just the scaling behavior or pick out dominant helicity amplitude, but also to calculate the actual normalization of some amplitude. This we will now do. The amplitudes we are able to calculate in the baryon electroproduction context are the leading ones for nucleon elastic scattering[1,2] (G_M) and for the N-Δ and N-S_{11} transitions[7] ($A_{1/2}$).

$$\left|\Delta^+(p,1/2)\right\rangle = \int \frac{[dx][dk_T]}{\sqrt{x_1 x_2 x_3}} \psi_\Delta(x_i, k_{iT}) \cdot color\ \ w.f.\ .$$

$$\cdot \left\{ \frac{1}{\sqrt{3}}\left|uud + udu + duu\right\rangle_{\uparrow\downarrow\uparrow} + \text{permutations} \right\}$$

The notation is that the momentum of the Δ is written in light front variables,

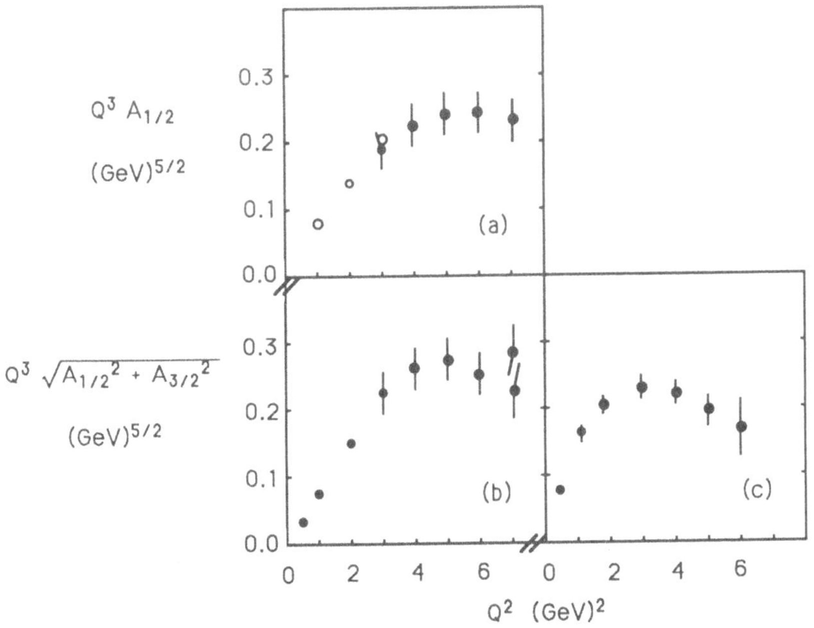

Fig. 8. Scaling for resonance electroproduction. The open circles come from data where the amplitudes were separated. All other points come from total cross section measurements. (a) is for the $S_{11}(1535)$. (There is no $A_{3/2}$ amplitude for this resonance.) (b) is for the bump at 1688 and (c) is for the delta(1232).

$$p = (p^+, p^-, p_T) = (p^0 + p^3, p^0 - p^3, p_T) = (p^+, m_N^2/p^+, 0_T)$$

and the momentum of each quark is given by

$$k_i = (x_i p^+, (m^2 + k_T^2)/x_i p^+, k_T) ,$$

so that the momentum fractions x_i and the transverse momenta k_{iT} are the arguments of the wave function. The momentum labels of the quarks are suppressed; otherwise, the first quark state would be written $u(x_1, k_{1T})$. The isospin state is I=3/2 as it should be and since the color wave function is antisymmetric and the spin wave function is symmetric in the first and third variables, the (momentum) spatial wave function must also be symmetric in the first and third variables.

There are two ways to combine the three quarks into I=1/2 wave functions, so that for the proton we get

$$\left| p(p, 1/2) \right\rangle = \int \frac{[dx][dk_T]}{\sqrt{x_1 x_2 x_3}} \cdot color\ w.f. \cdot$$

$$\cdot \{ \psi_A (x_i, k_{iT}) \frac{1}{\sqrt{2}} | uud - duu \rangle_{\uparrow\downarrow\uparrow} +$$

$$+ \psi_S (x_i, k_{iT}) \frac{1}{\sqrt{6}} | 2udu - uud - duu \rangle_{\uparrow\downarrow\uparrow} + \text{permutations} \ \} .$$

The subscripts A and S on the wave functions indicate that they are antisymmetric and symmetric, resp., when the first and third arguments are interchanged. There is also a normalization condition which we will state for the proton case,

$$\int [dx][d^2 k_T](|\psi_S|^2 + |\psi_A|^2) = P_{3q} ,$$

where P_{3q} is the probability of finding the three quark Fock component of the proton.

The S_{11} is a negative parity isospin 1/2 state, and its wave function looks the same as for the proton.

We may now think about the form factor calculation, and will write the formulas first for the pion, simply because the notation is easier to carry along. The form factor can be given as in Fig.9 or algebraically as

$$F(Q^2) = \int dx\, dy\, d^2k_T\, d^2l_T\, \psi^*(y, l_T) T (y, l_T, x, k_T, Q) \psi(x, k_T) .$$

Here y and l_T are the momentum fractions and transverse momenta for the quarks in the outgoing state. The diagram has been divided into three parts representing the initial and final wave functions and T, which is what happens in between. More formally, T is the two particle irreducible (meaning that the diagram cannot fall into two non-trivial pieces if the two quark lines are cut) two quark form factor.

Only the lowest order contribution to T is shown in the diagram, and note that in this order,

$$T = \tilde{T}\, \delta(x-y)\, \delta(l_T + y q_T - k_T) ,$$

where $\tilde{T}$ contains no delta functions or other singularities.

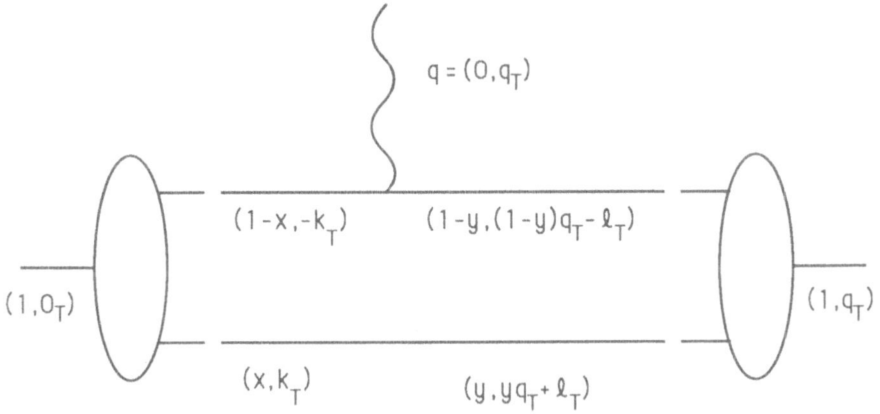

Fig. 9. The pion form factor. Momenta are labelled by their light cone momentum fractions and transverse momenta.

The interesting results are going to come from the high transverse momentum tail of the wave function, so we would like to separate the wave function into high and low transverse momentum parts. An extreme but good way to do this is to us a projection operator defined by

$$(P\psi)\,(x,k_T) = \delta^2(k_T)\int d^2l_T\;\psi(x,l_T) \equiv \delta^2(k_T)\;\phi(x)$$

and ϕ is given its own name: "distribution amplitude." Now we recall that the wave function satisfies an equation $\psi = GV\psi$, where G is the propagator and V is the binding interaction, and we can expand

$$\begin{aligned}\psi &= P\psi + (1-P)\psi \\ &= P\psi + (1-P)GV\psi \\ &= P\psi + (1-P)GV\,P\,\psi + \text{higher orders.}\end{aligned}$$

Keeping just the leading term in both the incoming and outgoing wave functions leads to a result that is too simple. To wit, calling the result F_0,

$$\begin{aligned}F_0(Q^2) &= \int dx\,dy\,d^2k_T\,d^2l_T\,\delta^2(l_T)\phi^*(y)\,\tilde{T}\,\delta(x-y)\delta^2(l_T-k_T+yq_T)\delta^2(k_T)\phi(x) \\ &= \phi^*(0)\;\tilde{T}\;\phi(0) \;\rightarrow\; 0\;,\end{aligned}$$

the last result following because x = 0 in the distribution amplitude corresponds to $k^z \rightarrow -\infty$ and the wave function vanishes.

The real leading terms in the form factor come from taking the first term in the expansion of one wave function and the next term in the other. Calling one of the possibilities F_{1a}, we have

$$F_{1a}(Q^2) = \int dx\, dy\, d^2k_T\, d^2l_T\, \delta^2(l_T)\, \phi^*(y)\, T\,(1-P)\, GV\, P\psi(x,k_T)$$
$$= \int dx\, dy\, \phi^*(y)\, \tilde{T}(y,0_T;y,q_T;Q)\, G(y,yq_T)\, V(y,yq_T;x,0_T)\, \phi(x) \quad .$$

The quantity between the two distribution amplitudes is graphically the first diagram in Fig. 10, and the sum of all the possibilities is what we call T_H. Hence,

$$F(Q^2) = \int dx\, dy\, \phi^*(y)\, T_H(y,x,Q)\, \phi(x).$$

Four diagrams contribute to T_H in lowest non-trivial order and none of them are zero. Only one requires independent calculation and the others can be gotten by interchanging quarks or by interchanging incoming and outgoing states. We can quote the result[2],

$$T_H = \frac{64\pi\,\alpha_s(Q^2)}{3Q^2}\left\{\frac{e_2}{xy} + \frac{e_1}{(1-x)(1-y)}\right\}$$

where e_1 and e_2 are the charges of the quarks.

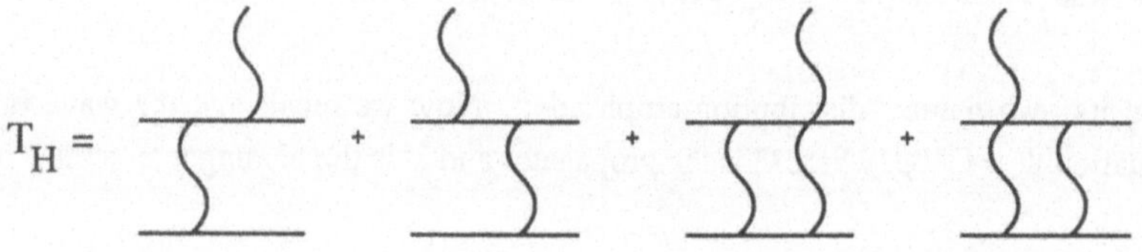

Fig. 10. The four diagrams that contribute in leading order to T_H for pions.

For the nucleon case, the procedure is similar. In the limit that we neglect the quark mass, G_E and F_2 are zero and we cannot calculate them easily. The generic result for F_1 or G_M is

$$G_M(Q^2) = F_1(Q^2) = \int [dx][dy]\, \phi^*(y_i)\, T_H(y_i,x_i,Q)\, \phi(x_i)$$

in the limit $Q^2 \to \infty$ and $[dx] = dx_1 dx_2 dx_2 \delta(1-x_1-x_2-x_3)$. Some of the diagrams for T_H are shown in Fig. 11. There are 42 of them (the number is somewhat held down because diagrams of the same order involving the triple gluon coupling are zero for color singlet initial and final states) but 28 are zero and only four require independent calculation.

$T_H =$ 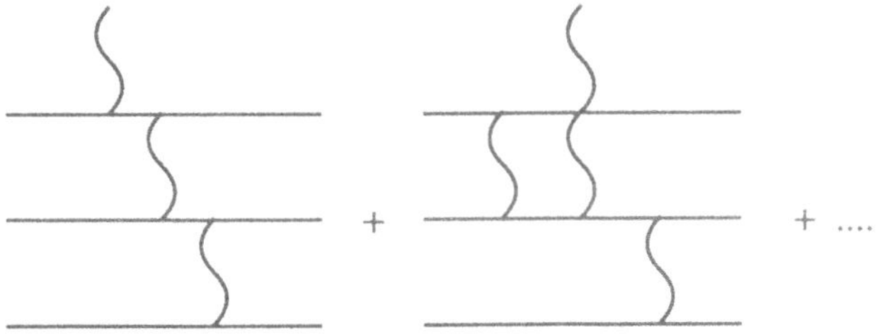

Fig. 11. Some of the diagrams for T_H for the case of electron-nucleon elastic scattering.

T_H can be looked up. The question becomes what distribution amplitude one should use. In the "old days" one choose some plausible form, and using another plausible guess for the transverse momentum distribution of the wave function one could use the wave function normalization condition to normalize the distribution amplitude. A non-relativistic model for the quarks in the proton would put each of the momentum fractions close to 1/3, or

$$\phi(x) \sim \delta(x_1-1/3)\,\delta(x_2-1/3) \quad ,$$

and this in turn gives a small G_{Mp}. On the other hand, using a rather broad distribution amplitude such as

$$\phi(x) \sim (x_1x_2x_3)^{0.6}$$

gives $Q^4G_{Mp} \approx 1\ (\mathrm{GeV})^4$ which is about what the data says. These comments indicate that, at least if perturbative QCD has anything to do with the observed form factor, the quarks in the proton are quite relativistic. However, we should note that T_H is fairly singular as we approach the kinematic limits of the x_i or y_i. For example, the first diagram in Fig. 11 is proportional to

$$\frac{\alpha_s^{\ 2}}{Q^4}\,\frac{e_1}{x_3(1-x_1)^2y_3(1-y_1)^2}$$

and using $\phi(x) \sim (x_1x_2x_3)^{0.5}$ gives an infinite form factor[14].

The "old days" being behind us, we should ask again what distribution amplitude we should use? Good models for distribution amplitudes can be made because we can calculate, more or less *ab initio*, some moments of the distribution amplitude using the QCD sum rule technique, which we will now attempt to explain.

As a preliminary, let us ensure that everyone knows what a moment is. A moment ϕ^{klm} of the distribution amplitude is

$$f_\Delta\varphi^{klm} = \int[dx]\,x_1^kx_2^lx_3^m\,\varphi(x_1,x_2,x_3) = \int[dx][dk_T]\,x_1^kx_2^lx_3^m\,\psi(x_i,k_{iT}) \quad ,$$

where f_Δ is a constant inserted for the convenience of having ϕ^{000} equal to one.

Recalling for Fourier transforms that z^- is the coordinate conjugate to $k^+ = xp^+$ gives for the coordinate space wave function

$$\tilde{\psi}(z_1 - z_2, z_2 - z_3) = \int [dx][dk_T] e^{-i \sum (z_i^- x_i p^+ - z_{iT} \cdot k_{iT})} \psi(x_i, k_{iT}) \quad .$$

(Because of translation invariance, the spatial wave function depends only on the relative coordinates.) Hence the spatial wave function at the origen is just the zeroth moment,

$$\tilde{\psi}(0) = f_\Delta \varphi^{000} = f_\Delta$$

and other moments are related to derivatives,

$$\frac{1}{(p^+)^N} (i\partial_1^+)^k (i\partial_2^+)^l (i\partial_3^+)^m \tilde{\psi}(0) = f_\Delta \varphi^{klm}$$

Here N = k+l+m. Thus the low moments correspond to the wave function at the origen and low derivatives thereof. Short distance properties are often calculable in QCD so we should not be too surprised that these moments are susceptible of calculation. Of course, if we can get all the derivatives, we can Taylor expand the wave function and get it everywhere, but the approximations that will be made lead to bigger errors with increasing numbers of derivatives and this will discourage our Taylor expanding.

Now we will get some information on the distribution amplitude using the QCD sum rule technique[1]. A vulgarized description will be given here. Among other things, Dirac indices will not be written. Consider

$$I = i \int d^4 y \, e^{iqy} \langle 0 | T \, V^{klm}(y) \, J(0) | 0 \rangle \quad .$$

If a name is desired, I may be called the "correlator." We will evaluate it twice, once by inserting a complete set of hadronic intermediate states and once by inserting a complete set of quarkic states.

We make J(0), the "auxiliary operator," from three quark field operators and give it some desired isospin and parity. For examplc

$$J = (\bar{u} \gamma^+ C \, \bar{u}^T) \, \bar{d} \, + \, permutations$$

is clearly isospin 3/2 (because of the total symmetry in flavor) and can easily enough be shown to have positive parity. Since J involves three quark fields at the same point, matrix elements of it with baryon states will be proportional to the quark wave function at the origen for those states. For our sample J(0),

$$\langle \Delta | J(0) | 0 \rangle \propto f_\Delta$$

and the corresponding matrix element for the nucleon would of course be zero. The operator V^{klm} is also made from three quark fields this time including derivatives,

$$V^{klm} = [(D^{+^k} u)^T C\gamma^+ (D^{+^l} u)]\,(D^{+^m} d) \ ,$$

so that

$$\langle 0 | V^{klm} | \Delta^+ \rangle \propto f_\Delta \phi^{klm} \ .$$

Thus the evaluation in terms of hadronic intermediate states will involve $f_\Delta{}^2\phi^{klm}$, as well as contributions from excited Δ's and the Δπ etc. continuum.

The quarkic evaluation of the correlator begins with a purely perturbative contribution involving only three quark intermediate states illustrated by Fig. 12a. The result requires doing two loop integrals if done in momentum space so requires a bit of labor but is otherwise straightforward, and we get

$$I_1^{klm} = \frac{c_1^{klm}}{\pi^4} (q^+)^{N+3} q^2 \ln(-q^2) \ .$$

The factor $(q^+)^{N+3}$ will cancel against a similar factor from the hadronic evaluation, and $c_1{}^{klm}$ is a number which is calculated and known. There are "non-perturbative" corrections to the above coming from the fact that the vacuum, by which we mean the ground state of QCD, is not a state which is free of particles -- at least not free of particles from the viewpoint of a theorist who does perturbative calculations. The main component of the ground state, the physical vacuum, is a dense collection of mutually interacting gluon pairs. Their interaction is so attractive that the energy density of this dense collection of gluon pairs is lower than that of the perturbative vacuum, the latter being a state with no gluons or quarks at all.

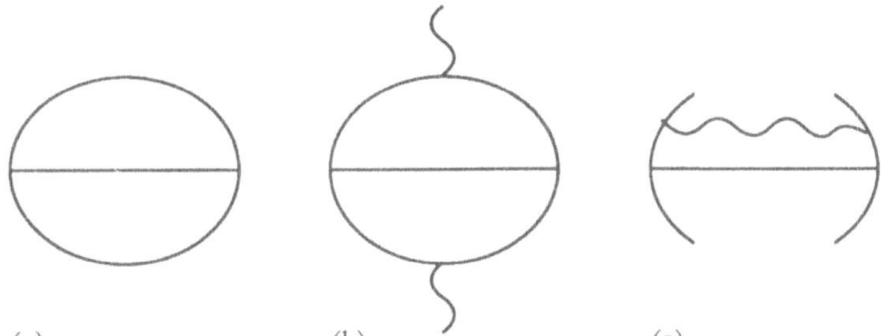

(a) (b) (c)

Fig. 12. Diagrams for the perturbative evaluation of the correlator. For (b) and (c) only one example of many possible is shown.

Now, quarks running through the physical vacuum can absorb gluons from or emit gluons into the vacuum, producing diagrams such as those in Fig. 12b. We parameterize the vacuum with a quantity which is roughly the energy density of the gluon pairs,

$$\left\langle 0 \left| \frac{\alpha_s}{\pi} G_{\mu\nu\, a} G^{\mu\nu}{}_a \right| 0 \right\rangle \equiv \left\langle \frac{\alpha_s}{\pi} G^2 \right\rangle$$

Using this parameter we can calculate the rest of diagrams 12b perturbatively and get

$$I_2^{klm} = \frac{c_2^{klm}}{\pi^2} (q^+)^{N+3} \frac{1}{q^2} \left\langle \frac{\alpha_s}{\pi} G^2 \right\rangle$$

where again c_2^{klm} is calculated and known. Finally, since gluon pairs can breed quark pairs, we also have diagrams such as Fig. 12c where quarks can be absorbed into or absorbed from the physical vacuum, and this gives

$$I_3^{klm} = \frac{c_3^{klm}}{\pi} (q^+)^{N+3} \frac{1}{q^4} \left\langle \sqrt{\alpha_s}\, \bar{q}q \right\rangle^2$$

where still again c_3^{klm} are calculated and known.

Then we should try to match the two evaluations of the correlator. If we take the imaginary parts for each case, we get

$$\mathrm{Im}\, I = (\#) f_\Delta^2 \phi^{klm} \delta(q^2 - m^2) + higher\ res. + continuum$$

$$= \mathrm{Im}\, \{ \frac{c_1^{klm}}{\pi^4} q^2 \ln(-q^2/\Lambda^2) + \frac{c_2^{klm}}{\pi^2} \frac{1}{q^2} \left\langle \frac{\alpha_s}{\pi} G^2 \right\rangle + \frac{c_3^{klm}}{\pi} \frac{1}{q^4} \left\langle \sqrt{\alpha_s}\, \bar{q}q \right\rangle^2 \}$$

where the number (#) is known. Matching as is is impossible because of the delta function on one side being unmatchable on the other side.

A new idea is that if we average over a wide enough range of q^2 we should get the same result from both evaluations. In addition to doing such averaging (or smoothing) we can weight the smoothing so that the lowest resonance is enhanced,

$$\mathrm{Im}\, I \longrightarrow \frac{1}{\pi} \int_0^\infty dq^2\, e^{-q^2/M^2}\, \mathrm{Im}\, I$$

(Some readers will recognize this as the Borel transform.) The value of M should be in the range of the lowest resonance mass. If M is very large, we are doing no averaging at all and if M is very small we will not be isolating the lowest resonance. Then before doing the integral for the hadronic evaluation, approximate the contributions of the higher resonances and continuum by saying that they contribute above some threshold and in amount roughly the same as the purely perturbative contribution. This leads to

$$(\#) f_\Delta^2 \phi^{klm} =$$

$$= e^{m_\Delta^2/M^2} \left\{ - \frac{c_1^{klm}}{\pi^4} M^4 [1 - continuum\ approx.] - \frac{c_2^{klm}}{\pi^2} \left\langle \frac{\alpha_s}{\pi} G^2 \right\rangle + \frac{c_3^{klm}}{\pi} \frac{1}{M^2} \left\langle \sqrt{\alpha_s}\, \bar{q}q \right\rangle^2 \right\}$$

where some terms have been moved from one side of the equation to the other.

The left hand side of the above equation should be constant in M^2 and if the approximations are good, the right hand side should also be independent of M^2. All we have to do to check both the quality of our approximation and obtain the value of ϕ^{klm} is to compute and plot the right hand side vs. M^2. The result should be more or less constant -- again, at very low or very high it M^2 will fail for reasons we understand -- and the value of the constant tells us the moment directly. A typical good case is shown in Fig. 13. The actual value of the right hand side is constant to ±1% for M^2 in the range 1 to 2 1/2 $(\mathrm{GeV})^2$.

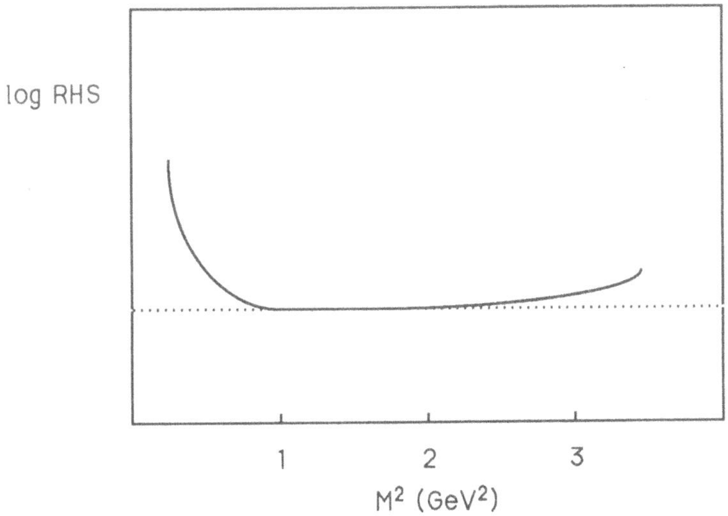

Fig. 13. Stability plot for QCD sum rule. The value of the right hand side in its constant region is proportional to the moment in question

We will close by summarizing the results of the actual analysis of the moments and distribution amplitudes, and give some justification for part of the procedure.

Nucleon. The QCD sum rule work in this context was begun by Chernyak and Zhitnitsky[1], with some corrections made by King and Sachrajda[15]. Relatively accurate moments were calculated up to the quadratic level (N=2) and the results show a significant asymmetry. That is, the size of the antisymmetric distribution amplitude ϕ_A is not small compared to ϕ_S. A model distribution amplitude was found by fitting to a quadratic polynomial, as in

$$\phi = x_1 x_2 x_3 \times (2^{nd} \ order \ polynomial)$$

and the results for measurable quantities are a good value for $Q^4 G_{Mp}(Q^2)$ and $G_{Mn}/G_{Mp} \approx -1/2$. Some justification for the polynomial expansion and the particular weighting function will be given below.

First we would like to remark that presently data[16] on electron-neutron elastic scattering at high Q^2 exists at only one scattering angle. This does not allow a Rosenbluth or angular separation to get G_E and G_M separately, although upper limits on each can be got and for G_M gives $|G_{Mn}/G_{Mp}| \leq 1/2$ at $Q^2 = 10$ GeV^2 (which is the highest momentum transfer for which there is data). However, the ratio of electron-proton and electron-neutron elastic cross sections is falling, more or less like $1/Q^2$, for Q^2 above 5 GeV^2. This allows what might be called a "true believers" separation, or a separation based on Q^2 dependence. If G_{Mn} and G_{Mn} both scaled according to the QCD expectation and neither was unnaturally small one would expect the cross section ratio to be constant. As it is not, one lays the blame on G_{Mn} being small. This argument has been suggested by Gari and Krümpelmann[17] and Gari and Stefanis[18] have given a modified distribution amplitude which fails to fit one of the (independent) QCD sum rule moments but give a good normalization for G_{Mp} and also $G_{Mn} \approx 0$. We will quote some results for the Gari-stefanis distribution amplitude as well as for the Chernyak-Zhitnitsky-King-Sachrajda distribution amplitude.

The justification for the polynomial expansion begins with noting that the distribution amplitude $\phi(x)$ is really also weakly a function of momentum transfer $\phi(x,Q^2)$ because what is seen, for example, a quark as opposed to a quark with a gluon very near by, depends on the resolution of the observation. The changes of the distribution amplitude with Q^2 are perturbatively calculable at high Q^2. The exists an evolution equation[2]

$$Q^2 \frac{\partial \phi(x_i, Q^2)}{\partial Q^2} = \alpha_s(Q^2) \times \ldots.$$

which is solved by separation of variables, $\phi \rightarrow (\log Q^2)^{-\gamma_n} \phi_n(x_i)$.

The resulting equation for ϕ_n is solvable only for discrete eigenvalues γ_n and only for ϕ_n being $x_1x_2x_3$ times a polynomial. Thus the general solution is

$$\phi(x_i, Q^2) = x_1x_2x_3 \sum_n b_n \tilde{\phi}_n(x_i) \left[\frac{\ln Q^2/\Lambda^2}{\ln Q_0^2/\Lambda^2}\right]^{-\gamma_n}$$

where the $\tilde{\phi}_n$ are polynomials called Appell polynomials, the g_n are known, and the b_n are constants to be determined; we determine them up to a certain order using the QCD sum rules.

Now we return to our catalog of results.

<u>Delta(1232)</u>. The QCD sum rule technique works best for the lightest state in a given category. Hence we consider the nucleon, which is the lightest baryon, but we could also consider the lightest isospin 3/2 baryon, the delta(1232). The QCD sum rules for this state have been worked out relatively recently[7,19], and indicate a distribution amplitude consistent with total symmetry. The results for the N-Δ transition amplitude depend on which of the nucleon distribution amplitudes discussed above we chose to use. We find

$$Q^3|A_{1/2}(p\rightarrow\Delta^+)| = \begin{cases} 0.02 \text{ GeV}^{5/2} & \text{CZ} \\ 0.03 \text{ -"-} & \text{KS} \\ 0.17 \text{ -"-} & \text{GS}\ . \end{cases}$$

There seems to be an anticorrelation between the size of the N-Δ transition amplitude and the size of G_{Mn}. The anticorrelation is more general than just these examples and makes still more interesting an experiment scheduled to run at SLAC in January 1989 to measure e-n elastic scattering over a range of angles at high momentum transfer to allow a Rosenbluth separation of G_{Mn} and G_{En}.

The S_{11}(1535). We can also consider the lightest negative parity baryon, which happens to be isospin 1/2. The $D_{13}(1520)$ and $S_{11}(1535)$ compete for this title and the state that we are able to calculate must be a linear combination of these. Data at lower Q^2 shows that as Q^2 increases the S_{11} comes to dominate the cross section[20] and we will call our state that. Since the S_{11} is a isospin 1/2 state, its wave function is like the nucleons. The detailed calculations show that the asymmetry is about half as great as for the nucleon[7]. It happens that the result for the N-S_{11} transition amplitude is not much dependent on which of the distribution amplitudes we choose for the nucleon,

$$Q^3|A_{1/2}(p\to S_{11}^+)| = \begin{cases} 0.11\ \mathrm{GeV}^{5/2} & \mathrm{CZ} \\ 0.14\ \text{-"-} & \mathrm{KS} \\ 0.12\ \text{-"-} & \mathrm{GS} \end{cases}$$

This is about one-half the experimental value of $A_{1/2}(p\to S_{11}^+)$. However the errors that creep into the theoretical evaluation of the moments propagate into factor of two or slightly more error in $A_{1/2}(p\to S_{11}^+)$. Hence, fortunately or unfortunately, if the theory is correct it agrees with the data as well as could be expected.

V. PERORATION

We close with a summary.

Hadron helicity conservation is one of the consequences of perturbative QCD. For the resonance electroproduction cases considered here, it works well enough given the sparse data. More data would of course be welcome, and it should be remembered that in other situations hadron helicity conservation is not successful.

The power law falloffs given by perturbative QCD do work. In the case of the power law falloffs, they seem to work qualitatively in general, not just for resonance electroproduction.

The normalized calculations are in the ballpark of the data. For the N-S_{11} there is just one answer. It is about half of what it should be to agree with the data, but the uncertainties in the evaluation accommodate the data.

Regarding the Δ(1232), we may say that it will have an interesting future. There are two results for the N-Δ transition, depending on what model distribution amplitude we choose for the nucleon. The result based on a pure QCD sum rule inspired distribution amplitude is much less than the total cross section data, and if it is right it means that the present data is dominated by non-leading (i.e., not $A_{1/2}$) helicity amplitudes. A modification by Gari and Stefanis gives a result that is in agreement with the total cross section data, if the data is mostly $A_{1/2}$. An experiment allowing separated measurements of the helicity amplitudes contributing to Δ production at moderately high momentum transfers would be very interesting. Also we should again note that there is an anticorrelation between the magnitude of $A_{1/2}(p\to\Delta^+)$ and G_{Mn} so that a measurement of both quantities would give some test of the applicability of perturbative QCD.

Incidentally, the cancellation that gives the small result for $A_{1/2}(p\rightarrow\Delta^+)$ for the Chernyak-Zhitnitsky or King-Sachrajda distribution amplitudes depends mainly on the relation between the symmetric and antisymmetric parts of the nucleon wave function, and if the cancellation works for the N-Δ(1232) transition it will also work for any Δ, where Δ now is a generic name for any isospin 3/2 baryon resonance. Hence if CZ-KS are correct in their distribution amplitudes, all N-Δ transitions will be small at high Q^2.

Finally, we may remark that there are also normalized results for the lightest isospin 3/2 negative parity baryon resonance, a putative Δ(1640). We have not mentioned it before because the result is small no matter what nucleon distribution amplitude is taken and there is no separated data at high Q^2 for the bump at around 1688 MeV.

ACKNOWLEDGEMENT

I wish to thank Stanley Brodsky, Gerry Brown, Volker Burkert, Manfred Gari, Franz Gross, Jenny Poor, and Nico Stefanis for many useful comments and suggestions. I also wish to thank the National Science Foundation for financial support, NATO for a collaborative research grant, and the organizers of this Advanced Sudy Institute in Dronten for a wonderful and productive time.

REFERENCES

1. V.L. Chernyak and A.R. Zhitnitsky, Phys. Rep. 112, 173 (1984); V.L. Chernyak and I.R. Zhitnitsky, Nucl. Phys. B246, 52 (1982).
2. G.P. Lepage and S.J. Brodsky, Phys. Rev. D 22, 2157 (1980).
3. S.J. Brodsky and G.P. Lepage, Phys. Rev. D 24, 2848 (1981).
4. C.E. Carlson and F. Gross, Phys. Rev. Lett. 53, 127 (1984).
5. C.E. Carlson, Phys. Rev. D 34, 2704 (1986).
6. S.J. Brodsky and G.R. Farrar, Phys. Rev. Lett. 31, 1153 (1973) and Phys. Rev. D 11, 1309 (1975); Y. Matveev, R. Muradyan, and A. Tavkhelidze, Nuovo Cimento Lett. 7, 719 (1973).
7. C.E. Carlson and J.L. Poor, Phys. Rev D 38, 2758 (1988).
8. P.Bosted *et al*, proposal to NPAS no. NE-11 (1987).
9. V. Burkert, Research Program at CEBAF (Report of the 1985 Summer Study Group), ed. F. Gross, p. 5-1 (CEBAF, Newport News, 1986).
10. C.E. Carlson, Research Program at CEBAF III (Report of the 1987 summer study group), ed. V. Burkert et al, p. 503 (CEBAF, Newport News, 1988).
11. C.R. Ji, A.F. Sill, and R.M. Lombard-Nielsen, Phys. Rev. D 36, 165 (1987).
12. R.G. Arnold *et al*, Phys. Rev. Lett. 57, 174 (1986).
13. Shown in F.W. Brasse *et al*, Nuclear Physics B110, 413 (1976) and V. Burkert, Research Program at CEBAF II (Report of the 1986 Summer Study Group), ed. V. Burkert *et al*, p. 161 (CEBAF, Newport News, 1987).
14. C.E. Carlson and F. Gross, Phys. Rev. D 36, 2060 (1987).
15. I.D. King and C.T. Sachrajda, Nucl. Phys. B279, 785 (1987).
16. S. Rock et al, Phys. Rev. Lett. 49, 1139 (1982).
17. M. Gari and W. Krümpelmann, Z. Phys A 322, 689 (1985) and Phys. Lett. 173B, 10 (1986).
18. M. Gari and N.G. Stefanis, Phys. Lett. B175, 462 (1986).
19. G.R. Farrar, H. Zhang, A.A. Ogloblin, and I.R. Zhitnitsky, Rutgers preprint RU-88-14 (1988).
20. See V. Burkert, ref.13.

SCATTERING MODELS IN NUCLEAR SYSTEMS

J.A. Tjon

Institute for Theoretical Physics
Princetonplein 5, P.O. Box 80.006
3508 TA Utrecht, The Netherlands

INTRODUCTION

Understanding the dynamical properties of nuclei and the underlying nuclear force are longstanding important issues in nuclear physics and clearly of central interest. Since the seminal work of Yukawa about the role of the pion as the mediator of the nuclear force, considerable work has been done to clarify in a quantitative way its basic nature. With increasing energies and momentum transfers a certain breakdown of an only nucleon picture will occur and effects of subnucleonic degrees of freedom such as of mesons and quarks are expected to be detectable in appropriately chosen measurements of the system. Evidence has indeed been presented that the dynamical behaviour of the nucleus cannot be described in terms of only nucleonic degrees of freedom. Also in the kinematic regions of medium and high energies effects of special relativity are expected to play a role and accordingly a proper microscopic description of the nucleus is needed.

One possible way to study these questions is to assume from the outset that the dynamics of the nucleons in the nucleus can be described by a non-relativistic quantum theory and then to examine the limits of validity of such a description. The few nucleon system is particularly suited for such studies since in principle an exact treatment of the dynamics can be carried out. Comparison of the predictions with the experimental data in these simple systems have strongly suggested a necessity to go beyond such a conventional non relativistic approach. Specifically, the elastic electron scattering data are found at higher momentum transfer to be different from the predictions of non-relativistic calculations. Effects of special relativity, treated in a perturbative way in terms of the socalled pair excitation contribution, were quite successful in explaining the discrepancies. However, since the electro magnetic (em) interaction is in principle related to the detailed nuclear dynamics through Ward identities, it is not apparent whether these calculations are done in a consistent way.

Given the above issues it is natural to search for a dynamical scheme in which both relativity and the treatment of the em interaction are included in a proper fashion. In these lectures we want to review some of the dynamical models, which have been studied and which are based on the assumption that the subnucleonic degrees of freedom are described by the mesonic ones. First a short introduction is given on the integral equation scattering formalism[1], which is used to study the three-body problem. The non relativistic results obtained for the trinucleon system is then discussed using these equations. Next we turn to two relativistic approaches, which have in common that the starting point is a relativistic field theory consisting of nucleons and mesons. One corresponds to a massive quantum electrodynamics theory, which in practice is treated in mean field approximation. The main virtue of this model is that it is renormalizable and in principle predictions can be made, once a certain finite number of parameters are given.

The other relativistic approach is much less ambitious and should be considered more as an effective theory. It is a relativistic extension of the one boson exchange (OBE) model and the problem of ultra violet divergences is eliminate by introducing phenomenological strong form factors in the meson nucleon vertices. To describe such a model relativistic scattering equations have to be formulated. In our case they are based on the field theoretical Bethe Salpeter equation[2,3] (BSE) and relativistic quasi potential equations derived from this. Within the relativistic OBE model the problem of consistency of nuclear dynamics and the em interaction will be discussed in the case of the elastic em form factors of the deuteron. In the last part of these lectures the microscopic description for more complex nuclei will be treated in terms of the Dirac analysis which is a natural extension to the N-body system of these relativistic models based on meson theory. Using the relativistic OBE models the Dirac optical potential for the case of elastic proton nucleus scattering can be constructed and shown to give remarkable good agreement with the experimental data.

NON-RELATIVISTIC INTEGRAL EQUATION APPROACH

Let us consider the scattering of two particles in a non relativistic Schrödinger theory. It is well known[1] that an alternative procedure for solving the time independent Schrödinger equation with the boundary condition of an incoming plane wave and a scattered outgoing spherical wave at large distances is to introduce the off shell two-body T-matrix operator

$$t(z) = v + v\, g(z)\, v \tag{1}$$

where v is the two-body potential and $g(z) = [z - H]^{-1}$ is the complete Green function, with z a complex c-number and $H = H_0 + v$, H_0 being the kinetic energy of the two particle system. For regular potentials it can readily be shown that the T-matrix satisfies the Lippmann-Schwinger (LS) equation

$$t(z) = v + v\, g_0(z)\, t(z) \tag{2}$$

where $g_0(z) = [z - H]^{-1}$ is the free Green function. Eq. (2) is an integral equation which possesses an unique solution for complex z. The on shell scattering amplitude at a given positive energy E can simply be obtained from the T-matrix by letting $z \longrightarrow E + i\,\epsilon$ ($\epsilon>0$, $\epsilon\to 0$) and taking the matrix elements between corresponding initial and final plane wave states, satisfying energy conservation. The above limiting procedure in ϵ automatically warrants that the proper causal boundary conditions are satisfied. As a function of the complex variable z the T-matrix is analytic except for a cut along the positive real axis, corresponding to the scattering region and poles for negative z, if the system supports bound states. The discontinuity in t(z) across the cut can in principle be found from

$$\mathrm{Disc}[g_0(z)] = 2\pi\,\delta(z-H_0) \tag{3}$$

and which leads to the unitarity condition, i.e. the optical theorem. A nice property of the off shell T-matrix is that it contains also the information about existence of boundstates in the system. They can simply be found as poles of t(z) at negative values $z = z_b$, where z_b are the energies of the boundstates. The boundstate wavefunctions can immediately be determined from the residue of the T-matrix at the poles z_b.

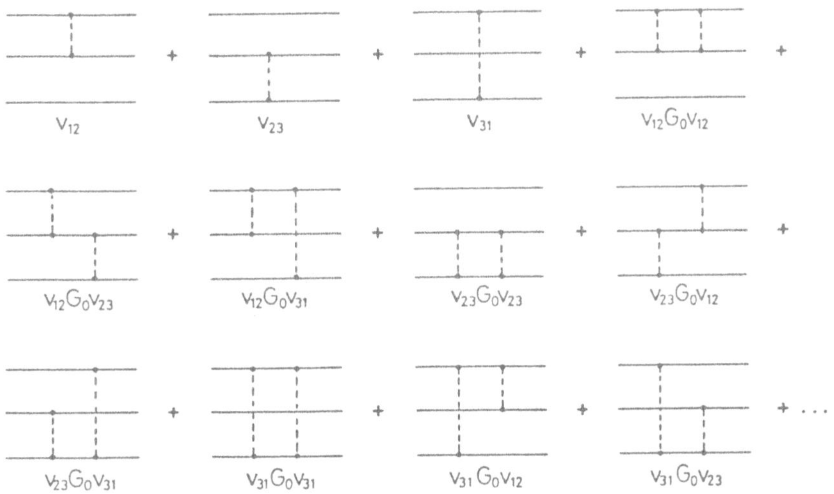

Fig. 1. Diagrammatic representation of the Born series solution for the three particle T-matrix. The potentials are represented by dashed lines

The solutions to the LS equation can be found by discretizing the integral equation and using direct matrix inversion techniques. A minor complication is the presence of singularities in the free Green function for z real and > 0 . They can be eliminated by regularizing the equation using for example the Kowalski-Noyes reduction[4, 5]. Another way to solve the LS equation is to generate first the perturbation series solution by iterating Eq. (2) and then using analytic continuation techniques such as Padé Approximants[6] to reconstruct the actual solution. The occurring singularities in the integrals can simply be removed by standard subtraction techniques. Although both methods are practical and efficient in the two particle case, the Padé method has a distinct advantage that it can be applied to more complicated problems such as in the case of the relativistic BSE and the Faddeev equations for the three-body problem where we are dealing with substantially larger matrices and complicated singularity structures.

Considering the case of three particle scattering one may attempt to generalize the above procedure to construct the scattering amplitude. Let us for convenience assume that the interaction is described by pair wise forces i.e.

$$V = v_{12} + v_{23} + v_{31} \tag{4}$$

where v_{ij} denotes the interaction between particles i and j. The presence of an additional three-body force doesnot lead to essential complications. Although one may write down a LS equation for the T-matrix of three particles, defined by

$$T(z) = V + V\,G(z)\,V \tag{5}$$

with $G(z) = [z - H]^{-1}$, the kernel of the resulting integral equation is not compact because of the presence of the δ-function corresponding to the free propagation of a third particle while the remaining pair is interacting. As a result the solution to the LS equation is not unique. To see how one possibly can get rid of this problem we may carry out an analysis of the perturbation series solution of the T-matrix. In Fig. 1 is shown a diagrammatic representation of the Born series, where the δ-function difficulty is reflected in the occurrence of disconnected parts in individual diagrams. This problem can fortunately be resolved by carrying out a resummation of diagrams, which results in the socalled multiple scattering series shown in Fig. 2. The series is now expressed in terms of only two-body t-matrices. The multiple scattering series can be obtained formally by writing down the T-matrix as

$$T = T^{12} + T^{23} + T^{31} \tag{6}$$

where T^{ij} represents the part of the T-matrix in which the first interaction in the sequence of collisions takes place between the pair ij. It can readily be seen that the perturbation series solution of

$$\begin{pmatrix} T^{12} \\ T^{23} \\ T^{31} \end{pmatrix} = \begin{pmatrix} t^{12} \\ t^{23} \\ t^{31} \end{pmatrix} + \begin{pmatrix} 0 & t^{12} & t^{12} \\ t^{23} & 0 & t^{23} \\ t^{31} & t^{31} & 0 \end{pmatrix} G_0 \begin{pmatrix} T^{12} \\ T^{23} \\ T^{31} \end{pmatrix} \tag{7}$$

corresponds precisely to the multiple scattering series solution. Eqs. (7) are the well known Faddeev equations. Due to the presence of the zero diagonal matrix elements one can show that the integral equations obtained

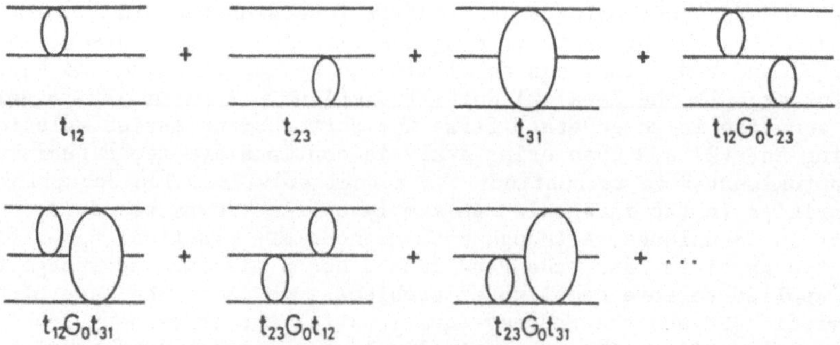

Fig. 2. Diagrammatic representation of the multiple scattering series solution for the three particle T-matrix. The series is expressed in terms of two body T-matrices, which are represented by blobs.

after iterating Eq. (7) a finite number of times leads to a compact kernel[7]. As a result these equations have an unique solution and they can in principle be used for numerical calculations.

APPLICATION TO THE THREE NUCLEON SYSTEM

In the study of the three nucleon system one is mostly interested in the question whether one can explain the various physical properties of the system assuming that the two nucleon interaction is known. In particular, as input to the Faddeev equations are usually taken realistic NN potentials, such as those of RSC[8], Paris[9], Nijmegen[10] and Bonn[11], which are obtained from fitting in an accurate way the two nucleon data. Trinucleon properties which one is often interested in determining are those of the groundstate, such as binding energy, charge radius and em form factors, and those of the continuum states like elastic and breakup reactions of nd scattering. In addition, more recently with the possibility to do more exclusive inelastic electron scattering such reaction processes are also being examined.

Table I. Quantum numbers of the five channels appearing in the Faddeev equations for the case that the NN interaction is given by the $^1S_0$ and $^3S_1$-$^3D_1$ waves and the total angular momentum is given by J=1/2.

NN	s_{12}	l_{12}	j_{12}	K	l_3
$^3S_1$-$^3D_1$	1	0	1	1/2	0
"	1	0	1	3/2	2
"	1	2	1	1/2	0
"	1	2	1	3/2	2
$^1S_0$	0	0	0	1/2	0

Using an angular momentum reduction the Faddeev equations have been solved both in momentum as well as in coordinate space. The complexity of the resulting equations arises from in addition to the two dimensional character of the integral equations, the presence of in general many possible isospin and angular momentum channels. A much employed angular momentum coupling scheme is given by $[\{\{(s_{12};l_{12})\, j_{12};s_{12}\}K;l_3\}J]$[12]. Using for the ground state analysis (J=1/2) only the $^1S_0$ and $^3S_1$-$^3D_1$ components of the two nucleon interaction, we already have to deal with a five channel problem (see Table I). Taking all the $j_{12} \leq 2$ components in the two nucleon interaction into account leads to a coupled set of 18 channel equations. In Fig. 3 a summary is plotted of some recent calculated results of the binding and charge radii for various realistic two nucleon interactions[13]. As is seen there is a clear correlation between these

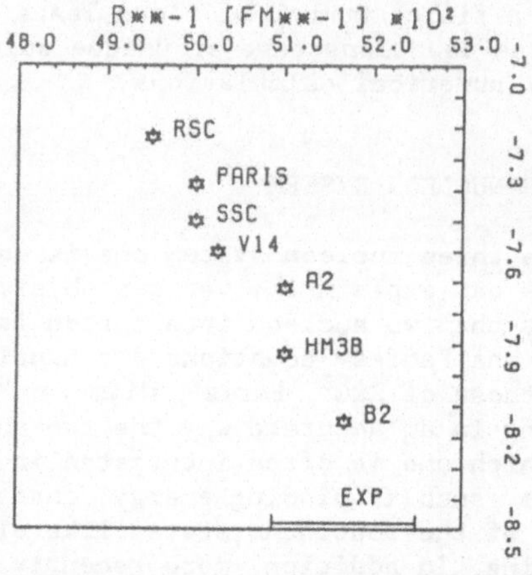

Fig. 3. Calculated results for the the triton binding energy and the charge radius for various realistic two nucleon interactions (from Ref. 13).

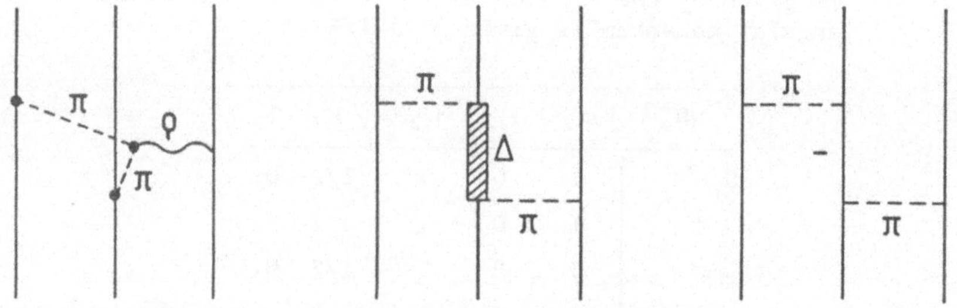

Fig. 4. Examples of effective three-body forces arising from meson theory.

observables, which shows that once the binding energy can be reproduced in a calculation in accordance with the experimental value, also agreement is reached for the charge radius. For most of the realistic two nucleon interactions underbinding of the triton is found of about one MeV. This discrepancy has been ascribed to the presence of three nucleon forces, arising from virtual mesons and isobar excitation. Three examples are shown of a three body force in Fig. 4. Estimates of the long range part have been made using various models for the three body force[14], showing a sizable effect. It should however be considered as indicative, since the result is very sensitive to the short range cutoff. It should also be noted that the triton underbinding is sensitive to the deuteron D-state probability[15]. Furthermore additional binding is expected from relativistic effects[16].

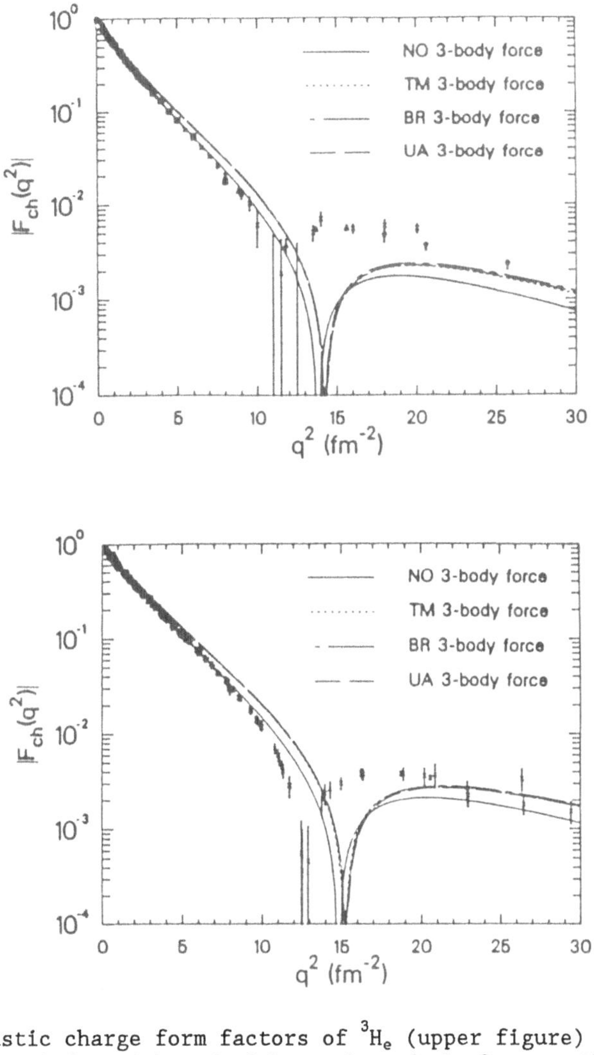

Fig. 5. Elastic charge form factors of ^3H_e (upper figure) and ^3H (lower figure) for with and without three body forces. The configurational approach has been used (from Ref. 17).

Once the trinucleon wavefunction is determined one may calculate the em form factors in the impulse approximation. The one body em operators for the charge is given in the non relativistic approximation by

$$\rho_{ch} = \sum_{i=1}^{3} \rho^{(i)} \tag{8}$$

with

$$\rho^{(i)} = f^{p}_{ch}\,(1-\tau_{iz})/2 + f^{n}_{ch}\,(1+\tau_{iz})/2 \tag{9}$$

and for the current by

$$J = \sum_{i=1}^{3} J^{(i)} \tag{10}$$

with

$$J^{(i)} = J_c + J_s = k_i\,\rho^{(i)} + i\,[\sigma_i \times q]\,\mu^{(i)} \tag{11}$$

In Eq. (11) J_c is the convection current with $\mathbf{k}_i$ the momentum of the nucleon i and J_s is the spin current with $\mathbf{q}$ the momentum of the photon. Furthermore μ is the intrinsic magnetic moment given by

$$\mu^{(i)} = \mu_p\, f^{p}_{magn}\,(1+\tau_{iz})/2 + \mu_n\, f^{n}_{magn}\,(1-\tau_{iz})/2 \tag{12}$$

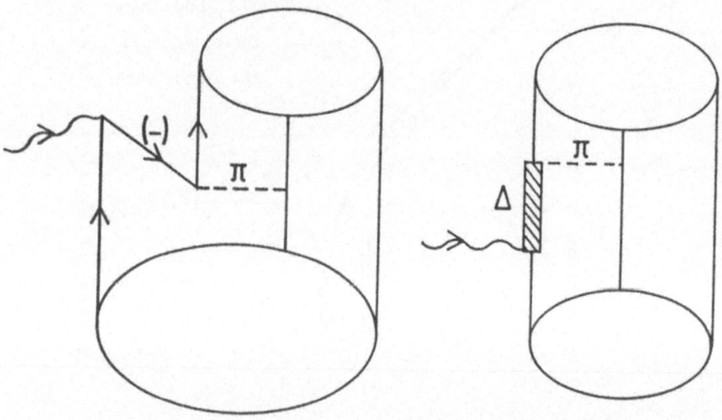

Fig. 6. MEC corrections to the em trinucleon form factors. The pair term (left diagram) corresponds to the excitation of an $N\bar{N}$ pair.

with $\mu_p = 2.793$ and $\mu_n = -1.913$. Using these expressions the charge and magnetic form factors of ^3H and ^3H_e can be calculated, where the one nucleon em form factors are assumed to be given by the on shell ones determined from electron nucleon scattering. Some typical results are shown in Fig. 5 for the case of the charge form factor[17]. In this case the trinucleon wavefunctions have been calculated using the coordinate space representation. As can be seen the calculated dip is too far away and the secondary maximum is too low as compared to the experiment.

Possible reasons for this discrepancy are corrections to the non relativistic impulse approximation due to mesonic exchange currents (MEC). Examples are the socalled pair term and the isobar current shown in Fig. 6. Calculations of these diagrams in the limit of large nucleon masses leads to effective local em two body currents. The dominant correction to the trinucleon form factors comes from the pair term[18-20], resulting into a substantial improvement with regard to the experimental data. In Fig. 7 the results are shown the effect of including the pair correction terms for the charge and magnetic form factors[13] of ^3H. Although these calculations have been carried out using mesons and nucleons as the degrees of freedom, it is worth noting that similar results can be obtained in a model with quarks and mesons[21].

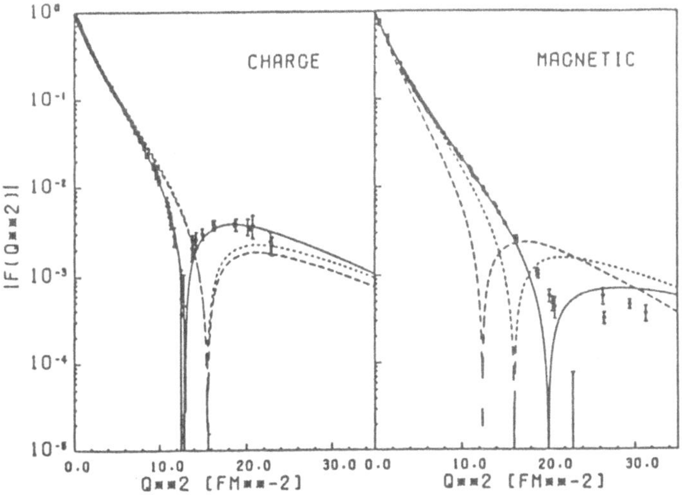

Fig. 7. Elastic charge and magnetic form factors of ^3H for the Paris potential with (solid line) and without (broken lines) MEC corrections (from Ref. 13).

The problem of neutron deuteron scattering has also been studied in much detail. Both elastic scattering and break up processes into three free nucleons have been calculated. In contrast to the trinucleon boundstate situation continuum calculations have mostly been done in the momentum representation. One of the major difficulties in rendering a coordinate space analysis successful is to impose the proper boundary conditions for above the breakup threshold. In this energy region the scattered part of the asymptotic wavefunction consists of an elastic part

$$\Psi_{el} \simeq A_{el} \frac{e^{ikR_n}}{R_n^{3/2}} \tag{13}$$

with n = 1-3 and a breakup part

$$\Psi_{inel} \simeq A_{inel} \frac{e^{i\sqrt{E}\rho}}{\rho^{5/2}} \tag{14}$$

where ρ is the hyperspherical radius given by $\rho = [r_n^2 + R_n^2]^{1/2}$, R_n being the relative coordinate of particle n with respect to the cm coordinate of the other two particles, while r_n is the relative coordinate in this pair. The elastic part, Eq. (13), is present in the region where r_n is finite and of the order of the size of the deuteron. Slightly away from this region the behavior of the asymptotic wavefunction can be complicated. In addition it has been suggested that true asymptotics may set in at prohibitive large distances of the order of 10^4 fermis[23, 24].

As an example how successful continuum calculations can be, in Fig. 8 are shown the results for the elastic nd differential cross section at 31 MeV and 46.3 MeV[24], using a local S-wave two nucleon interaction in the $^1S_0$ and $^3S_1$ channels[25]. It is of the form

$$V(r) = \lambda_1 \frac{e^{-\mu_1 r}}{r} + \lambda_2 \frac{e^{-\mu_2 r}}{r} \tag{15}$$

Except for the angular region where the cross section reaches a minimum the agreement is reasonable. Introducing non S-wave components in the nuclear force fills in this minimum, thereby improving the agreement with data. Continuum calculations with more realistic two nucleon interactions have been done, using a perturbative treatment of the non S-wave components[12], separable expansions for the two nucleon interaction[26] and more recently in an exact way by solving the two dimensional version of

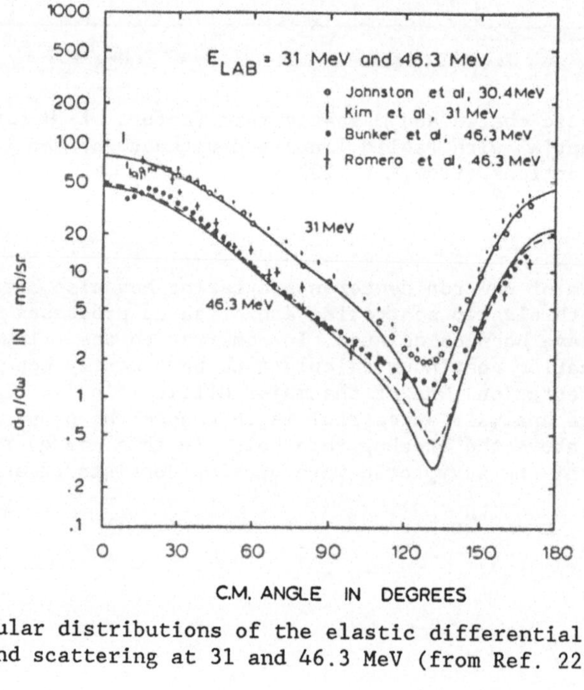

Fig. 8. Angular distributions of the elastic differential cross section of nd scattering at 31 and 46.3 MeV (from Ref. 22).

the Faddeev equations[27, 28], showing that although the gross features of the data are reproduced detailed differences exist with experiment. In most calculations to date the Coulomb force has not been included. Because of the long range character some conceptual problems remain about the treatment of the Coulomb singularities[29].

INELASTIC ELECTRON SCATTERING

Information on the half off shell continuum wavefunctions is essential in the calculation of final state interaction (FSI) effects in inelastic electron scattering. Inclusive electron scattering experiments in the deep inelastic region have yielded interesting results on the y-scaling behaviour of nuclei. For a discussion of this we refer to the lectures of West in this summerschool[30]. The y-scaling behaviour can essentially be understood using the plane wave impulse approximation (PWIA). However, in the actual experiments the kinematics is such that it is not apparent that FSI effects can be neglected.

Also for the (e,e',p) reaction FSI is expected to play an important role. Below one pion production threshold one may distinguish in the trinucleon case between two- and three body breakup processes, corresponding to a final state with a free outgoing nucleon and deuteron and three free outgoing nucleons respectively. From relativistic covariance and gauge invariance follows that the unpolarised (e,e',p) reactions can be characterized by four structure functions[31]. To extract physical information about the nuclear structure from such experiments two main complications arise. The first one is, although the em interaction is well known, that we are dealing with off mass shell electron nucleon scattering. This can already be seen in the PWIA, which is shown schematically in Fig. 9 for the two processes. In this approximation the structure and electron nucleon em part factorizes explicitly as[32]

$$\frac{d^6\sigma}{de'\, d\Omega_{e'}\, dE_{p'}\, d\Omega_{p'}} = p'\, E_{p'}\, \sigma_{ep}\, \rho_n\, (p_m) \qquad (16)$$

where e, e' are the energy of the initial and scattered electron and p' is the momentum of measured outgoing proton. Furthermore, σ_{ep} is the electron

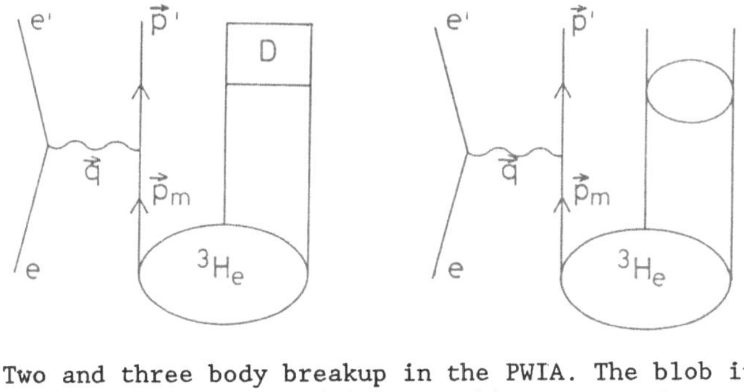

Fig. 9. Two and three body breakup in the PWIA. The blob in the three body breakup diagram (right graph) corresponds to the distortion of the spectator pair of outgoing nucleons.

proton cross section and ρ_n is the spectral distribution function depending on the missing momentum $\mathbf{p}_m = \mathbf{p}' - \mathbf{q}$, $\mathbf{q}$ being the three momentum transfer. The spectral function ρ_n with n= 2, 3 represents the combined probability to find a nucleon with momentum $\mathbf{p}_m$ and having the final residual system be a deuteron or two free nucleons respectively. Since energy conservation holds for the initial and final state, we have

$$e + m(^3H_e) = e' + [p'^2+m^2]^{1/2} + [(p'-q)^2+ m_d^2]^{1/2} \qquad (17)$$

where m, m_d and $m(^3H_e)$ are the nucleon, deuteron and ^3H_e groundstate mass respectively. Since in a non relativistic treatment it is implicitly assumed that the particles are real, we know that the proton before it was hit, being initially in the nucleus with momentum $\mathbf{p}_m$, has an energy of $E_{p_m} = [p_m^2+m^2]^{1/2}$. Therefore from Eq. (17) we see immediately that there is no energy conservation in the ep collision process and hence σ_{ep} is an off shell cross section. This ambiguity has been studied in some detail by de Forest[33] using two forms of em currents, one given by the on shell form

$$J_\mu = i\,\bar{u}(p')[\,F_1(Q^2)\,\gamma_\mu + F_2(Q^2)\,\frac{\kappa}{2m}\,\sigma_{\mu\nu}\,Q_\nu]u(p) \qquad (18)$$

with Q = (e'-e, **q**) and the second one given by

$$J_\mu = i\,\bar{u}(p')[\,F_1(Q^2)\,\gamma_\mu + F_2(Q^2)\,\frac{\kappa}{2m}\,\sigma_{\mu\nu}\,\bar{Q}_\nu]u(p) \qquad (19)$$

The only difference with Eq. (18) is in the four momentum $\bar{Q} = (E_{p'} - E_{p_m}, \mathbf{q})$ in the anomalous magnetic term. None of the two choices satisfies gauge invariance

$$Q_\mu\,J_\mu = 0 \qquad (20)$$

This is imposed ad hoc on the structure functions by eliminating the longitudinal component J_q of the current using

$$J_q = \omega\,\rho_0/q \qquad (21)$$

where $\omega = e - e'$ is the energy loss of the scattered electron. In so doing, his results indicate an ambiguity of about 10 % in the kinematic regions studied by him.

The second complication, which prevents a simple interpretation of inelastic electron scattering on nuclei are the rescattering effects between the nucleons after the photon has been absorbed. For the trinucleon system they can in principle be determined by solving the Faddeev equations for 3⟶2 and 3⟶3 scattering. In Fig. 10 are shown the various diagrams which have to be computed for the case of two body breakup. Various studies have indicated that the resulting FSI effects are important and that they should be included before being able to draw correct physical conclusions from such experiments. As an example in Fig. 11 is shown the calculated results for the NIKHEF experimental setup[34], using the two nucleon interaction given in Eq. (15). In this kinematic region the electron deuteron contribution is dominant. A simple phenomenological factorizable form similar to Eq. (16), but σ_{ep} replaced by σ_{ed} is well in accordance with the data. However, this result is fortitius, as can be seen if we calculate the γpn contribution. It should be noted that contrary to the PWIA the ed part in this diagram doesnot factorize. Only after the inclusion of the FSI the data are reproduced. We

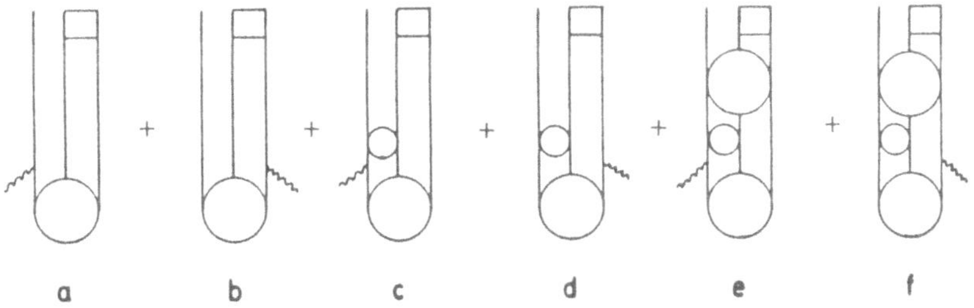

Fig. 10. The class of contributions to the electrodisintegration process. (a) is the PWIA and (b) is the γpn contribution. The connected diagrams describing FSI are given by the multiple scattering series given by (c-f), c and d are the first term in this series.

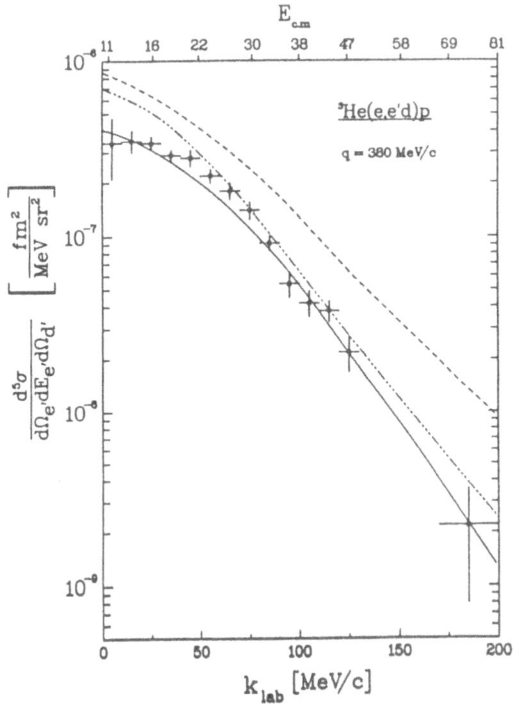

Fig. 11. Two body breakup cross section of the (e,e',p) reaction in the anti parallel kinematics at a fixed momentum transfer as a function of missing momentum. γpn----, complete FSI ———, phenomenological factorization...–...–. Experimental data are from Ref. 34.

are involved in Utrecht[35] in a FSI analysis of the various kinematic regions explored experimentally at BATES[36], NIKHEF[37] and SACLAY[38]. In most cases the kinematics is such that a non relativistic description of the dynamics may be correct. However with the future facilities with higher electron beam energies such as planned at BATES and CEBAF this may not be any longer true and a relativistic formulation will be needed to describe the dynamics correctly.

QUANTUM HADRON DYNAMICS

When the kinetic energies of the particles become comparable to their rest masses aspects of special relativity cannot be neglected any more. Several attempts have been made to construct a relativistic dynamical theory of hadrons, including the em interaction with the hadrons. Apart from approaches based on field theory also relativistic constrained Hamilton formalism[39] have been investigated. Starting point in these approaches are considerations on the generators of the Poincaré group. An example of this is the light front dynamics[40, 41] which has been used successfully to describe the deuteron properties and the EMC effect[42]. Here we shall concentrate on the field theoretical approaches.

One of the interesting theoretical attempts to formulate a theory of strongly interacting hadrons is to start from a relativistic field theory. At not too high energies we expect that a theory of hadrons and mesons as the effective degrees of freedom may be reasonable. To be able to have in principle unambiguous predictive power the requirement of renormalizibilty can be imposed. A possible candidate for such a theory is that of a massive quantum electrodynamics consisting of a scalar and vector meson field ϕ respectively V_μ, in addition to a nucleonic field ψ. It has been studied extensively by the Stanford group and sometimes called QHD. For a review we refer to Ref. 43. Here we treat only some of the essential ingredients. The Lagrangian is given by

$$\mathcal{L} = \bar{\Psi}\,[\gamma_\mu(i\partial^\mu - g_V V^\mu) - (m - g_s\phi)\,]\Psi + \tfrac{1}{2}(\partial_\mu\phi\,\partial^\mu\phi - m_s^2\,\phi^2) - (\tfrac{1}{4}F_{\mu\nu}\,F^{\mu\nu} - \tfrac{1}{2}m_V^2\,V_\mu\,V^\mu) \tag{22}$$

with

$$F_{\mu\nu} = \partial_\mu\,V_\nu - \partial_\nu\,V_\mu \tag{23}$$

The Euler Lagrange equations are given by

$$[\partial_\mu\,\partial^\mu + m_s^2]\;\phi = g_s\;\bar{\Psi}\Psi \tag{24a}$$

$$\partial_\mu\,F_{\mu\nu} + m_v^2\,V_\nu = g_v\;\bar{\Psi}\gamma_\mu\Psi \tag{24b}$$

$$[\gamma^\mu(\partial_\mu - g_v\,V_\mu) - (m - g_s\phi)]\;\Psi = 0 \tag{24c}$$

Using the antisymmetry property of F and the condition

$$\partial_\mu\,V^\mu = 0 \tag{25}$$

we obtain from Eq. (24.b) the conservation of baryon current

$$\partial_\mu\,B^\mu = \partial_\mu\,\bar{\Psi}\gamma^\mu\Psi = 0 \tag{26}$$

Due to Eq. (26) it can be shown that we have a renormalizable theory. Since we are interested in a theory of strong interactions we have to look for non perturbative solutions of these equations. An explicit solution can be found using the mean field or Hartree approximation[44]. For strong coupling it is reasonable to assume that the meson fields behave classical and as a result may be replaced by their expectation value taken with respect to the state we are interested in. Looking for a spatially uniform and time independent ground state for infinite nuclear matter, we have

$$\phi \longrightarrow \langle\phi\rangle \equiv \phi_0 \qquad\qquad V_\mu \longrightarrow \langle V_\mu\rangle \equiv \delta_{\mu 0} V_0 \tag{27}$$

where $\langle \vec{V}\rangle = 0$ because of rotational invariance of the groundstate. Using Eqs. (27) in Eqs. (24) we get

$$\phi_0 = \frac{g_s}{m_s^2}\langle\bar\Psi\Psi\rangle \equiv \frac{g_s}{m_s^2}\rho_s \qquad\qquad V_0 = \frac{g_v}{m_v^2}\langle\bar\Psi\gamma^0\Psi\rangle \equiv \frac{g_s}{m_s^2}\rho_v \tag{28}$$

and

$$[\gamma^\mu \partial_\mu - g_v \gamma^0 V_0) - (m - g_s\phi_0)]\,\Psi = 0 \tag{29}$$

Since the scalar and vector densities ρ_s and ρ_v are constants, we see that Eq. (29) is a Dirac equation for a free particle with a mass

$$m^* = m - g_s\,\phi_0 \tag{30}$$

Hence its solution is completely known and as a result the nuclear matter groundstate can be written down explicitly as being a Fermi sphere filled with nucleons with effective mass m^*. Consequently ϕ_0 can be determined from Eq. (28), which on substitution in Eq. (30) leads to a nonlinear equation for m^* in terms of $C_s = g_s^2 m^2/m_s^2$ and the fermi momentum k_f. The energy density of the ground state can also be determined using the energy momentum tensor. Two parameters only appear in the theory, C_s and $C_v = g_v^2 m^2/m_v^2$, which can be used to calculate the saturation curve for nuclear matter. The experimental binding energy and saturation density can be fitted using a value of $C_s = 267.1$ and $C_v = 195.9$. The effective mass in the mean field approximation is found to be about 0.5m, considerably smaller than the free nucleon mass, indicating very strong meson fields.

The above results can readily be extended to finite nuclei by looking at spatially non uniform solutions. In momentum space Eqs. (24a-b) leads to scalar and vector potentials in the Dirac equation (24.c) of the form

$$S(k) \equiv g_s\phi(k) = \frac{g_s^2}{k^2+m_s^2}\,\bar\Psi\Psi \qquad\qquad V(k) \equiv g_v V_0(k) = \frac{g_v^2}{k^2+m_v^2}\,\bar\Psi\gamma^0\Psi \tag{31}$$

The resulting nonlinear equations can be solved numerically. Relativistic orbitals for spherical nuclei have been obtained and used to calculate charge densities in good agreement with experiment[45]. As an example in Fig. 12 is shown the case of $^{208}P_b$. Extensions to the Hartree calculation have also been studied such as the inclusion of the vacuum polarisation[46]. Although the results are very encouraging some intrinsic problems exist, which have to be clarified. Although the predictive power is appealing, it is not clear whether one will be able to calculate for example the meson-nucleon strong form factors in a reliable way and the outcome will be medium dependent. Moreover, the meson propagators will also be modified by the medium. No attempt has been made up to date to study these

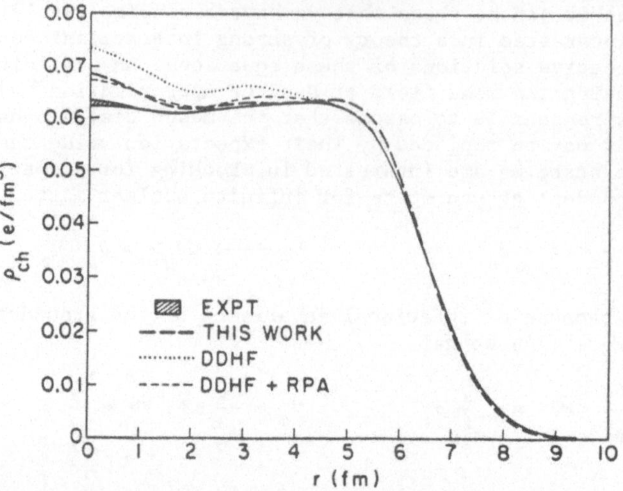

Fig. 12. Charge density distributions for ^{208} Pb as calculated in the Hartree approximation (long dashed curve). Other curves correspond to density dependent Hartree-Fock type of calculations (from Ref. 43).

problems. With regard to quantum corrections, since we are in a strong interaction regime the quantum effects due to the Dirac sea cannot be simply calculated using a perturbational approach. Using an effective action analysis estimates have been made on the one loop level[47]. However on this level instability of the groundstate appears for high momentum fluctuations[48, 49].

RELATIVISTIC DYNAMICS

A less ambitious approach is to study the nuclear interaction based on the one boson exchange model. To regularize the high momentum behaviour strong form factors in the meson nucleon vertices are employed. As a consequence the type of couplings of the mesons to the nucleons need not be restricted to renormalizable ones. A main ingredient in the study of quantum dynamics is the formulation of relativistic dynamical equations. They should satisfy general principles such as causality, unitarity and clustering property. The latter implies that if subclusters in a N particle system are infinitely far apart in coordinate space and scattering takes only place between the particles within each subcluster, the N particle S-matrix should separate out into the S-matrices of the individual subclusters. Also the treatment of the em interaction should be incorporated in a consistent way, satisfying gauge invariance.

For the two nucleon system this has been studied in some detail using as a starting point the field theoretical Bethe Salpeter equation (BSE). In terms of the four point function

$$G(x_1',x_2';x_1,x_2) = \langle 0|T\{\bar{\Psi}(x_1')\bar{\Psi}(x_2')\Psi(x_1)\Psi(x_2)\}|0\rangle \qquad (32)$$

we may introduce the T-matrix as

$$G = G_0 + G_0 \, T \, G_0 \tag{33}$$

where G_0 is the free two nucleon Green function. In the momentum space representation it is given by the product of the propagators of the two nucleons

$$G_0 = S_F(k_1) \, S_F(k_2) \tag{34}$$

with $S_F(k) = [k_\mu \gamma^\mu + m] \, [k^2 - m^2 + i\epsilon]^{-1}$, $\epsilon > 0$.

A Feynman diagram analysis can in principle be written down for the four point function. Let us introduce the notion of irreducible graphs as being those Feynman graphs which only become disconnected if at least three lines, two of them being the nucleons, are cut internally. Then one can readily show that the T-matrix satisfies the BSE, given formally by

$$T = V + V \, G_0 \, T \tag{35}$$

where V is the set of all irreducible graphs. In Fig. 13 a graphical representation is shown of the BSE. From the Cutkowski cutting rules[50] it can readily be shown that two particl unitarity is satisfied when we are below one particle production threshold. Although Eq. (35) has formally

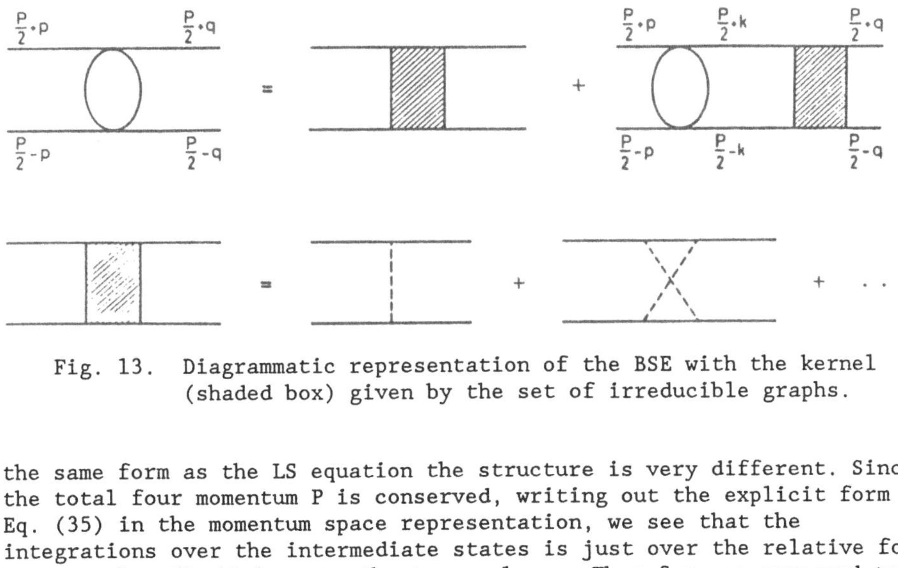

Fig. 13. Diagrammatic representation of the BSE with the kernel (shaded box) given by the set of irreducible graphs.

the same form as the LS equation the structure is very different. Since the total four momentum P is conserved, writing out the explicit form of Eq. (35) in the momentum space representation, we see that the integrations over the intermediate states is just over the relative four momentum $k = (k_0, \mathbf{k})$ between the two nucleons. Therefore as compared to the LS equation the relative energy k_0 appears as an additional integration variable, resulting into a four dimensional integral equation for Eq. (35). Because of the occurrence of the relative energy variable the singularity structure of the BSE is much more complicated than the LS equation. In the cm system $P = (\sqrt{s}, 0)$ we have for the scalar part of the two nucleon free Green function Eq. (34)

$$S_0(k_0, \mathbf{k}) = \left[\{ (\frac{\sqrt{s}}{2} - k_0)^2 - E_k^2 \} \, \{ (\frac{\sqrt{s}}{2} + k_0)^2 - E_k^2 \} \right]^{-1} \tag{36}$$

From this we see that there are four poles in the complex k_0 plane. Due to the $i\epsilon$ prescription in the propagators, two of these singularities can pinch the path of integration when the three momentum variable **k** is varying. It is precisely this pinching which leads to the two particle unitarity condition. Although the two nucleons are in the BSE off the mass shell i.e. $k_n^2 \neq m_n^2$, the discontinuity of the free two nucleon propagator is obtained from the condition that both nucleons are on the mass shell. We have

$$\mathrm{Disc}[S_0(k_0,\mathbf{k})] = 4\,\pi^2\,\delta^{(+)}(k_1^2-m^2)\,\delta^{(+)}(k_2^2-m^2) \tag{37}$$

Since it is in practice very hard to construct solutions to the BSE, it is appealing to look for relativistic equations, which have a similar complexity as the non relativistic LS equation, but where special relativity has properly been built in. For the T-matrix one writes down a quasi potential equation with a properly chosen Green function G_{pq} and where in the intermediate states only integrations take place over the relative three momentum. It has the form

$$T = V_{qp} + V_{qp}\,G_{qp}\,T \tag{38}$$

where V_{qp} is chosen such that it gives the same result as the T-matrix obtained as a solution of the BSE. It can easily be verified that V_{qp} is related to the driving force of the BSE through

$$V_{qp} = V + V\,[G_0 - G_{qp}]\,V_{qp} \tag{39}$$

It should be noted that Eq. (39) in general doesnot have an unique solution and that it should only be considered as a formal relation, which can be used to calculate perturbatively higher corrections to V_{qp}. It is clear that there are essentially unlimited possibilities for G_{qp}. The conditions we would like to impose on the choice of such a Green function is that it would satisfy the general principles of relativistic covariance, unitarity and causality. Various popular choices exist in literature. One is due to Blankenbecler, Sugar[51], Logunov and Tavkhelidze[52] (BBSLT), where a dispersion relation is written down for the Green function with the same discontinuity as G_0. In the cm system we have

$$G_{qp} = \frac{1}{\pi}\int \frac{ds'}{s - s'}\,4\pi^2\,\delta[(\sqrt{s'}/2 + k_0)^2 - E_{\mathbf{k}}^2]\,\delta[(\sqrt{s'}/2 - k_0)^2 - E_{\mathbf{k}}^2] \tag{40}$$

or

$$G_{qp} = 2\,\pi\,\delta(k_0)\,\frac{1}{E_{\mathbf{k}}}\,[s - 4\,E_{\mathbf{k}}^2]^{-1} \tag{41}$$

Note that Eq. (41) is the same as the non relativistic Green function except for the phase space factor $1/E_{k'}$. Also the two nucleons are treated in a symmetric way (k_0=0). Another choice is due to Gross[53] where one of the particles is put on the mass shell and which has extended by him for more particle systems. It is especially suited to discuss the em interaction. Due to the asymetric treatment of the nucleons the Pauli principle is violated, although one can repair this by explicit symmetrization. Also non physical singularities arise in calculating higher order contributions to V_{qp}.

MESON THEORETICAL DESCRIPTION WITH EFFECTIVE INTERACTIONS

In studying for NN scattering the relativistic equations as described in the previous section it is clear that some reasonable approximation has to be made for the driving force. In view of the success of the non relativistic OBE model, it is natural to assume that we may parameterize the kernel in the BSE by a sum of meson exchanges. Specifically, we have taken as driving force the exchange of π, σ, ω, ρ, δ and η mesons. For the pion nucleon interaction we may use either the pseudo-scalar, pseudo-vector or an admixture i.e.

$$L_{\pi NN} = ig_{\pi NN} [\lambda \bar{\Psi}\gamma_5\tau\Psi\phi_\pi + (1-\lambda)/2m \Psi\gamma_5\gamma \tau\Psi\partial_\mu\phi_\pi] \tag{42}$$

For the other meson nucleon interactions standard type of couplings are taken. To regularize the short distance behaviour strong form factors are used in the meson nucleon vertices of a monopole type. Using this OBE model the BSE and QP equations have been studied in the region up to 250 MeV lab energy[54]. It should be noted that in these relativistic models in addition to the physical positive energy spinor states also negative energy spinor states are present. Using the γ_5 coupling for the pion we were unable to get any qualitative good fits to the experimental phase shifts. The main reason is that there is a large coupling between the positive and negative energies states in this case. Using the pseudo-vector coupling which has a substantially smaller coupling we succeeded in getting reasonable phase shifts. The pair suppression effect in the pseudo-vector case is also clearly favoured in photo pion production experiments and chiral symmetry arguments. Of course a certain admixture of pseudo-scalar is in principle not excluded. In fact, a 25 % admixture was recently used with success to describe the NN interaction[55].

Having a relativistic model for the NN interaction we may study the em properties of the deuteron in the model. As mentioned before MEC corrections have been studied in a perturbative treatment. One of the important contributions comes from the pair excitation graph[56]. It can be considered of relativistic origin since it arises from the Dirac structure of the nucleon in the intermediate state. In the conventional treatment of these corrections it is implicitly assumed that the non relativistic dynamics is not affected and that as a consequence we do not have to go beyond the non relativistic wavefunction framework concerning the dynamics. This aspect we can study in our relativistic model. The em interaction can simply be included in our description by taking as the current operator Eq. (18). Gauge invariance is satisfied[57].

In the one photon exchange approximation the elastic differential cross section of electron deuteron scattering is given by the well known Rosenbluth formula

$$\frac{d\sigma}{d\Omega} = \frac{d\sigma_{Mott}}{d\Omega} [A(Q^2) + B(Q^2) \tan^2(\theta_e,/2)] \tag{43}$$

where the electric and magnetic formfactors can be expressed as[58]

$$A(Q^2) = F_C^2 + \frac{8}{9}\eta^2 F_Q^2 + \frac{2}{3}\eta F_M^2 \tag{44}$$

$$B(Q^2) = \frac{4}{3}\eta(1+\eta) F_M^2 \tag{45}$$

with $\eta = -Q^2/4m_d^2$. The elastic em form factors F, can most conveniently be computed from the deuteron current by going to the Breit system. In the impulse approximation we need in addition to the nucleon em current, the deuteron vertex function, which is determined in the two nucleon cm system. As a consequence we have to deal with the major technical problem of the boost transformations to the Breit system. This has been done by shifting these boosts to the em current operator. For details we refer to Ref. 59. The result is shown in Fig. 14 for the charge form factor. Contrary to the pair excitation contribution estimate, this result shows

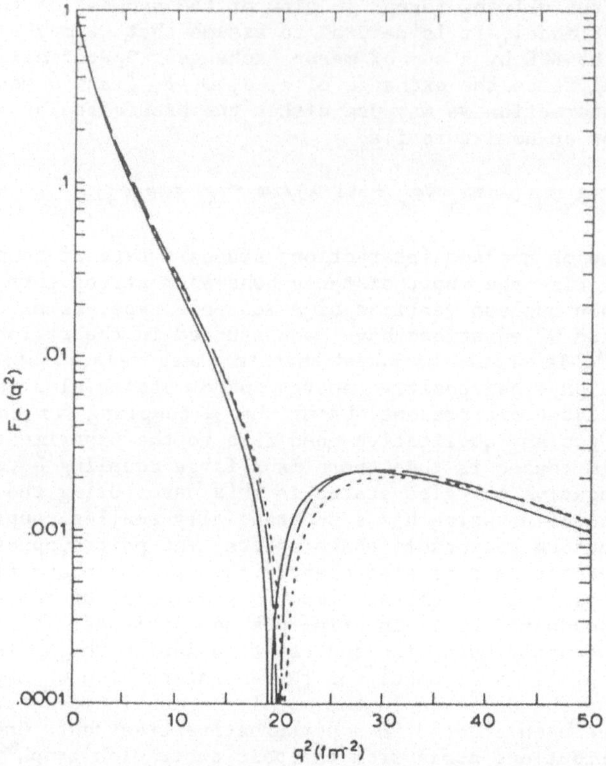

Fig. 14. Charge form factor F_C of deuteron obtained from the BSE for the relativistic OBE model (——). Also are shown the RSC result (---) and the static approximation (...), obtained by neglecting boost effects and negative energy spinor states (from Ref. 59).

that the relativistic effects seem to be small. Since in our calculation the pair graph is automatically included because of the presence of the negative energy states in our equations, clearly additional effects have been included in the model. One important contribution which has been neglected is of dynamical nature. One easy way to see its origin is to use the Gross QP equation framework. The various corrections to the non relativistic impulse approximation can be studied using a perturbational treatment[57]. The diagrammatical analysis is shown in Fig. 15. Since the deuteron vertex function satisfy the homegeneous QP equation we may replace it in the relativistic impulse approximation by the once iterated vertex function. The resulting graph can be rewritten in three pieces, namely (i) the non relativistic contribution where all the nucleons are on mass shell, (ii) the pair excitation contribution and (iii) a dynamical contribution which is connected to the negative energy state component in the deuteron. Calculations of the contributions (ii) and (iii) show (see Fig. 16) that the dynamical correction is of the same order of magnitude as the pair term, but opposite in sign, sothat a cancellation takes place. From this study we see that a consistent analysis has to be done both for the dynamics and the em interaction to get a reliable prediction.

Much attention has been paid recently to the magnetic form factor of deuteron. The experimental results exhibit a dip at high momentum transfer[60] and at intermediate momentum transfer region[61] they fall considerably below non relativistic calculations (see Fig. 17). Although corrections from the pair term and the $\pi\rho\gamma$ MEC contribution[62] brings the

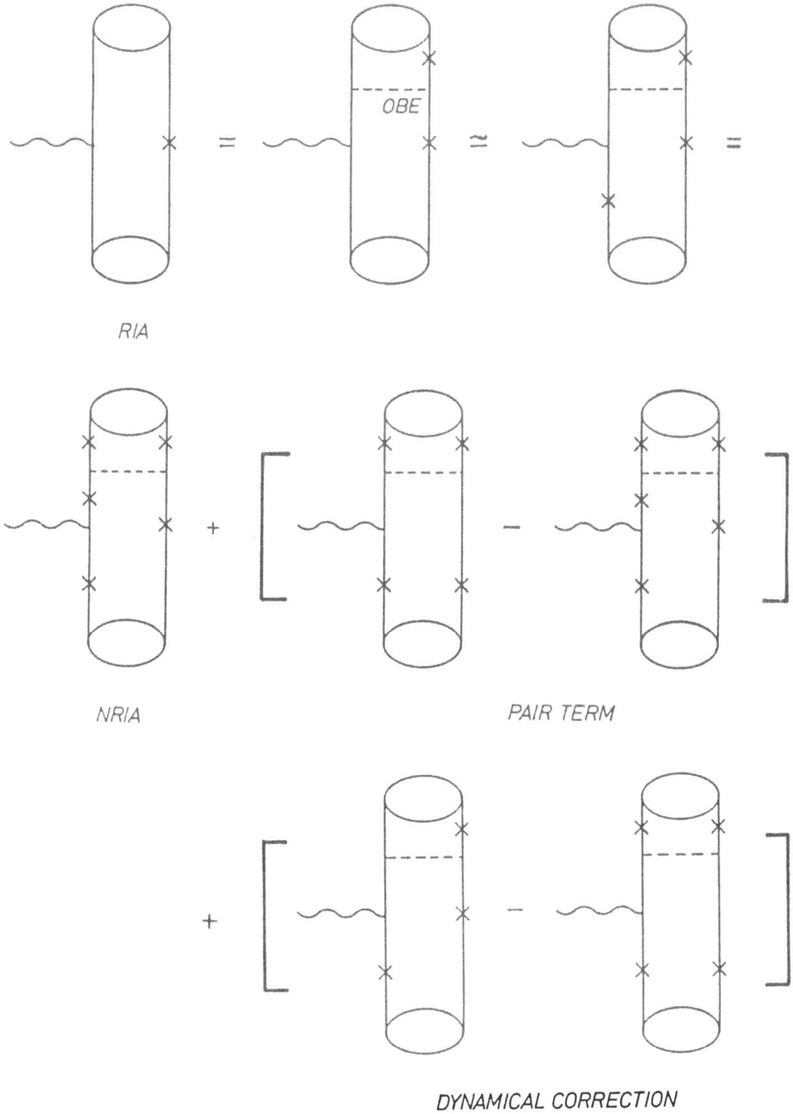

Fig. 15. Perturbational analysis of relativistic corrections to the non relativistic impulse approximation using the Gross QP equations. For explanation see text. In the first line use is made of the fact that the deuteron wavefunction satisfies the homegeous BSE and that we are calculating first order corrections to the non relativistic result. The remaining part of the figure is an identity.

non relativistic prediction close to the experimental results at intermediate momentum transfer, some remarks are in order. First as discussed above the pair term contribution is cancelled largely by a dynamical relativistic correction, moving the non relativistic impulse approximation away from the experimental data. Furthermore, some question arises in how far the $\pi\rho\gamma$ contribution will fill the dip at high momentum transfer. Calculations of the MEC currents are usually done assuming that m is large, resulting into a local two body current operators. The resulting em operator has a rather smooth behaviour with sizable

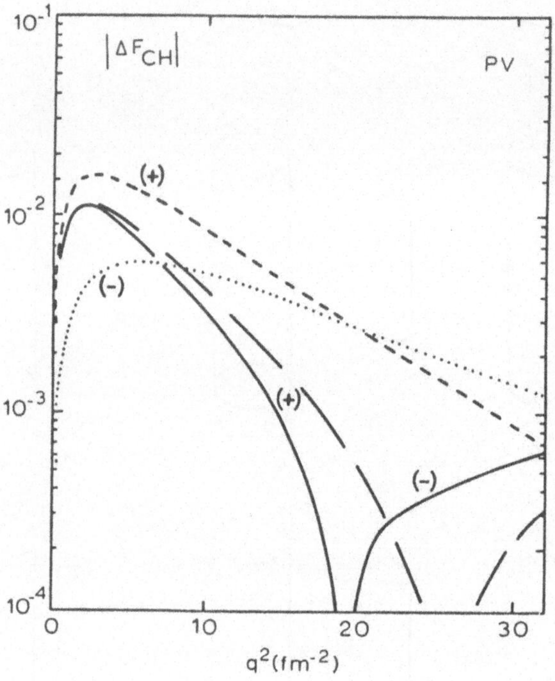

Fig. 16. The absolute values of the pair term (dotted line) and dynamical correction (dashed line) to the ^{3}H charge form factor. In the figure (±) designates the sign of the contribution. Also are shown the final perturbational result (solid line) and the difference between the full relativistic calculation and the non relativistic result.

contributions at large momentum transfer, sothat there is indeed a tendency to fill in the dip. However it is clear that the local approximation doesnot hold at these momentum transfers. Carrying out an exact calculation[62] of the two loop $\pi\rho\gamma$ diagram in our relativistic OBE model show that complete current operator falls off much stronger. As a result the MEC effects are considerably smaller at high momentum transfer due to the recoil effects in the nucleus. It should be pointed out that there is also an important sensitivity of the magnetic form factor predictions[40, 65] on the choice of the neutron form factor[66, 67].

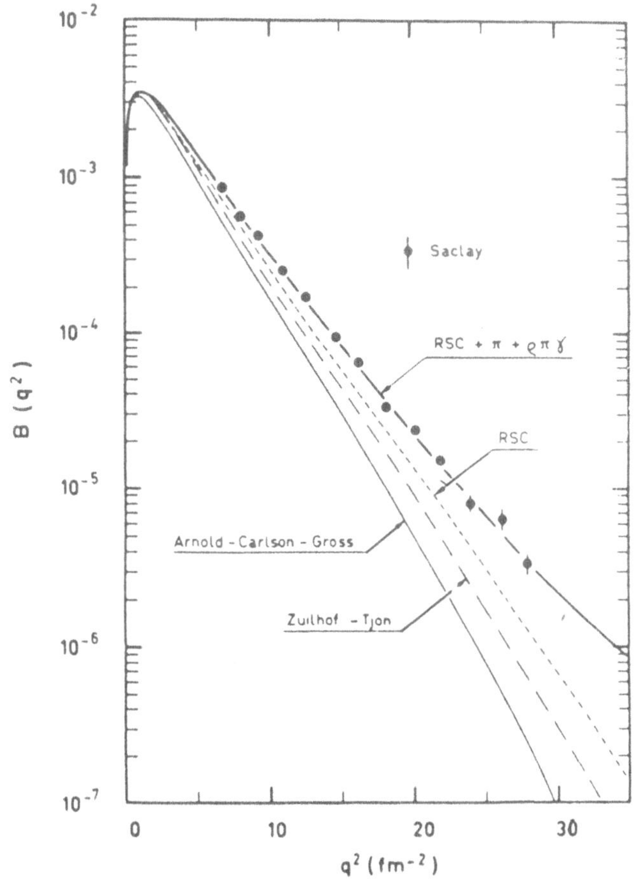

Fig. 17. Magnetic form factor $B(Q^2)$ of the deuteron. The lowest two curves are relativistic results using QP[63] and BSE[57] (from Ref. 61).

NN INTERACTION AT INTERMEDIATE ENERGY

With increasing energy pion production processes become possible in NN scattering. Experimentally[68] resonant structures were found in polarised pp scattering in the region around 600 MeV lab energy. Phase shift analysis[69, 70] of these data indicated that the $^1D_2$ and $^3F_3$ channels exhibited looping behaviour in the Argand plot. Although originally suggested that these structures were signals of exotic dibaryon resonances, they could also be explained partially with more conventional models one of which we shall describe below. The physical mechanism is essentially a combined effect of threshold behaviour of opening up of inelastic channels, leading to the socalled pseudo-resonance behaviour and coupled channel resonances. The models which have been studied are Faddeev like ones with relativistic kinematics and two particle isobar type of models. For a review of these models we refer to Ref. 71.

Since the kinetic energies of the particles become comparable with their rest masses at medium energies, say up to 1 GeV, a relativistic description is needed. Obviously our relativistic OBE model should be extended to also allow for inelastic processes. In the energy region of interest much of the inelastic processes proceeds via the production of P_{33} πN resonance. So it is natural to add to our model, the Δ isobar

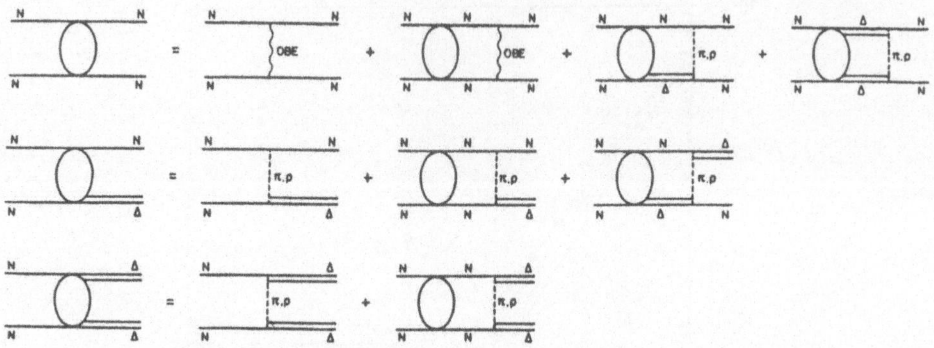

Fig. 18. Diagrammatical representation of relativistic OBE with Δ degrees of freedom.

degrees of freedom as additional channels in the BSE[72]. The diagrammatic representation of the coupled set of integral equations to be solved is shown in Fig. 18. For the description of the Δ we have used the Rarita Schwinger formalism[73] for spin 3/2 particles, keeping only the positive energy part of the propagator i.e.

$$S_\Delta = \left[p_0 - \sqrt{p^2 + m_\Delta^2}\right]^{-1} \sum_\sigma \Delta^\mu(p,\sigma)\Delta^\nu(p,\sigma) \qquad (46)$$

where the mass m_Δ is taken to be complex and Δ^μ are the positive energy 3/2 spinors. The superscript μ is a Lorentz index while σ characterizes the spin with $\sigma = \pm 1/2, \pm 3/2$. Using a $N\Delta\pi$ and $N\Delta\rho$ coupling of the form

$$L_{N\Delta\pi} = -\frac{f_{N\Delta\pi}}{m_\pi} \bar{\psi}\, \vec{T}\, \psi^\mu \partial_\mu \vec{\phi}$$

$$L_{N\Delta\rho} = -i\frac{f_{N\Delta\rho}}{m_\rho} \bar{\psi}\, \gamma^5\gamma^\mu\, \vec{T}\, \psi^\nu \left(\partial_\mu \vec{\phi}_\nu - \partial_\nu \vec{\phi}_\mu\right) \qquad (47)$$

the transition interactions between NN, NΔ and ΔΔ states was constructed. In Eq. (47) $\vec{\phi}$, $\vec{\phi}_\mu$ and Ψ^μ are the π,ρ and Δ fields respectively. With this model the phase shifts δ and inelasticity parameters ρ were calculated. For uncoupled channels the scattering amplitude is given by[70]

$$A = [\cos^2(\rho)\, e^{2i\delta} - 1]/2i \qquad (48)$$

As an example in Fig. 19 is shown the dependence of the phase parameters on $f_{N\Delta\pi}$ for the $^1D_2$ channel, when the coupling of the ρ in the transition interaction is neglected. The resonant structure, reflected as a fast decrease of the phase shift is well reproduced for a $f^2_{N\Delta\pi}/4\pi = 0.23$, predicted by the quark model[74]. The model has been improved in various respects. Inclusion of the ρ exchange in the transition interaction was used to get a better state dependence in the P waves and an instable Δ particle model in terms of πN bubble graphs has been considered[75]. In

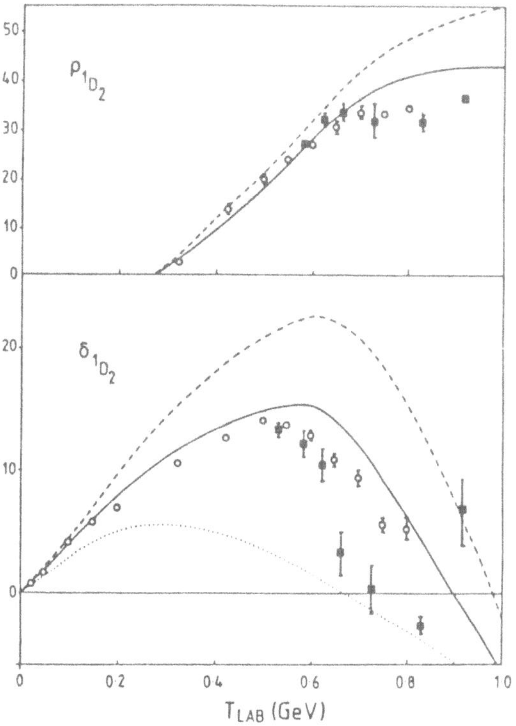

Fig. 19. Calculated phase shifts δ and inelasticities ρ for some chosen strengths of $f_{N\Delta\pi}$ using the relativistic OBE model with Δ degrees of freedom for the $^1D_2$ channel. $f^2_{N\Delta\pi}/4\pi$ = 0.23 (——), = 0.35 (----), = 0 (....).

these improved models a $f^2_{N\Delta\pi}/4\pi=0.35$ was used, which gives a good description of the P_{33} πN phase shifts. The overall agreement of the phase parameters are qualitatively reasonable, especially since no χ^2 fit was attemped. More recently effects of coupling to the π deuteron channels have been studied[76].

DIRAC ANALYSIS OF PROTON NUCLEUS SCATTERING

Considerable attention has been paid in recent years to the role of special relativity in elastic proton nucleus scattering. Assuming that the proton can be described as spin 1/2 Dirac particle, a remarkably good description was found for the polarisation observables in elastic proton $^{40}C_a$ scattering[77], using a phenomenological analysis based on the Dirac equation, whereas a Schrödinger description was not successful. For a spin zero target the amplitude for a proton with initial momentum **k** scattered elastically to a final state with momentum **k'** can be written as

$$A = f(\theta) + g(\theta)\ \sigma.[\mathbf{k} \times \mathbf{k'}] \qquad (49)$$

Observables which can be measured are the differential cross section

$$\frac{d\sigma}{d\Omega} = |f|^2 + |g|^2 \tag{50}$$

the analyzing power

$$A_y = \frac{2\,\mathrm{Re}(fg^*)}{|f|^2 + |g|^2} \tag{51}$$

and spin rotation function

$$Q = \frac{2\,\mathrm{Im}(fg^*)}{|f|^2 + |g|^2} \tag{52}$$

The Dirac optical potential which is used has the form

$$U^{\mathrm{Dirac}} = S + \gamma^0 V \tag{53}$$

where a Wood Saxon parameterisation has been used for the scalar and vector potentials. In the actual fits they were found to be very strong, of the order of 500 MeV. The proton is assumed to be described by the Dirac equation

$$[E\gamma^0 - \vec{\gamma}.\vec{p} - m - U^{\mathrm{Dirac}}]\Psi(\vec{r}) = 0 \tag{54}$$

The main difference in the results obtained from the Dirac and Schrödinger description can be ascribed to the pair excitation graph contribution, which is present in the Dirac approach due to the negative energy states.

Instead of doing pure phenomenology, one could attempt to obtain a more microscopic description of the optical potential. In analogy with the non relativistic KMT[78] theory where the optical potential is in a good approximation given by the non relativistic impulse approximation, one may assume that the Dirac optical potential is given by the relativistic impulse approximation (IA), shown diagrammatically in Fig. 20. The two ingredients needed to construct the optical potential are the relativistic orbitals in the nucleus and the NN interaction. In the actual calculations

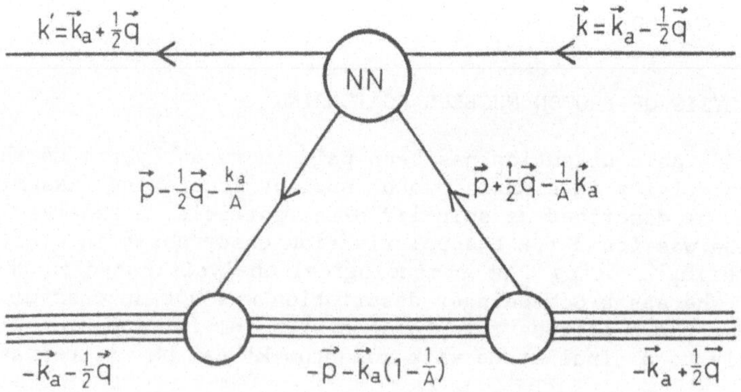

Fig. 20. Dirac optical potential in the impulse approximation for elastic proton nucleus scattering.

the loop integral in the IA is approximated by the socalled factorized $t\rho$ approximation. For the orbitals the Hartree results from quantum hadron dynamics are used.

In the original IA[79] (to be called IA1) the NN interaction in the full Dirac space was constructed assuming that it can written as

$$T_{NN} = F_1 S + F_2 V + F_3 T + F_4 P + F_5 A \tag{55}$$

where $S = 1$, $V = \gamma_1 \cdot \gamma_2$, $T = \sigma_1^{\mu\nu} \sigma_{2\mu\nu}$, $P = \gamma_1^5 \gamma_2^5$ and $A = P \gamma_1^{\mu} \gamma_{2\mu}$ and F_n are invariant functions depending only on the relativistic invariants s, t and u. The F_n functions can in principle be calculated using the physical S-matrix elements between positive energy states. Although the predicted proton nucleus observables were good for medium energies, the strengths of the scalar and vector potentials were found to become extremely large (for example about 2 GeV at 10 MeV lab energy)[78]. It should be realized that there is an ambiguity in the choice of the representation Eq. (55), since it doesnot constitute a complete set of invariants. The term F_4 tends to favour a pseudo-scalar coupling for the pion, resulting into very large potentials for $E_{Lab} \longrightarrow 0$. A complete set of invariants has been constructed by us in accordance with parity, time reversal invariance and charge conjugation.

To determine the set of invariants the physical NN scattering

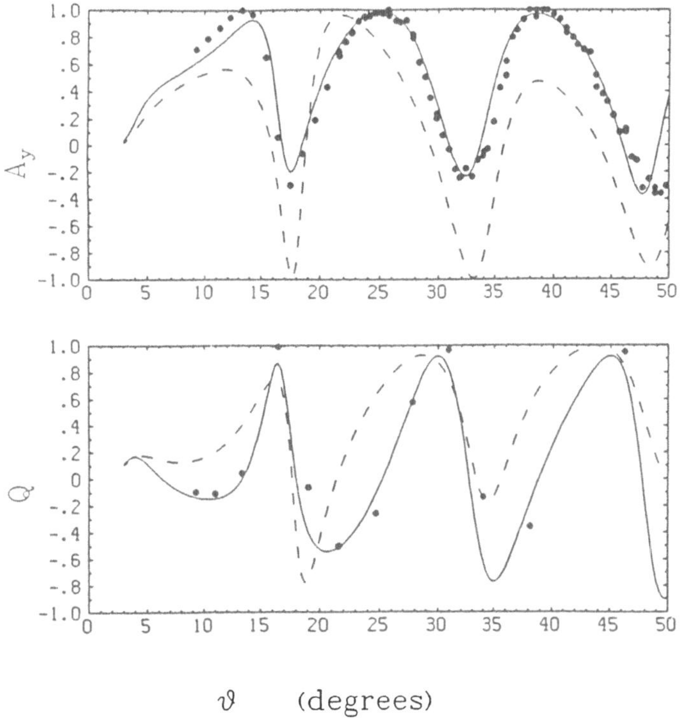

Fig. 21. Analysing power and spin rotation functions for ^{40}Ca at 200 MeV, using IA1 (----) and IA2 (——) (from Ref. 80).

information is not sufficient, but a relativistic dynamical model for the NN interaction is needed to obtain the full amplitude in Dirac space. The NN model as discussed in the previous section has been used as dynamical input (IA2)[80]. Calculations are carried out within the quasi potential approach with the BBSLT propagators. Using the computed on energy shell NN S-matrix elements in the full Dirac space a localized approximation is made to reconstruct the Dirac optical potential. The resulting description of elastic p nucleus scattering is considerably better than IA1 at energies of 200 MeV lab and comparable at higher energies where the role of the pion is expected to be smaller. Moreover, in general our potentials are substantially smaller than those obtained from IA1. In Fig. 21 are shown the polarisation and spin rotation function for p-^{40}Ca scattering at 200 MeV using IA1 and IA2. Recently a systematic analysis has been carried out for some nuclei, where effects of vacuum polarisation and Pauli blocking have been studied[81]. The corrections are found to have the tendency to enhance the agreement between theory and experiment. As an example in Fig. 22 is shown the dependence of the polarisation observables in elastic proton scattering on vacuum polarisation corrections in the case of ^{208}Pb.

The issue of how sensitive the p-nucleus observables are for a certain admixture of pseudo-scalar coupling of the pion has been addressed by us[82]. Two sets of relativistic OBE interactions have been constructed

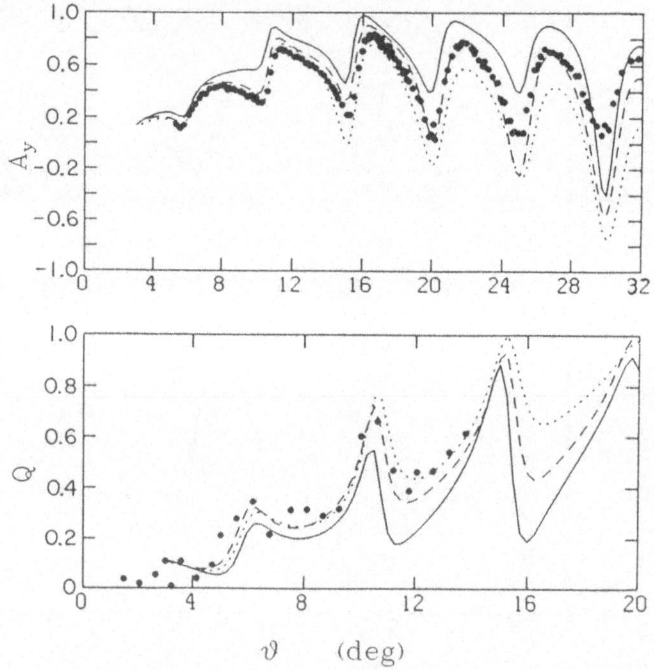

Fig. 22. Sensitivity of polarisation observables on the fraction x of vacuum polarisation contribution for 500 MeV proton scattering from ^{208}Pb. Solid, dashed and dotted lines are for x = 0, 0.5, 1 respectively.

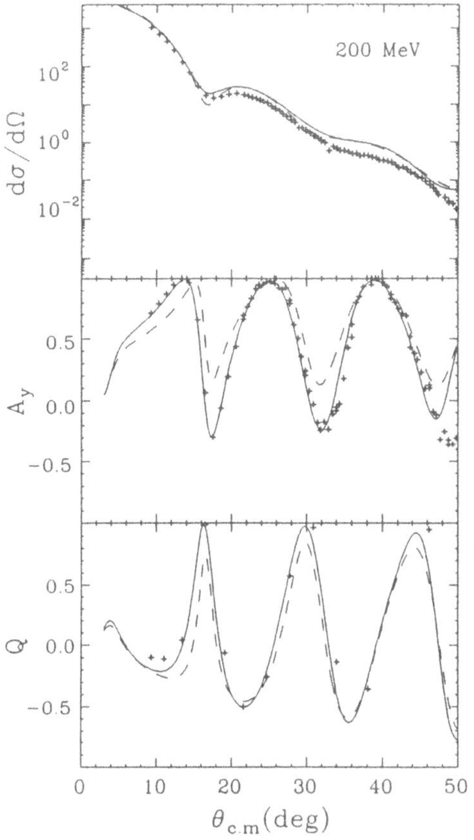

Fig. 23. Sensitivity of elastic p-^{40}Ca observables on admixtures of γ^5 coupling for the pion. Solid line is for the model with λ=0.25, while dashed line is for λ=0.

which equally well fits the NN data, one contains only pseudo-vector coupling whereas the other has a 25% admixture of γ^5 coupling for the pion[55]. QP equations have been used with the Gross prescription for the two nucleon propagator and explicit anti-symmetrisation has been done to satisfy the Pauli principle. The results are shown in Fig. 23 for p-^{40}Ca scattering at 200 MeV. From this we see that the mixed coupling case is in closer agreement with experiment. Although other contributions like Pauli blocking and vacuum polarisation corrections are equally important at this energy and they should also be included, the results show that even an admixture of γ^5 coupling as large as 25 % doesnot lead to such dramatic changes in the polarisation observables that it should be excluded because of that.

CONCLUDING REMARKS

We have discussed various relativistic scattering models based on meson theoretical interactions. One of the major difficulties in a relativistic theory is the proper inclusion of boost transformations when more than two particles are involved. Therefore in considering the em interaction we are faced with this problem because of the presence of the photon. Using the Bethe Salpeter equation a consistent treatment of both the dynamics as well as the em interaction could be carried out for the deuteron in a relativistic OBE model. A remarkable cancellation takes place between the pair term and the dynamical effect, that the deuteron vertex function also has negative energy state components. This shows that the conventional perturbational treatment of MEC effects does lead to the wrong answer in this case. It obviously suggests that the problem of MEC corrections to the em form factors of the trinucleon system should be considered critically.

Regarding the three particle system a limited number of studies has been carried out on relativistic effects. Some of them have used quasi potential equations where essentially relativistic kinematics is built in. Relativistic corrections to the binding energy of the trinucleon system have been considered using the Blankenbecler Sugar prescription for three particles[16, 81-83]. Since the change to relativistic propagators also directly affects the two particle dynamics care should be taken to do the calculation consistently i.e. the parameters in the two nucleon interaction should be adapted for the new propagators to yield the same two nucleon observables as the non relativistic results. In so doing an additional attraction is found for the triton of 0.25-0.5 MeV. Also the effects on the em form factors have been examined using the relativistic OBE model with only the positive energy states. This study shows that with the increase of binding the secondary maximum in the charge form factor becomes smaller, contrary to the finding of an earlier study[84]. More recently within a field theory these questions are being considered, using the BSE approach for three nucleons[85]. In particular, separable representations are used to parameterize the NN interaction.

Having an underlying relativistic two nucleon interaction the Dirac approach has been employed to study the effects of the pair excitation graph contribution to elastic proton nucleus scattering. The results are very encouraging, but it should be stressed that the calculations still miss some essential ingredients. For example, they are not entirely consistent because Hartree relativistic orbitals are used, whereas a Hartree-Fock-Dirac calculation of these orbitals with the same model is clearly more preferable. Furthermore, off shell effects have been neglected by only assuming the information of the on energy shell T-matrix. Calculations are now under way to study the resulting non-localities in the Dirac optical potential. On the formal side contrary to the non relativistic formulation, no multiple scattering theory exists as the basis for the relativistic IA. This as well applies for QHD. It is clear that much work is needed in the future to clarify these issues.

REFERENCES

1. See for example R.G. Newton, "Scattering Theory of Waves and Particles", Mc Graw-Hill,New York (1966).
2. E.E. Salpeter and H.A. Bethe, Phys. Rev. **84**, 1232 (1951).
3. For a review and other references see N. Nakanishi, Prog. Theor. Phys., Suppl. **43**,1 (1969).
4. K. Kowalski, Phys. Rev. Lett. **15**, 798 (1965).
5. H.P. Noyes, Phys. Rev. Lett. **15**, 538 (1965).
6. G.A. Baker Jr., "Essentials of Padé Approximants", Academic Press, New York (1975).
7. L.D. Faddeev, "Mathematical Aspects of the Three Body Problem in Quantum Scattering Theory" (Israel Program for Sci. Transl., Jerusalem (1965).
8. R.V. Reid, Ann. Phys. **50**, 411 (1968).
9. M. Lacombe et al., Phys. Rev. **C21**, 861 (1980).
10. M.M. Nagels et al., Fortschr. Phys. **28**, 215 (1978); Proc. European Workshop on Few-Body Physics, Rome, Springer Verlag, p. 1 (1986).
11. R. Machleidt, K. Holinde and Ch. Elster, Phys. Rep. **149**, 1 (1987).
12. C. Stolk and J.A. Tjon, Nucl. Phys. **A319**, 1 (1979).
13. P.U. Sauer, Proc. XI-th International IUPAP Conference on few Body Systems in Particle and Nuclear Physics, Tokyo and Sendai, Nucl. Phys. **A463**, 273c (1986).
14. For a progress report and references see B.F. Gibson and B.H.J. McKellar, Few Body Systems **3**, 143 (1988).
15. R.A. Malfliet and J.A. Tjon, Ann. Phys. **61**, 425 (1970).
16. J.A. Tjon, Proc. of the IX-th International Conference on the Few Body Problem, Oregon 1980, Nucl.Phys. **A363**, 47c (1980).
17. J.L. Friar, Proc. European Workshop on Few-Body Physics, Rome, Springer Verlag 94 (1986).
18. W.M. Kloet and J.A. Tjon, Phys. Lett.**61B**, 356 (1976).
19. M Haftel and W.M. Kloet, Phys. Rev.**C15**, 404 (1977).
20. E. Hadjimichael, R. Bornais and B. Goulard, Phys. Rev. **C27**, 831 (1983).
21. M. Beyer, D. Drechsel and M.M. Giannini, Phys. Lett. **122B**, 1 (1983).
22. W.M. Kloet and J.A. Tjon, Ann. Phys. **79**, 407 (1973); Nucl Phys. **A120**, 380 (1973).
23. C. Kuruoglu and F.S. Levin, Phys. Rev. **C36**, 49 (1987).
24. W. Glöckle, Phys. Rev. **C36**, 49 (1987).
25. R.A. Malfliet and J.A. Tjon, Nucl. Phys.**A127**, 161 (1969).
26. Y. Koike, J. Haidenbauer and W. Plessas, Phys. Rev. **C35**, 396 (1987).
27. R.A. Brandenburg, Few Body Systems **3**, 59 (1987).
28. H. Witała, T. Cornelius and W. Glöckle, Few Body Systems **3**, 123 (1980).
29. For references see C. Chandler, Proc. XI-th International IUPAP Conference on few Body Systems in Particle and Nuclear Physics, Tokyo and Sendai, Nucl. Phys. **A463**, 181c (1986).
30. G.B. West, Lectures in this summerschool.
31. T. de Forest Jr., Ann. Phys. **45**, 365 (1967).
32. S. Frullani and J. Mougey, Adv. Nucl. Phys. **14**, 122 (1984).
33. T. de Forest Jr., Nucl. Phys. **A392**, 232 (1983).
34. P.H.M. Keizer et al., Phys. Lett. **197B**, 29 (1987).

35. E. van Meijgaard and J.A. Tjon, Phys.Rev.Lett. **57**, 3011 (1986); Proc. 1987 CEBAF Summer Workshop, Eds. F. Gross and C. Williamson, p. 101 (1987).
36. A.M. Bernstein, Proc. 3rd Workshop on Perspectives in Nuclear Physics at Intermediate energies, Editors S. Boffi et al., World Scientific, p. 511 (1987).
37. G.van der Steenhoven et al., Phys. Rev. Lett. **57**, 182 (1986); Phys. Rev. Lett. **58**, 1727 (1986).
38. C. Marchand et al., Phys. Rev. Lett. **60**, 1703 (1988); D Reffay-Pikeroen et al., Phys. Rev. Lett. **60**, 776 (1988).
39. P.A.M. Dirac, Rev. Mod. Phys. **17**, 195 (1945); ibid **21**, 392 (1949).
40. P.L. Chung et al., Phys. Rev. **C37**, 2000 (1988).
41. L.L. Frankfurt and M.I. Strikman, Phys. Rep. **76**, 215 (1981).
42. E.L. Berger et al., Phys. Rev. **D29**, 398 (1984).
43. B.D. Serot and J.D. Walecka, "The relativistic Nuclear Many-Body Problem", Advances in Nuclear Physics, eds. J.W. Negele and E. Vogt, Vol. **16** (1986).
44. A.L. Fetter and J.D. Walecka, "Quantum Theory of Many Particle Systems", McGraw-Hill (1971).
45. C.J. Horowitz and B.D. Serot, Nucl. Phys. **A368**, 503 (1981).
46. S.A.Chinn, Ann. Phys., **108**, 301 (1977).
47. R.J. Perry, Phys. Lett. **182B**, 269 (1986).
48. T. Cohen, Phys. Rev. **C36**, 1653 (1987).
49. R.J. Perry, Phys. Lett.**199B**, 489 (1987).
50. R.E. Cutkowski, J. Math. Phys. **1**, 429 (1960).
51. R. Blankenbecler and R. Sugar, Phys. Rev. **142**, 1051 (1966).
52. A.A. Logunov and A.N. Tavkhelidze, Nuovo Cim. **29**, 380 (1963).
53. F. Gross, Phys. Rev. **186**, 1448 (1969); Phys. Rev. **C26**, 2203 (1984).
54. J. Fleischer and J.A. Tjon, Nucl. Phys. **B84**, 375 (1975); Phys. Rev. **D21**, 87 (1980).
55. F. Gross, K. Holinde and J.W. van Orden, to be published.
56. A.D. Jackson, A. Landé and D.O. Riska, Phys. Lett. **55B**, 23 (1975).
57. J.A. Tjon and M.J. Zuilhof, Phys. Lett. **84B**, 31 (1979).
58. M. Gourdin, Diffusion des Électrons de Haute Énergies (Masson & Cie Paris (1966).
59. M.J. Zuilhof and J.A. Tjon, Phys. Rev. **C22**, 2369 (1980).
60. R.C. Arnold et al., Phys. Rev. Lett.**58**, 1723 (1987).
61. S. Auffret et al., Phys. Rev. Lett. **54**, 649 (1985).
62. M. Gari and H. Huyga, Nucl. Phys. **A264**, 409 (1976).
63. R.C. Arnold, C.E. Carlson and F. Gross, Phys. Rev. **C21**, 1426 (1980).
64. E. Hummel and J.A. Tjon, to be published.
65. W.P. Sitarski, P.G. Blunden and E.L. Lomon, Phys. Rev. **C36**, 2479 (1987).
66. G. Höhler et al., Nucl. Phys. **B114**, 505 (1976).
67. M. Gari and W. Krümpelmann, Zeit. Phys. **322**, 689 (1985).
68. A. Yokosawa, Phys. Rep. **64**, 47 (1980).
69. N. Hoshizaki, Progr. Theor. Phys. **61**, 129 (1979).
70. R.A. Arndt et al., Phys. Rev. **D28**, 97 (1983).
71. J. Tomusiak et al., Plenum Press, New York p. 431 (1986).
72. J.A. Tjon and E.E. van Faassen, Phys. Lett. **120B**, 39 (1983).
73. W. Rarita and J. Schwinger, Phys. Rev. **59**, 436 (1941).
74. G.E. Brown and W. Weise, Phys. Rep. **22C**, 281 (1975).
75. E.E. van Faassen and J.A. Tjon, Phys. Rev **C28**, 2354 (1983); ibid C30,285 (1984)
76. E.E. van Faassen and J.A. Tjon, Phys. Lett. **186B**, 276 (1987).
77. B.C. Clark et al., Phys. Rev. Lett. **50**, 1644 (1983).
78. A.K. Kerman, H.McManus and R. Thaler, Ann. Phys. **8**, 551 (1959).
79. J.A. McNeil, L. Ray and S.J. Wallace, Phys. Rev. Lett. **50**, 1439 (1983); ibid **50**, 1443 (1983).

80. J.A. Tjon and S.J. Wallace, Phys. Rev. Lett. **54, 1357** (1985); Phys. Rev. **C32**, 267 (1985); ibid **C36,** 1085 (1987).
81. N. Ottenstein, S.J. Wallace and J.A. Tjon, Phys. Lett.**197B**, 493 (1987); Phys. Rev. C, in press (1988).
82. F. Gross et al., to be published.
83. A.D. Jackson and J.A. Tjon, Phys. Lett. **32B**, 9 (1970).
84. E. Hammel, H. Baier and A.S. Rinat, Phys. Lett. **85B**, 193 (1979).
85. G. Rupp and J.A. Tjon, Phys. Rev. **C37**, 1729 (1988).

GIANT RESONANCES IN THE RANDOM PHASE APPROXIMATION

Nguyen Van Giai

Division de Physique Théorique [1]
Institut de Physique Nucléaire
F-91406 Orsay Cedex

I Introduction

The study of giant resonances is an important corner stone of our knowledge of nuclear structure. These collective excitations, which appear in all kinds of nuclei, reflect a specific aspect of the dynamics of many-nucleon systems interacting through short range forces. It is therefore quite important to have a theoretical framework for understanding the giant resonance properties.

Soon after the first observation of a nuclear giant resonance, namely the Giant Dipole Resonance [1], successful macroscopic models where neutron and proton fluids are oscillating again each other were proposed [2,3]. Since then, the fluid-dynamical approach [4] has been thoroughly studied and applied to a great variety of resonances. There is an abundant literature on this subject [5], to which we refer the interested reader. In these lectures, however, our interest is more oriented towards a microscopic approach. Our goal is to lay out a general framework where the starting point is an effective nucleon-nucleon interaction which should describe static as well as dynamical properties of nuclei. This effective interaction contains all the phenomenological input of the theory and it is generally determined by an overall fit to bulk properties of nuclear matter as well as nuclear ground states. One can the use this interaction in conjunction with various approximation schemes appropriate to the nuclear many-body problem. The two main approximations we shall need here are the Hartree-Fock (HF) and the Random Phase approximations (RPA). It must be stressed that, contrarily to the fluid-dynamical approach, the microscopic theory does not assume the existence of collective excitations beforehand. Collective states such as giant resonances, when they exist, must emerge naturally as a result of the nuclear dynamics described by the effective interaction and the RPA.

It is not our aim here to review the whole subject of microscopic theory of giant resonances. Many important and interesting aspects will be left aside. One of them is the sum rule approach, which is quite useful because of its simplicity and its ability to show systematic trends of giant resonances [6]. This method also provides a link between microscopic and fluid-dynamical approaches. A recent review of sum rule applications can be found in ref.[7]. Another important aspect of giant resonances is the spreading mechanism by which they acquire a damping width, which represents the dominant part of their total width. This spreading is due to the coupling of the simplest configurations (doorway configurations) to the more and more complex ones, and it is discussed in detail in ref.[8]. Even in the restricted framework of RPA, we shall not dwell at length on the numerous applications to giant resonances, but we shall only mention a few of them to illustrate the RPA method. Further

[1] Laboratoire associé au C.N.R.S.

discussions of RPA calculations, as well as surveys of the experimental situation, can be found in refs.[9,10].

Here, we shall put particular emphasis on the self-consistency of the RPA approach. This means that both single-particle spectra and residual particle-hole interaction are derived from the same starting interaction. This requires that the Hartree-Fock problem has been solved first. We do not discuss this preliminary step in these lectures, but details on Hartree-Fock calculations with Skyrme effective interactions are given in refs.[11,12] whereas a review of ground state properties in the Hartree-Fock approach can be found in ref.[13]. For the sake of simplicity, we restrict ourselves to the case of spherical nuclei and assume that pairing correlations can be neglected.

We shall begin with general considerations on the linear response of a system submitted to a weak external field. Then, we show how the response function can be calculated in RPA and its connection with the time-dependent Hartree-Fock (TDHF) approach. The use of simple but nevertheless reasonable effective interactions of the Skyrme type enables one to carry out calculations in coordinate representation and to fully account for continuum effects. This scheme can be extended in a straightforward manner to the case of giant resonances at finite temperature, i.e. collective modes built on excited states at high excitation energies.

Of particular current interest is the question of particle decay of giant resonances. This type of data can provide very useful information on wave functions and thus allows for detailed tests of microscopic models. As results of exclusive measurements where the emitted particles are detected in coincidence with the scattered projectile become available, one needs a theoretical framework to extract the relevant spectroscopic quantities such as neutron and proton partial widths. Therefore, the second part of these lectures will be devoted to a discussion of the problem of nucleon emission by RPA states.

II Linear response function in nuclei

II.1 General definitions

Let us consider a system of N interacting nucleons governed by the time-independent Hamiltonian H_0. We denote by ω_n its eigenvalues and by $|n>_t$ its eigenvectors in Schrödinger representation. The time-dependent Schrödinger equation is :

$$i\hbar\frac{\partial}{\partial t}|n>_t = H_0|n>_t \qquad (1)$$

In the Heisenberg representation, the state vectors are time-independent and will be denoted by $|n)$:

$$|n) = e^{iH_0t/\hbar}|n>_t \ . \qquad (2)$$

If Q is a time-independent one-body operator, and $\tilde{Q}$ its Heisenberg representation :

$$\tilde{Q} = e^{iH_0t/\hbar}Qe^{-iH_0t/\hbar} \ , \qquad (3)$$

the expectation values of Q can be evaluated in any representation and are, of course, time-independent :

$$q_n \equiv <n|Q|n> = (n|\tilde{Q}|n) \ . \qquad (4)$$

If we now add an external field $Af(t)$ where A is a one-body operator and $f(t)$ is a real function of t, the modified Hamiltonian is :

$$H = H_0 + Af(t) \ , \qquad (5)$$

and its eigenvectors $|\Phi_n>$ obviously obey the equation :

$$i\hbar\frac{\partial}{\partial t}|\Phi_n>_t = H|\Phi_n>_t \ . \qquad (6)$$

In the representation defined by eqs.(2-3) :

$$
\begin{aligned}
|\Phi_n) &= e^{iH_0t/\hbar}|\Phi_n> \;, \\
\tilde{A} &= e^{iH_0t/\hbar} A\, e^{-iH_0t/\hbar} \;,
\end{aligned} \tag{7}
$$

the relation (6) becomes :

$$
i\hbar\frac{\partial}{\partial t}|\Phi_n) = \tilde{A}f(t)|\Phi_n) \; . \tag{8}
$$

We define the response of the system as the change in the ground state expectation value of Q at time t caused by the perturbing field $Af(t)$:

$$
q(t) \equiv (\Phi_0|\tilde{Q}|\Phi_0)_t - (0|\tilde{\Phi}|0) \; . \tag{9}
$$

Let us expand $|\Phi_0)$ in a power series of the field A :

$$
|\Phi_0) = |\Phi_0^{(0)}) + |\Phi_0^{(1)}) + |\Phi_0^{(2)}) + \ldots, \tag{10}
$$

and insert this expansion into (8). We obtain :

$$
\begin{aligned}
& i\hbar\frac{\partial}{\partial t}|\Phi_0^{(0)}) = 0 \;, \\
& i\hbar\frac{\partial}{\partial t}|\Phi_0^{(1)}) = \tilde{A}f(t)|\Phi_0^{(0)}) \;, \\
& i\hbar\frac{\partial}{\partial t}|\Phi_0^{(2)}) = \tilde{A}f(t)|\Phi_0^{(1)}) \;, \\
& \vdots
\end{aligned} \tag{11}
$$

whose solution is :

$$
\begin{aligned}
& |\Phi_0^{(0)}) = |0) \;, \\
& |\Phi_0^{(1)}) = [-\frac{i}{\hbar}\int_{-\infty}^{t} \tilde{A}(t')f(t')dt']|0) \;, \\
& \vdots
\end{aligned} \tag{12}
$$

If the perturbing field is small, we can keep only terms up to first order in A and express the response $q(t)$ as :

$$
q(t) = -\frac{1}{\hbar}\int_{-\infty}^{+\infty} R(t-t')f(t')dt' \;, \tag{13}
$$

where the linear response function R is :

$$
R(t-t') = \begin{cases} 0 & \text{if } t \leq t' \\ -i(0|[\tilde{A}(t'),\tilde{Q}(t)]|0) & \text{if } t > t' \end{cases} \tag{14}
$$

It is easy to relate the function R to the particle-hole Green's function $G(\vec{r},\vec{r}';t-t')$ which describes the propagation of a particle-hole pair from $x' = (\vec{r}',t')$ to $x = (\vec{r},t)$. This propagator is [14] :

$$
G(\vec{r},\vec{r}';t-t') = -i(0|T(\psi^\dagger(x)\psi(x)\psi^\dagger(x')\psi(x'))|0) \;, \tag{15}
$$

where $\psi^\dagger(x), \psi(x)$ are field operators which respectively create and annihilate a nucleon at point x, and T denotes the time-ordered product. In terms of the field operators, the second-quantized forms of A and Q are :

$$
\begin{aligned}
A &= \textstyle\int d^3r A(\vec{r})\psi^\dagger(\vec{r})\psi(\vec{r}) \;, \\
Q &= \textstyle\int d^3r Q(\vec{r})\psi^\dagger(\vec{r})\psi(\vec{r}) \; .
\end{aligned} \tag{16}
$$

Then, eq.(14) becomes :

$$
\begin{aligned}
R(t-t') &= \textstyle\int d^3r d^3r' A(\vec{r})Q(\vec{r}') \\
& \quad i\theta(t-t')(0|[\psi^\dagger(x)\psi(x),\psi^\dagger(x')\psi(x')]|0) \; .
\end{aligned} \tag{17}
$$

The second line of this expression is the retarded part G^R of the particle-hole Green's function. This retarded propagator is also called the density-density correlation function. The reason for this is that if we want to calculate the density change $\delta\rho(\vec{r}_0)$ at $\vec{r}_0$ caused by the field A, we would find, using eq.(17) with $Q(\vec{r}') = \delta(\vec{r}' - \vec{r}_0)$:

$$\delta\rho(\vec{r}_0) = -\int d^3r G^R(\vec{r}_0, \vec{r}; t - t')A(\vec{r}) \ . \tag{18}$$

The spectral decomposition of the linear response function is obtained by taking the Fourier transform of eq.(17). Inserting a complete set of eigenstates $|n)$ of the Hamiltonian H_0 in the commutator of (17), and using the relation :

$$\theta(t - t') = -i \int_{-\infty}^{+\infty} \frac{d\omega}{2\pi} \frac{e^{-i\omega(t-t')}}{\omega + i\eta} \ , \tag{19}$$

the Fourier transform of $R(t - t\prime)$ is :

$$R(\omega) = \int d^3r d^3r' A(\vec{r})Q(\vec{r}')$$
$$\sum_n < 0|\psi^\dagger(\vec{r})\psi(\vec{r})|n >< n|\psi^\dagger(\vec{r}')\psi(\vec{r}')|0 > \left[\frac{1}{\omega_{no} - \omega - i\eta} + \frac{1}{\omega_{no} + \omega + i\eta}\right] \ . \tag{20}$$

The poles of $R(\omega)$ are on the real axis at $\pm\omega_{no}$, where $\omega_{no} = \omega_n - \omega_0$ are the excitation energies. If we choose $A = Q$ (hermitian), the residues of $R(\omega)$ are the transition probabilities $| < 0|Q|n > |^2$. The distribution of transition strength $S(\omega)$, a very important quantity for characterizing the excitation spectrum, is very simply related to the imaginary part of $R(\omega)$. For $\omega > 0$, we have indeed :

$$S(\omega) \equiv \sum_n | < 0|Q|n > |^2\delta(\omega - \omega_{no}) = \frac{1}{\pi}\Im m R(\omega) \ . \tag{21}$$

Notice that, in all expressions like (20-21) where $\sum_n$ appears, this summation means a discrete sum over normalizable states as well as an integral over the continuous part of the spectrum.

In summary, the linear response function $R(\omega)$ can be calculated if one knows the retarded particle-hole Green's function G^R, since they are related by the Fourier transform of eq.(17), namely :

$$R(\omega) = \int d^3r d^3r' A(\vec{r})G^R(\vec{r}, \vec{r}'; \omega)Q(\vec{r}') \ . \tag{22}$$

In practice, it is more convenient to work with the full particle-hole Green's function G, which is related to G^R by [14]

$$\begin{aligned} \Re e G^R(\vec{r}, \vec{r}'; \omega) &= \Re e G(\vec{r}, \vec{r}'; \omega) \ , \\ \Im m G^R(\vec{r}, \vec{r}'; \omega) &= Sgn(\omega)\Im m G(\vec{r}, \vec{r}'; \omega) \ . \end{aligned} \tag{23}$$

II.2 RPA as small amplitude limit of TDHF

The exact particle-hole Green's function G obeys a chain of coupled integral equations involving the full set of many-body Green's functions [15]. For the restricted purpose of studying small amplitude vibrations, one generally uses the RPA as an approximation scheme to calculate G. There are many ways to introduce the RPA [16], all leading to the same set of equations. The most pedagogical one is perhaps the linearized TDHF method. This approach will allow us to see clearly the connection between RPA and the Hartree-Fock approximation, and at the same time it shows explicitly that RPA is just the small amplitude limit of TDHF, a property which is not so obvious if one derives the RPA equations by other means like the quasi-boson or Green's function methods. Here, we follow the derivation of Bertsch and Tsai [17] which is well adapted to interactions of the Skyrme type [11,12].

If the starting effective interaction contains delta functions of the coordinates, as it is the case for Skyrme forces, the corresponding static Hartree-Fock Hamiltonian H_0 is a functional of local densities [11]. For simplicity of notations, we write explicitly the dependence of H_0

on nuclear density ρ_0 only, but the dependence on kinetic energy density, spin density, etc ... can be treated in the same way. The Hamiltonian H_0 is :

$$H_0 = H(\rho_0) = K + U(\rho_0) \ , \tag{24}$$

where K is the nucleon kinetic energy and U is the static Hartree-Fock potential. The local nuclear density is :

$$\rho_0(\vec{r}) = \sum_i \varphi_i^*(\vec{r})\varphi_i(\vec{r}) \ , \tag{25}$$

where φ_i is a single-particle eigenstate of H_0 with eigenvalue ε_i, and the sum runs over all occupied states of the Hartree-Fock ground state. Thus, H_0 must be determined self-consistently. Notice that H_0 denotes here a one-body Hamiltonian while in the previous subsection the same notation was used for a many-body Hamiltonian, but this should not cause too much confusion.

Adding now a small perturbation $A(\vec{r})(e^{-i\omega t} + e^{i\omega t})$, the TDHF approximation tells us that the wave function of the perturbed system is a Slater determinant built on modified wave functions ϕ_i :

$$\phi_i(\vec{r},t) = \varphi_i(\vec{r}) + \lambda_i(\vec{r})e^{i\omega t} + \chi_i(\vec{r})e^{-i\omega t} \ , \tag{26}$$

such that $< \lambda_i|\varphi_i > = < \chi_i|\varphi_i >= 0$. The $\phi_i's$ are solutions of the TDHF equations :

$$i\frac{\partial}{\partial t}\phi_i = (H(t) - \varepsilon_i)\phi_i \ . \tag{27}$$

The nuclear density becomes :

$$\begin{aligned} \rho(t) &= \textstyle\sum_i \phi_i^*\phi_i \\ &= \rho_0 + \delta\rho e^{-i\omega t} + \delta\rho^* e^{i\omega t} \ , \end{aligned} \tag{28}$$

whereas the Hamiltonian $H(t)$ is, assuming that the density change is small enough to allow the neglect of terms beyond first order in $\delta\rho$:

$$H(t) = H_0 + [(A(\vec{r})e^{-i\omega t} + \frac{\partial U}{\partial \rho}\delta\rho e^{-i\omega t}) + \text{h.c.}] \ . \tag{29}$$

From eqs.(26-29) we obtain for χ_i and λ_i the formal solutions :

$$\begin{aligned} \chi_i &= \frac{1}{\omega - H_0 + \varepsilon_i + i\eta}(A + \frac{\partial U}{\partial \rho}\delta\rho)\varphi_i \ , \\ \lambda_i &= -\frac{1}{\omega + H_0 - \varepsilon_i + i\eta}(A + \frac{\partial U}{\partial \rho}\delta\rho^*)\varphi_i \ . \end{aligned} \tag{30}$$

This leads to the following integral equation for the density change :

$$\delta\rho(\vec{r}) = -\int d^3r' G^{(0)}(\vec{r},\vec{r}';\omega)[A(\vec{r}') + \frac{\partial U}{\partial \rho}\delta\rho(\vec{r}')] \ , \tag{31}$$

where we have introduced the non-interacting particle-hole Green's function $G^{(0)}$:

$$\begin{aligned} G^{(0)}(\vec{r},\vec{r}';\omega) \ &\equiv \sum_i \varphi_i^*(\vec{r}) < \vec{r}|\frac{1}{H_0 - \varepsilon_i - \omega - i\eta} \\ &+ \frac{1}{H_0 - \varepsilon_i + \omega - i\eta}|\vec{r}' > \varphi_i(\vec{r}') \ . \end{aligned} \tag{32}$$

Comparing eq.(31) with the Fourier transform of eq.(18) we see that the full Green's function G satisfies the integral equation :

$$G(\vec{r},\vec{r}';\omega) = G^{(0)}(\vec{r},\vec{r}';\omega) + \int d^3r'' G^{(0)}(\vec{r},\vec{r}'';\omega)\frac{\partial U(\vec{r}'')}{\partial \rho}G(\vec{r}'',\vec{r}';\omega) \ . \tag{33}$$

Eq.(33) is identical to the RPA equation derived by the quasi-boson or Green's function methods, with the functional derivative $\partial U/\partial\rho$ playing the role of the antisymmetrized particle-hole interaction. By iterating the r.h.s. of eq.(33), we can see that the RPA Green's function G sums up the infinite series of ring diagrams [14].

II.3 Self-consistency

As we have mentioned before, the starting point is an effective nucleon-nucleon interaction of a simple analytical form and yet realistic enough to describe satisfactorily bulk properties of nuclear ground states in the Hartree-Fock approximation. A very successful interaction of this kind is the Skyrme force [11,12]. It is relatively easy to handle because it contains $\delta(\vec{r}_1-\vec{r}_2)$ factors, but it can mock up to some extent finite range effects by its velocity-dependent terms. Somehow, it can be considered as a phenomenological substitute to a Brueckner G-matrix [18].

The general form of a Skyrme force is :

$$\begin{aligned} v(1,2) &= t_0(1+x_0P_\sigma)\delta(\vec{r}_1-\vec{r}_2)+\frac{t_1}{2}(1+x_1P_\sigma)[\delta(\vec{r}_1-\vec{r}_2)k^2+k'^2\delta(\vec{r}_1-\vec{r}_2)] \\ &+t_2(1+x_2P_\sigma)\vec{k}'.\delta(\vec{r}_1-\vec{r}_2)\vec{k}+iw_0(\vec{\sigma}_1+\vec{\sigma}_2).(\vec{k}'\times\delta(\vec{r}_1-\vec{r}_2)\vec{k}) \\ &\frac{t_3}{6}(1+x_3P_\sigma)\rho^\alpha(\vec{R})\delta(\vec{r}_1-\vec{r}_2)\ , \end{aligned} \tag{34}$$

where $\vec{R}=(\vec{r}_1-\vec{r}_2)/2$, and $\vec{\sigma}_1$ and $\vec{\sigma}_2$ are the spin Pauli matrices, $P_\sigma=(1+\vec{\sigma}_1.\vec{\sigma}_2)/2$ is the spin-exchange operator, $\vec{k}=(\vec{\nabla}_1-\vec{\nabla}_2)/2i$ and $\vec{k}'$ is the hermitian conjugate of $\vec{k}$. This interaction depends on the set of adjustable parameters $\{t_i,x_i,w_0,\alpha\}$. The t_0 term is a usual zero-range force, the t_1 and t_2 terms contain all the velocity dependence and govern the non-locality of the Hartree-Fock mean field as well as the surface properties of finite nuclei, the w_0 term is a two-body spin-orbit force of zero range. The last term t_3 contains the density dependence of the force, a feature which could be related to the density dependence of the Brueckener G-matrix itself.

We have seen that the residual particle-hole interaction appearing in the RPA equation (33) is $\partial U/\partial\rho$, where U is the Hartree-Fock mean potential. This particle-hole force is just the quasi-particle interaction in the Landau-Migdal theory of fermion systems [19]. To see the connection between $\partial U/\partial\rho$ and the starting effective interaction $v(1,2)$, let us calculate the expectation value in the Hartree-Fock ground state $|0>$ of

$$H=\sum_{i=1}^{A}K_i+\sum_{i<j}^{A}v(i,j)\ , \tag{35}$$

where $K_i=-\hbar^2\nabla_i^2/2M$ is the kinetic energy of nucleon i. Denoting by $\{\alpha\}$ a complete set of single-particle states and by $\rho_{\alpha\beta}=<0|a_\alpha^\dagger a_\beta|0>$ the one-body density matrix, we have :

$$\begin{aligned} E\equiv<0|H|0> &= \sum_{\alpha\gamma}<\alpha|-\frac{\hbar^2\nabla^2}{2M}|\gamma>\rho_{\alpha\gamma} \\ &+\frac{1}{2}\sum_{\alpha\beta\gamma\delta}<\alpha\beta|v(1,2)(1-P_{12})|\gamma\delta>\rho_{\alpha\gamma}\rho_{\beta\delta}\ , \end{aligned} \tag{36}$$

where P_{12} is the operator interchanging particles 1 and 2. In the general case where $v(1,2)$ has a density dependence, like in the Skyrme case, the matrix elements of the Hartree-Fock Hamiltonian are given by :

$$\begin{aligned} <\alpha|K+U|\gamma> &= \frac{\partial E}{\partial\rho_{\alpha\gamma}} \\ &=<\alpha|-\frac{\hbar^2\nabla^2}{2M}|\gamma>+\sum_{\beta\gamma}<\alpha\beta|v(1-P_{12})|\gamma\delta>\rho_{\beta\delta} \\ &+\frac{1}{2}\sum_{\alpha'\gamma'\beta\gamma}<\alpha'\beta|\frac{\partial v}{\partial\rho_{\alpha\gamma}}(1-P_{12})|\gamma'\delta>\rho_{\alpha'\gamma'}\rho_{\beta\delta}\ . \end{aligned} \tag{37}$$

The last term of the r.h.s. of eq.(37) is a rearrangement contribution to the Hartree-Fock potential $U_{\alpha\gamma}$ coming from the explicit density dependence of $v(1,2)$. Let us first examine the simple case where $v(1,2)$ does not have this density dependence. Then, the quasi-particle interaction would be :

$$\frac{\partial U_{\alpha\gamma}}{\partial \rho_{\beta\delta}} = <\alpha\beta|v(1,2)(1-P_{12})|\gamma\delta> \ . \tag{38}$$

i.e., it is identical to the antisymmetrized starting interaction, as it should. In a more general case, there will be an additional contribution to eq.(38) due to the derivative of the last term of (37) with respect to $\rho_{\beta\delta}$.

From the above discussion, we can deduce the particle-hole interaction one must use if one starts from a Skyrme force. For the density-independent part, one simply uses $v(1-P_{12})$ and take direct matrix elements only, since exchange is already included by P_{12}. For the density-dependent part, the differentiation of U with respect to density gives :

$$\begin{aligned} v_{ph}(1,2) &= \frac{t_3}{24}\rho^\alpha \delta(\vec{r}_1-\vec{r}_2)\Big\{\frac{3}{2}(\alpha+1)(\alpha+2)+\frac{\alpha}{2}(1-\alpha)(1+2x_3)(\frac{\rho_n-\rho_p}{\rho})^2 \\ &-(1-2x_3)\vec{\sigma}_1.\vec{\sigma}_2-(1+2x_3)\vec{\tau}_1.\vec{\tau}_2-\vec{\sigma}_1.\vec{\sigma}_2\vec{\tau}_1.\vec{\tau}_2\Big\} \ , \end{aligned} \tag{39}$$

where ρ_n and ρ_p are neutron and proton densities, respectively ($\rho = \rho_n + \rho_p$), and all densities are taken at $\vec{R} = (\vec{r}_1+\vec{r}_2)/2$. Again, one must take only direct matrix elements of interaction (39). Actually, this part of the particle-hole matrix element is not antisymmetric under exchange of the two interacting particles.

The enforcement of self-consistency in RPA calculations leads to several RPA sum rules which would not be valid otherwise. For instance, the well-known Thouless theorem which relates the RPA energy-weighted sum rule to a double commutator expectation value in the Hartree-Fock ground state requires that the single-particle spectrum and the residual interaction derive from the same starting force. Detailed discussions of sum rule methods in RPA can be found in Refs.[6,7].

II.4 Inclusion of continuum effects

The main advantage of calculating the response function in coordinate space is that one does not have to discretize the continuous part of the single-particle spectrum, nor to truncate the particle-hole space. Thus, effects of the single-particle continuum are fully included. The calculated response function appears as a continuous function of excitation energy in the region above particle emission threshold, with resonance-shaped structures having natural widths. The interpretation of these widths will be discussed in section III. Below particle emission threshold, the response function only consists, of course, of discrete lines having zero width (delta functions) and corresponding to bound states of infinite lifetime.

The practical task at hand is how to calculate the non-interacting Green's function $G^{(0)}$ introduced in (32), without approximating the continuum. Once this is done, it is not very difficult to solve the integral eq.(33) by making a multipole decomposition and transforming this three-dimensional equation into a number of uncoupled one-dimensional equations in the radial coordinate. In eq.(32), the summation over occupied states i causes no problem since it contains a finite number of terms and all the wave functions φ_i are known. There remains to express quantities like $<\vec{r}|(z+i\eta-H_0)^{-1}|\vec{r}'>$ where z is a real parameter varying continuously ($z = \varepsilon_i \pm \omega$). Let us make the multipole expansion :

$$<\vec{r}|(z+i\eta-H_0)^{-1}|\vec{r}'> = \frac{1}{rr'}\sum_{\ell jm} \mathcal{Y}_{\ell j}^{m*}(\hat{r}) g_{\ell j}(r,r';z)\mathcal{Y}_{\ell j}^{m}(\hat{r}') \ . \tag{40}$$

The Green's function $g_{\ell j}$ is the resolvent of the radial Skyrme-Hartree-Fock Hamiltonian:[12]

$$H_0^{\ell j} = -\frac{d}{dr}(\frac{\hbar^2}{2m^*})\frac{d}{dr}+\frac{\hbar^2}{2m^*}\frac{\ell(\ell+1)}{r^2}+U_{\ell j}(r) \ , \tag{41}$$

where the Hartree-Fock potential $U_{\ell j}$ is the sum of a central term and a spin-orbit term, and $m^*(r)$ is an r-dependent effective mass arising from the velocity-dependence of the Skyrme force. Notice that $H_0^{\ell j}$ is a purely differential operator in the Skyrme case, in contrast to more general interactions of finite range which would lead to an integro-differential operator. This property of the Hamiltonian (41) enables one to express [20] $g_{\ell j}$ in terms of two linearly independent solutions, v and w, of the differential equation $(H_0^{\ell j} - z)v = 0$. These solutions must satisfy the following boundary conditions :

a) at the origin, v and w are respectively regular and irregular,

$$v \underset{r \to 0}{\longrightarrow} r^{\ell+1} \ , \quad w \underset{r \to 0}{\longrightarrow} r^{-\ell} \ .$$

b) at infinity, and for positive values of z, $v(r)$ behaves like a standing wave whereas $w(r)$ has a radially outgoing wave behaviour. If z is negative, $v(r)$ is exponentially increasing and $w(r)$ is exponentially decreasing, asymptotically.

The closed form expression of $g_{\ell j}$ is :

$$g_{\ell j}(r, r'; z) = \frac{2m^*}{\hbar^2} \frac{1}{W(w, v)} v(r_<) w(r_>) \ , \tag{42}$$

where $W(w,v) = w(r)v'(r) - v(r)w'(r)$ is the Wronskian of the two solutions, $r_<$ and $r_>$ are respectively the smaller and the larger of r and r'. The quantity $(\hbar^2/2m^*(r))W(w,v)$ is independent of r.

The Green's functions $g_{\ell j}(r, r'; z)$ is a continuous and symmetric function of r and r'. Its first derivative has a discontinuity at $r = r'$:

$$\frac{\partial g}{\partial r}(r' + \varepsilon, r'; z) - \frac{\partial g}{\partial r}(r' - \varepsilon, r'; z) \underset{\varepsilon \to 0}{\longrightarrow} \frac{2m^*(r')}{\hbar^2} \ . \tag{43}$$

This discontinuity must be taken into account when one solves numerically the RPA equation (33) with velocity-dependent interactions such as Skyrme forces, since higher order derivatives of $g_{\ell j}$ will appear [21].

II.5 Applications

It is not our purpose to review here the applications of the self-consistent RPA approach, and especially the response function calculations done with Skyrme-type interactions. However, it may be useful to list a few references where the reader can find illustrative examples of the methods described in these lectures.

Early calculations performed in coordinate space and using Skyrme interactions are those of Bertsch and Tsai [17], and Liu and Brown [22]. Response functions were calculated for isoscalar as well as isovector giant resonances of various multipolarities and in doubly-closed shell nuclei. In these works, the continuum is not treated, but it is instead discretized by calculating the single-particle spectrum with a box boundary condition. To obtain the multipole strength distributions as continuous functions of excitation energy, a Lorentzian energy averaging is made, so that all RPA states acquire an artificial width which is the Lorentzian width one has introduced.

The first calculations of response functions including continuum effects and without particle-hole space truncation are those of refs.[21,23]. The collective states above particle threshold now appear as giant resonances with their natural widths. Part of these widths is due to the finite lifetimes of the states, since they can decay by particle emission. Another part may come from the so-called Landau damping, an apparent widening of the line shape due to the fact that the states are not well isolated but they may overlap. The question of how to disentangle the particle escape width and the Landau spreading will be treated in section III. In any case, the RPA model alone cannot account for the total widths of giant resonances, because the spreading mechanism due to the coupling of simple RPA states to more complicated configurations (2particle-2hole and more) generally gives large spreading widths [8].

The response function method has been used to study isoscalar giant resonances in detail. For instance, monopole and dipole compression modes have been calculated in ref.[24]. In ref.[25], detailed properties of quadrupole modes, such as transition densities and transition currents, are studied in the RPA model. It is found that the transition current of the giant quadrupole resonance corresponds to irrotational flow, thus giving some microscopic support to its description in terms of fluid-dynamical models. On the other hand, this conclusion does not hold for the low-lying quadrupole state which also exists in closed-subshell nuclei like ^{208}Pb.

There are several applications of the response function method to isovector resonances. Early works include the study of isovector monopole and isobaric analog resonances [26]. The same method has been used for studying effects of RPA correlations on the giant dipole resonance [27], and on the total rates of μ-capture by nuclei [28]. More recently, Auerbach and Klein [29,30] have performed detailed calculations of giant resonances excited in charge-exchange reactions. All these works lead to quantitative predictions which compare rather well with existing data.

II.6 Extension to finite temperature

The question of giant resonances built on states at high excitation energies, i.e. at temperatures of several MeV, has become recently of great interest after the experimental observations of giant dipole resonances built on states above the yrast line. The RPA method we have presented so far lends itself to the study of the response function at finite temperature, with very little modifications. This generalization to finite temperature T has been done by Sagawa and Bertsch [31], and we briefly sketch it here.

First, the zero temperature Hartree-Fock ground state where occupation probabilities are just 0 or 1 must be extended to the $T \neq 0$ case by letting these probabilities to be continuous functions of single particle energies :

$$f_i(T) = \frac{1}{1+\exp[(\varepsilon_i - \varepsilon_F)/T]} , \tag{44}$$

where the chemical potential ε_F (more precisely, one chemical potential for each kind of particle) is determined by particle number conservation

$$\sum_i f_i(T) = A . \tag{45}$$

Note that there is no longer a sharp distinction between occupied and unoccupied states, and all summations run in principle over the complete spectrum. The Hartree-Fock equations become :

$$< \varphi_i|K|\varphi_j > + \sum_k f_k(T) < \varphi_i\varphi_k|v(1,2)(1-P_{12})|\varphi_j\varphi_k >= \varepsilon_i\delta_{ij} . \tag{46}$$

This defines the Hartree-Fock Hamiltonian $H_0(T) = K + U(\rho_0(T))$ analogous to the one introduced in eq.(24). The only difference is that the local density (25) is now modified by the occupation factors :

$$\rho_0(T) = \sum_{\text{all } i} f_i(T)\varphi_i^*(\vec{r})\varphi_i(\vec{r}) . \tag{47}$$

From this point, all the derivation of subsection II.2 can be repeated. Again, one obtains an integral equation formally identical to eq.(33), with a T-dependent Green's function $G^{(0)}$ which generalizes [31] eq.(32) :

$$\begin{aligned} G^{(0)}(\vec{r},\vec{r}';\omega,T) &\equiv \sum_{\text{all } i} f_i(T)\varphi_i^*(\vec{r}) \\ &\times < \vec{r}|\frac{1}{H_0-\varepsilon_i-\omega-i\eta} + \frac{1}{H_0-\varepsilon_i+\omega-i\eta}|\vec{r}' > \varphi_i(\vec{r}') . \end{aligned} \tag{48}$$

In ref.[31], the response function in ^{40}Ca has been calculated for the isovector dipole and isoscalar quadrupole modes at various temperatures between zero and 6 MeV. Notice that in this calculation, the particle-hole residual interaction $\partial U/\partial \rho$ depends (slightly) on T. It is found that the main resonance peaks are little affected by the temperature increase in the isovector dipole case, while the isoscalar quadrupole resonance is slightly shifted upwards and broadened when T is of the order of 3 to 6 MeV. The experimental data show a tendency for the isovector dipole to become broader as T gets larger. However, it would be wrong to oppose this experimental observation to the RPA prediction. Indeed, as we have already stressed, the RPA width is only a fraction of the total observed width since it does not contain the spreading width.

A striking result of ref.[31] is that, for increasing values of T, the response functions tend to have more and more strength at low excitation energies. This is particularly true in the isoscalar quadrupole case. An explanation of this phenomenon has been given by Barranco et al. [32] who have studied the isoscalar monopole response using a time-dependent Thomas-Fermi method. They argue that, at finite temperature, the static Hartree-Fock solution does not represent a stable state. Since unbound orbitals have non-zero probabilities for being occupied, this solution can evaporate nucleons and thus corresponds to a nucleus embedded in a nucleon bath. The calculations of ref.[32] show that one can understand the low energy component of the response function as the response of this outer nucleonic gas to the external field, and therefore this part of the response function is kind of spurious as far as the nucleus itself is concerned. If one is interested in a quantity like the polarizability of the heated nucleus, which is proportional to the inverse energy-weighted moment of the strength distribution, it is clear that RPA calculations of the kind of ref.[31] would give the wrong answer since the outer gas would give a large, unwanted contribution. Perhaps the giant resonance itself is not too much affected by the presence of the gas and the RPA response function would still be meaningful in the giant resonance region. This question deserves further investigation.

III Particle decay of giant resonances

Physical giant resonances are unnormalizable states located above particle threshold and therefore they must decay. One possible type of decay consists of electromagnetic transitions, with a corresponding width Γ_γ which is only a small fraction of the total width. Indeed, most of the decay width must come from strong interaction processes, namely particle emission. Although composite particle channels may sometimes be important, we shall concentrate here on nucleon channels. Nucleons can be emitted in a great variety of ways after a giant resonance has been formed, say, in an inelastic scattering experiment. The incident projectile produces a coherent superposition of one particle-one hole configurations modelized by a continuum-RPA state, and a nucleon can escape directly from this state. We call doorway state this model state reached by the one-step process, and direct escape width $\Gamma^\uparrow$ this nucleon decay width. A competing mechanism is the coupling of the doorway state to more and more complicated configurations. At each stage of complexity, nucleons can also be emitted and one can talk about various kinds of precompound emission until compound nucleus emission is reached down the line. These processes are gathered under the name of damping or spreading mechanism, and the corresponding width $\Gamma^\downarrow$ is the so-called damping width (see ref.[8]).

Although the escape width $\Gamma^\uparrow$ is generally small compared $\Gamma^\downarrow$, it is particularly interesting because it depends sensitively on the wave function of the doorway state and therefore it contains valuable spectroscopic information on the giant resonance. This is the reason why we devote this section to the question of escape widths of RPA states. Following ref.[33], we use projection operator techniques [34] to split the configuration space into a discrete subspace and a continuum subspace. Particle emission results from the coupling between the two subspaces. For simplicity of presentation, we neglect all configurations outside the RPA particle-hole space and therefore $\Gamma^\downarrow$ is absent from the present discussion. We refer the reader to the paper of Yoshida and Adachi [35] for a formal treatment including a larger configuration space, in the framework of the Tamm-Dancoff approximation.

III.1 One-body case

Let us start with the simple situation of a nucleon moving in a potential well, in order to explain how discrete and continuum subspaces can be constructed. The Hamiltonian is :

$$H = -\frac{\hbar^2}{2M}\nabla^2 + U(r) \ . \tag{49}$$

We choose a finite, discrete orthonormal basis of arbitrary functions :

$$\{q\} = \{\varphi_i, i = 1, 2, \ldots, N\} \ , \tag{50}$$

which span the N-dimensional subspace $\{q\}$. The projection operator onto $\{q\}$ is denoted by q. We call ψ_i, ε_i the orthonormalized eigenvectors and eigenvalues of the restriction of H to $\{q\}$:

$$(qHq - \varepsilon_i)\psi_i = 0 \quad i = 1, 2, \ldots, N \ . \tag{51}$$

If $\{q\}$ is sufficiently large, the lowest eigenstates of qHq will be excellent approximations of the bound states of H. If H has quasi-bound states, i.e. narrow single-particle resonances, they will also be well approximated by some of the ψ_i. Enlarging more and more $\{q\}$ will not affect appreciably those ψ_i corresponding to bound and quasi-bound states, but others will, of course, change considerably.

Our goal is now to build the complementary subspace $\{p\}$ orthogonal to $\{q\}$, such that $\{p\} + \{q\}$ is the complete space. We denote by $u_E^{(+)}$ the states of $\{p\}$ (they are scattering states), and by p the projection operator onto $\{p\}$:

$$\begin{aligned} p = 1 - q \ &= 1 - \textstyle\sum_{i=1}^{N} |\varphi_i><\varphi_i| \\ &= 1 - \textstyle\sum_{i=1}^{N} |\psi_i><\psi_i| \ . \end{aligned} \tag{52}$$

The projectors p and q satisfy :

$$\begin{aligned} &p = p^\dagger \ , \quad q = q^\dagger \\ &p^2 = p \ , \quad q^2 = q \ , \quad pq = 0 = qp \ . \end{aligned} \tag{53}$$

The states $u_E^{(+)}$ are solutions of :

$$\left\{ \begin{aligned} &(pHp - E)u_E^{(+)} = 0 \\ &<\psi_i|u_E^{(+)}> = 0 \quad i = 1, 2, \ldots, N \ . \end{aligned} \right. \tag{54}$$

Using the relations (52, 53), eq.(54) can be transformed into :

$$(H - E)u_E^{(+)} = qHu_E^{(+)} \tag{55}$$

The formal solution of this equation satisfying the boundary condition of spherically outgoing waves at infinity is :

$$u_E^{(+)} = v_E^{(+)} + (H - \varepsilon + i\eta)^{-1} qHu_E^{(+)} \ , \tag{56}$$

where $v_E^{(+)}$ is the spherically outgoing solution of the l.h.s. of eq.(55). We have seen in subsection II.4 how to express the resolvent $(H - E + i\eta)^{-1}$ in coordinate space. Projecting eq.(56) on the state ψ_i, we obtain :

$$<\psi_i|u_E^{(+)}> = 0 = <\psi_i|v_E^{(+)}> + \sum_{j=1}^{N} <\psi_i|\frac{1}{H - E + i\eta}|\psi_j><\psi_j|H|u_E^{(+)}> \ . \tag{57}$$

This algebraic system of linear equations can be solved for the unknowns $<\psi_j|H|u_E^{(+)}>$, and finally we have constructed explicitly the state $u_E^{(+)}$ as :

$$u_E^{(+)}(\vec{r}) = v_E^{(+)}(\vec{r}) + \sum_{i=1}^{N} \int d^3r' <\psi_i|H|u_E^{(+)}><\vec{r}|\frac{1}{H - E + i\eta}|\vec{r}'> \psi_i(\vec{r}') \ . \tag{58}$$

Suppose now that we want to calculate the response to an external field A. According to eq.(20) we have :

$$R(E) = <\psi_0|A^\dagger \frac{1}{E - H + i\eta} A|\psi_0> \ , \tag{59}$$

where we have identified the exact ground state to its approximation in $\{q\}$ - space. Using the projectors p and q, it is straightforward to show that :

$$R(E) = <\psi_0|A^\dagger q \frac{1}{E - \tilde{H} + i\eta} qA|\psi_0> \ , \tag{60}$$

where we have defined an effective Hamiltonian acting only in $\{q\}$-space [34] :

$$\tilde{H} = qHq + qHp\frac{1}{E - pHp + i\eta}pHq \ . \tag{61}$$

Thus, it is equivalent to solve the original Hamiltonian H in the full $\{p\} + \{q\}$ space, or to solve the effective Hamiltonian $\tilde{H}$ in the simpler $\{q\}$ space. The price to pay for it is that $\tilde{H}$ is more complicated than H. In particular, $\tilde{H}$ now depends on the energy E, and it is complex.

III.2 RPA in discrete space

We now go back to the many-body case. The one particle-one hole space can be divided into two classes of configurations. The first class consists of configurations where the hole is in an occupied state ψ_i while the particle is in an unoccupied state ψ_m, with both ψ_i and ψ_m belonging to $\{q\}$. We call $\{d\}$ this discrete subspace spanned by state vectors $|\psi_m\psi_i^{-1}>$, and d its projector. The second class consists of configurations like $|u_E^{(+)}\psi_i^{-1}>$, i.e. the particle is now in a continuum state orthogonal to $\{q\}$. The subspace $\{P\}$ spanned by all possible state vectors $|u_E^{(+)}\psi_i^{-1}>$ is the continuum subspace, whose projector is denoted by P. Any vector of $\{P\}$ is orthogonal to any vector of $\{d\}$, and the sum of $\{d\}$ and $\{P\}$ gives the complete one particle-one hole space. Having split the complete space into two orthogonal subspaces, we can proceed to define an energy-dependent, complex Hamiltonian $\tilde{H}$ as in the preceding subsection and solve it in the $\{d\}$ subspace within RPA. We shall perform this task in two steps.

In the first step, we solve the RPA problem with the starting Hamiltonian H and within the discrete $\{d\}$ space. We write H as :

$$H = H_0 + V \ , \tag{62}$$

where H_0 is the Hartree-Fock Hamiltonian and V is the residual interaction which, for RPA, must be taken as $\partial U/\partial\rho$ (see subsection II.3). Expanding the discrete RPA states in the usual way as :

$$|d_\alpha> \equiv d_\alpha^\dagger|\tilde{0}> = (\sum_{mi} X_{mi}^{(\alpha)} a_m^\dagger a_i - Y_{mi}^{(\alpha)} a_i^\dagger a_m)|\tilde{0}> \ , \tag{63}$$

where $a_m^\dagger$, a_i are creation and annihilation operators in states m and i, respectively, and $|\tilde{0}>$ is the RPA correlated ground state, one finds for (X, Y) the well-known RPA equations [16] :

$$\begin{pmatrix} A & B \\ -B & -A \end{pmatrix} \begin{pmatrix} X^{(\alpha)} \\ Y^{(\alpha)} \end{pmatrix} = \omega_\alpha \begin{pmatrix} X^{(\alpha)} \\ Y^{(\alpha)} \end{pmatrix} \ , \tag{64}$$

where A and B are real, symmetric matrices in $\{d\}$ space whose matrix elements are :

$$\begin{aligned} A_{mi,nj} &= (\varepsilon_m - \varepsilon_i)\delta_{mn}\delta_{ij} + <mj|V|ni> \ , \\ B_{mi,nj} &= <mn|V|ji> \ . \end{aligned} \tag{65}$$

The properties of the solutions of eq.(64) are well-known [16]. We recall that these solutions occur in pairs. For each solution $|d_\alpha>$ characterized by an eigenvalue ω_α and amplitudes $(X^{(\alpha)}, Y^{(\alpha)})$, there is a solution $|\bar{d}_\alpha>$ with eigenvalue $-\omega_\alpha$ and amplitudes $(Y^{(\alpha)}, X^{(\alpha)})$. The normalization of these states is :

$$\begin{aligned} &< d_\alpha|d_{\alpha'} >= \sum X_{mi}^{(\alpha)*} X_{mi}^{(\alpha')} - Y_{mi}^{(\alpha)*} Y_{mi}^{(\alpha')} = \delta_{\alpha\alpha'} , \\ &< \bar{d}_\alpha|\bar{d}_{\alpha'} >= -\delta_{\alpha\alpha'} , \\ &< d_\alpha|\bar{d}_{\alpha'} >=< \bar{d}_\alpha|d_{\alpha'} >= 0 . \end{aligned} \tag{66}$$

The set of states $\{|d_\alpha >, |\bar{d}_\alpha >\}$ forms a complete basis for the discrete RPA particle-hole space.

III.3 Coupling of discrete to continuum space : complex RPA states

According to subsection III.1, the complete RPA problem will be solved if we find the RPA solutions of an effective Hamiltonian $\tilde{H}$ acting only in $\{d\}$ space. This Hamiltonian is (see eq.(61) :

$$\begin{aligned} \tilde{H} &= dHd + dHP\frac{1}{E - PHP + i\eta}PHd \\ &= dHd + W^\uparrow(E) , \end{aligned} \tag{67}$$

where H is defined in eq.(62).

Let us denote by $|D_\alpha >$ and $\Omega_\alpha = \tilde{\omega}_\alpha - i\Gamma_\alpha^\uparrow/2$ the (complex) RPA eiggenvectors and eigenvalues of $\tilde{H}$. We can use the basis of $\{|d_\alpha >, |\bar{d}_\alpha >\}$ states instead of the particle-hole basis to expand the $|D_\alpha >$ states :

$$|D_\alpha > \equiv D_\alpha^\dagger|\tilde{0}> = \sum_{\beta=1}^{N}(F_\beta^{(\alpha)} d_\beta^\dagger - G_\beta^{(\alpha)}\bar{d}_\beta^\dagger)|\tilde{0}> , \tag{68}$$

where $d_\beta^\dagger, \bar{d}_\beta^\dagger$ are quasi-boson operators creating the states $|d_\beta >, |\bar{d}_\beta >$ (see eq.(63)) whereas D_α^+ creates the complex excitation $|D_\alpha >$. The correlated ground state $|\tilde{0} >$ is the vacuum for RPA excitations, and we have therefore :

$$d_\alpha|\tilde{0}>= \bar{d}_\alpha|\tilde{0}>= D_\alpha|\tilde{0}>= 0 . \tag{69}$$

The RPA equations for the amplitudes $(F^{(\alpha)}, G^{(\alpha)})$ can be obtained by using, for instance, the commutation relation method [16]. We thus find a set of equations analogous to (64) :

$$\begin{pmatrix} \mathcal{A} & \mathcal{B} \\ -\mathcal{B} & -\mathcal{A} \end{pmatrix} \begin{pmatrix} F^{(\alpha)} \\ G^{(\alpha)} \end{pmatrix} = \Omega_\alpha \begin{pmatrix} F^{(\alpha)} \\ G^{(\alpha)} \end{pmatrix} \tag{70}$$

Here, $\mathcal{A}$ and $\mathcal{B}$ are $N \times N$ complex, symmetric matrices whose energy-dependent matrix elements are defined by :

$$\begin{aligned} \mathcal{A}_{\alpha\beta} &= \omega_\alpha\delta_{\alpha\beta} + < \tilde{0}|[d_\alpha, [W^\uparrow(E), d_\beta^\dagger]]|\tilde{0}> , \\ \mathcal{B}_{\alpha\beta} &= - < \tilde{0}|[d_\alpha, [W^\uparrow(E), \bar{d}_\beta^\dagger]]|\tilde{0}> . \end{aligned} \tag{71}$$

The coupling betweeen discrete and continuum spaces is described by the $W^\uparrow$ part of $\tilde{H}$, and this coupling gives the possibility for infinitely long-living RPA states $|d_\alpha >$ to emit nucleons and to acquire a width which is the direct escape width. This is the meaning of the quantity $\Gamma_\alpha^\uparrow$ appearing in the imaginary part of the new eigenvalue Ω_α. The operator $W^\uparrow(E)$ itself is very complicated (see eq.(67)). We now introduce a simplifying assumption and approximate it by :

$$W^\uparrow(E) \equiv dHP\frac{1}{E - PHP + i\eta}PHd \simeq dH_0P\frac{1}{E - PH_0P + i\eta}PH_0d . \tag{72}$$

We can justify this approximation by the fact that neglected contributions of the type dVP are expected to be small. Indeed, they are two-body matrix elements where three single-particle states are in $\{q\}$ space while the fourth one is in $\{p\}$ space, and since $\{q\}$ and $\{p\}$ wave functions are essentially non-zero in different regions, these matrix elements cannot be large if V is short-ranged. With approximation (72), we can now calculate the $\mathcal{A}$ and $\mathcal{B}$ matrices. Following Yoshida and Adachi [35] we introduce an operator M which is the inverse in $\{d\}$ space of $d(E-H_0+i\eta)^{-1}d$. The matrix elements of M are easy to calculate, and $W^\dagger$ can be expressed in terms of them since one can show that :

$$W^\dagger(E) = E - H_0 - M(E) \,. \tag{73}$$

If we perform the usual linearization of commutators [16] appearing in eq.(71), i.e. we keep only terms linear in the particle-hole operators, we obtain the following expressions for $\mathcal{A}$ and $\mathcal{B}$:

$$\begin{aligned}\mathcal{A}_{\alpha\beta} &= \omega_\alpha\delta_{\alpha\beta} + \sum_{mi}(E-\varepsilon_m+\varepsilon_i)(X^{(\alpha)}_{mi}X^{(\beta)}_{mi} + Y^{(\alpha)}_{mi}Y^{(\beta)}_{mi}) \\ &\quad - \sum_{\substack{mi\\nj}}(ni|M(E)|mj)\delta_{ij}(X^{(\alpha)}_{nj}X^{(\beta)}_{mi} + Y^{(\alpha)}_{nj}Y^{(\beta)}_{mi}) \,,\end{aligned}$$

$$\mathcal{B}_{\alpha\beta} = \sum_{\substack{mi\\nj}}[(-E+\varepsilon_m-\varepsilon_i)\delta_{mn}\delta_{ij} + (ni|M(E)|mj)\delta_{ij}](X^{(\alpha)}_{nj}Y^{(\beta)}_{mi} + Y^{(\alpha)}_{nj}X^{(\beta)}_{mi}) \,. \tag{74}$$

Because of the structure of eq.(70), the complex RPA solutions also appear in pairs, each state $|D_\alpha>$ with eigenvalue Ω_α and amplitudes $(F^{(\alpha)}, G^{(\alpha)})$ having its counterpart $|\bar{D}_\alpha>$ with eigenvalue $-\Omega_\alpha$ and amplitudes $(G^{(\alpha)}, F^{(\alpha)})$. The set $\{|D_\alpha, |\bar{D}_\alpha>\}$ is related to the set $\{d_\alpha>, |\bar{d}_\alpha>\}$ by a complex orthogonal transformation [35]. One can obtain a bi-orthognal basis if one introduces the adjoints of $|D_\alpha>$ and $|\bar{D}_\alpha>$:

$$\begin{aligned}(D_\alpha| &= \sum_{\beta=1}^{N} F^{(\alpha)}_\beta < d_\beta| - G^{(\alpha)}_\beta < \bar{d}_\beta| \,, \\ (\bar{D}_\alpha| &= \sum_{\beta=1}^{N} G^{(\alpha)}_\beta < d_\beta| - F^{(\alpha)}_\beta < \bar{d}_\beta| \,.\end{aligned} \tag{75}$$

The normalization of the complex states is :

$$(D_\alpha|D_\alpha >= -(\bar{D}_\alpha|\bar{D}_\alpha >= \sum_\beta (F^{(\alpha)}_\beta)^2 - (G^{(\alpha)}_\beta)^2 = 1 \,. \tag{76}$$

Using the following spectral representation of $(E-\tilde{H})^{-1}$:

$$\frac{1}{E-\tilde{H}} = \sum_{\alpha=1}^{N} \frac{|D_\alpha>(D_\alpha|}{E-\Omega_\alpha} - \frac{|\bar{D}_\alpha>(\bar{D}_\alpha|}{E+\Omega_\alpha} \,, \tag{77}$$

we can write the response function (60) in the form :

$$R(E) = \sum_{\alpha=1}^{N} <\tilde{0}|A|D_\alpha>^2 \left[\frac{1}{E-\tilde{\omega}_\alpha + i\Gamma^\uparrow_\alpha/2} - \frac{1}{E+\tilde{\omega}_\alpha - i\Gamma^\uparrow_\alpha/2}\right] , \tag{78}$$

where the transition matrix elements are :

$$\begin{aligned}<\tilde{0}|A|D_\alpha> &= \sum_{\beta=1}^{N}(F^{(\alpha)}_\beta + G^{(\alpha)}_\beta) < \tilde{0}|A|d_\beta> \,, \\ <\tilde{0}|A|d_\beta> &= \sum_{mi} X^{(\beta)}_{mi} < i|A|m> - Y^{(\beta)}_{mi} < m|A|i> \,.\end{aligned} \tag{79}$$

The response function (78) and the strength distribution deduced from its imaginary part are completely equivalent to the corresponding quantities calculated in continuum RPA by the method discussed in section II. A discussion of numerical results obtained by different methods (TDHF, continuum-RPA, complex RPA states) can be found in ref.[36]. Although expression (78) looks simple, one must remember that all the quantities $|D_\alpha>, \tilde{\omega}_\alpha, \Gamma_\alpha^\uparrow$ depend on E. For collective states, however, this dependence is weak [33] so that it is meaningful to talk about these collective RPA excitations centered at $E = \tilde{\omega}_\alpha$ and having an escape width $\Gamma_\alpha^\uparrow$. The advantage of the formulation of the response function in terms of complex RPA states is that one can anlyze the underlying structure of the response function, and make a clear distinction between purely nucleon escape effects and the spreading of the strength distribution due to Landau damping [33].

III.4 Escape widths

The complex RPA states $|D_\alpha>$ act as doorway states in reactions where giant resonances are excited, for instance in inelastic scattering processes. Let us consider an experiment of the type $A(a,a'b)B^*$ where a doorway state $|D_\alpha>$ is excited in nucleus A by the incoming projectile a. This state $|D_\alpha>$ can either decay directly by emitting a nucleon b which will be observed in coincidence with the scattered particle a', or it can spread out over more and more complicated configurations ($2p-2h, 3p-3h$, etc ...), and at each stage of complexity nucleons again can be emitted, leading to the various stages of pre-compound and compound emission processes. Here, we shall consider only the direct emission process. More general expressions of the transition amplitude including pre-compound nucleus decays can be found in refs.[35,37]. For simplicity, we assume that the doorway state $|D_\alpha>$ is isolated. The generalization of the scattering amplitude to the case of several overlapping doorway states is straightforward, but it would be more delicate to define partial escape widths. This point is touched upon in ref.[38]. Also, we do not write the direct knock-out part of the scattering amplitude, since it is always possible to choose kinematical conditions such that the knock-out contributions are negligible.

Let us denote by $\vec{k}_i, \vec{k}_f$ the incoming and outgoing momenta of particle a, and by E, $\vec{q}$ the energy and momentum transferred to the target A in the inelastic collision :

$$\begin{aligned} E &= \frac{\hbar^2}{2m_a}(k_i^2 - k_f^2) , \\ \vec{q} &= \vec{k}_i - \vec{k}_f . \end{aligned} \tag{80}$$

In the final state, the energy E is divided into :

$$E = \omega_c + \varepsilon , \tag{81}$$

where ε is the energy of the escaping nucleon whereas ω_c is the energy of the residual nucleus B^* in a state φ_c. The scattering amplitude for the process $A(a,a'b)B^*$ going through the doorway state $|D_\alpha>$ is [35,37] :

$$T_c(E,\hat{k}_f,\hat{k}) = \mathcal{K}\frac{\gamma_{\alpha c}(\hat{k})T_\alpha^{\text{exc.}}(E,\hat{k}_f)}{E - \tilde{\omega}_\alpha + \frac{i}{2}\Gamma_\alpha^\uparrow} , \tag{82}$$

where $\mathcal{K}$ is an appropriate kinematical factor, $\hat{k}_f$ and $\hat{k}$ being unit vectors pointing to the directions of the outgoint particle a' and b. In Distorted wave Born Approximation (DWBA), the excitation amplitude $T_\alpha^{\text{exc.}}$ from ground state $|\Psi_0>$ to excited state $|D_\alpha>$ is :

$$\begin{aligned} T_\alpha^{\text{exc.}}(E,\hat{k}_f) &= (\chi_f^{(-)}D_\alpha|V_{aA}|\Psi_0\chi_i^{(+)}> \\ &= \int d^3r d^3r_i \rho_{\alpha 0}(\vec{r}_i)\chi_f^{(-)*}(\vec{r})V_{aA}(\vec{r}-\vec{r}_i)\chi_i^{(+)}(\vec{r}) . \end{aligned} \tag{83}$$

Here, $\rho_{\alpha 0}$ is the complex transition density of $|D_\alpha>$ and $\chi(\pm)$ is the distorted wave of particle a. As a simplification, let us assume that the DWBA expression (83) is proportional to the Plane Wave Born Approximation (PWBA) amplitude. In this case, we have :

$$T_\alpha^{\text{exc.}}(E, \hat{k}_f) = \lambda(q)\tilde{V}_{aA}(q)S_\alpha(q) , \tag{84}$$

where $\lambda(q)$ is the proportionality factor between DWBA and PWBA amplitudes, $\tilde{V}_{aA}$ is the Fourier transform of V_{aA}, and S_α is the matrix element $(D_\alpha|e^{i\vec{q}.\vec{r}}|\Psi_0>$. In eq.(82), the quantity $\gamma_{\alpha c}(\hat{k})$ is the escape width amplitude of state $|D_\alpha>$ into channel c :

$$\gamma_{\alpha c}(\hat{k}) = <\varphi_c u_\varepsilon^{(-)}(\hat{k})|H|D_\alpha> . \tag{85}$$

This escape width amplitude can be easily calculated once we know $|D_\alpha>$.

The coincidence cross-section has the form :

$$\begin{aligned} \frac{d^2\sigma_c}{dE d\Omega_k} &= |T_c(E, \hat{k}_f, \hat{k})|^2 \\ &= |K\lambda\tilde{V}_{aA}|^2 \frac{|S_\alpha(q)|^2|\gamma_{\alpha c}(\hat{k})|^2}{|E - \tilde{\omega}_\alpha + \frac{i}{2}\Gamma_\alpha^\uparrow|^2} , \end{aligned} \tag{86}$$

while the angle-integrated cross-section is :

$$\begin{aligned} \frac{d\sigma_c}{dE} &= \int \frac{d^2\sigma_c}{dE d\Omega_k} d\Omega_k \\ &= |K\lambda\tilde{V}_{aA}|^2 \frac{|S_\alpha(q)|^2\Gamma_{\alpha c}^\uparrow}{|E - \tilde{\omega}_\alpha + \frac{i}{2}\Gamma_\alpha^\uparrow|^2} , \end{aligned} \tag{87}$$

where

$$\Gamma_{\alpha c}^\uparrow \equiv \int d\Omega_k |\gamma_{\alpha c}(\hat{k})|^2 \tag{88}$$

is the partial escape width into channel c. On the other hand, the excitation cross-section for state $|D_\alpha>$ is :

$$\sigma_\alpha^{\text{exc.}} = |K\lambda\tilde{V}_{aA}|^2 \frac{|S_\alpha(q)|^2}{|E - \tilde{\omega}_\alpha + \frac{i}{2}\Gamma_\alpha^\uparrow|^2} . \tag{89}$$

Thus, the partial escape width $\Gamma_{\alpha c}^\uparrow$ is simply the ratio of the coincidence cross-section $d\sigma_c/dE$ to the excitation cross-section $\sigma_\alpha^{\text{exc.}}$.

It should be noted that the relationship between the partial widths $\Gamma_{\alpha c}^\uparrow$ and the quantity $\Gamma_\alpha^\uparrow$ appearing in the imaginary part of the complex eigenvalues $\Omega_\alpha = \tilde{\omega}_\alpha - i\Gamma_\alpha^\uparrow/2$ is not a simple one. Indeed, it can be shown that [35], due to the fact that the transformation (68) leading from states $\{|d_\alpha>, |\bar{d}_\alpha>\}$ to states $\{|D_\alpha>, |\bar{D}_\alpha>\}$ is a complex orthogonal transformation, one has the following relation :

$$\sum_c \Gamma_{\alpha c}^\uparrow = N_\alpha \Gamma_\alpha^\uparrow , \tag{90}$$

where

$$N_\alpha = \sum_{\beta=1}^{N} |F_\beta^{(\alpha)}|^2 - |G_\beta^{(\alpha)}|^2 \geq 1 . \tag{91}$$

The proton decay widths of isobaric analog resonances have been studied by Adachi and Yoshida [39] in the framework of the present method restricted to Tamm-Dancoff approximation (TDA) but with the inclusion of $2p-2h$ configuration space . In this case, precise data concerning partial widths are available. In ref.[39], it was concluded that the TDA model can give a reasonable understanding of the data.

The direct escape widths of neutrons from the isoscalar monopole resonance have been experimentally studied in the last few years . In ^{208}Pb, for instance, there are data from

$(\alpha, \alpha' n)$ coincidence experiments [40] indicating that direct escape must be small, on the grounds that most of the measured spectrum could be reproduced by a statistical model calculation. Clearly, such an indirect and model-dependent method is not satisfactory, and one needs more detailed data. In particular, no information was obtained on branching ratios of various decay channels. In ref.[41], progress into this direction has been made by observing in coincidence the γ-decay of the residual nucleus ^{207}Pb, thus allowing a signature of the neutron emission channel. Calculations of partial escape widths in this case have been performed using the RPA approach in ref.[42]. It is found that the results depend strongly on the model. A phenomenological RPA model with empirical single-particle energies and an adjusted particle-hole interaction gives a reasonable total escape width although some of the experimental branching ratios are not well reproduced. On the other hand, a more consistent model based on a Skyrme interaction, like in ref.[24], grossly overestimates the escape width. If we look at the wave function of the complex RPA state corresponding to the isoscalar monopole resonance in ^{208}Pb, we observe that the phenomenological model gives a state built on particle-hole configurations which mostly involve the bound orbitals of the first unoccupied shell, thus leading to relatively small escape widths. In contrast, the Skyrme model gives a state distributed over a much larger number of particle-hole configurations also involving positive energy single-particle orbitals, from which neutrons can easily fly out and have larger escape widths. It would be interesting to see if a more elaborated calculation including damping effects due to more complicated configurations could improve this situation. In any case, the fact that particle decay depends sensitively on the model wave function gives us a powerful tool to explore the detailed structure of giant resonances.

IV Conclusion

In these lectures, we have sketched a theoretical approach to a microscopic study of giant resonances. We have adopted a limited framework, namely the RPA description of collective excitations. This should be considered as a starting point from which one can add more complexity to the picture in order to gain better insight into the properties of giant resonances. For instance, a step into that direction is to study how RPA states are coupled to states consisting of pairs of RPA states (two-phonon states), or to configurations made of particle-hole plus a vibration, a mechanism which leads to the spreading of giant resonances. This is an important aspect of giant resonance studies, but it lies beyond the scope of the present lectures.

In the first part, we have seen explicitly the close relationship between RPA and the Hartree-Fock approximation by deriving the RPA equations as the small amplitude limit of time-dependent Hartree-Hock equations. This tells us that, in principle, a consistent RPA model should be built on a single-particle spectrum and with a particle-hole interaction which are not independent but must be derived from the same starting interaction between nucleons in the medium. In practice, many applications of RPA simply ignore this consistency requirement and use empirical single-particle energies and adjusted particle-hole interactions. However, it is quite possible to perform consistent RPA calculations, for instance by using the methods discussed here. It is rather gratifying to see that effective interactions which have been adjusted to give good ground state properties in the Hartree-Fock approximation also lead to a satisfactory description of overall properties of collective excitations in the framework of self-consistent RPA calculations.

In the second part, a formalism for studying particle decays of giant resonances is presented. Again, the discussion is restricted to the RPA framework and therefore only direct decays are treated, but this formalism can be generalized to include delayed emission if one extends the model space beyond the RPA space. This type of decay studies, along with γ decays, is particularly needed if one wants to gain insight into the microscopic structure of giant resonances. In the past decade, the main effort was to determine experimentally, and to understand theoretically, the energies and the strength distributions of giant resonances in nuclei throughout the mass table. Now, the next task is to know in greater detail the structure of these collective excitations. In this respect, the study of decay processes is a very powerful tool. Such an exploration has already begun, and no doubt that it will grow up rapidly in the near future.

References

1. G.C. Baldwin and G.S. Klaiber, Phys. Rev. **73** (1948) 1156.
2. M. Goldhaber and E. Teller, Phys. Rev. **74** (1948) 1046.
3. H. Steinwedel, J. Jensen and P. Jensen, Phys. Rev. **79** (1950) 1019.
4. A. Bohr and B.R. Mottelson, Nuclear Structure, Vol.2, Benjamin (New York) 1975.
5. see, e.g., Phase Space Approach to Nuclear Dynamics, Editors M. Di Toro, W. Nörenberg, M. Rosina and S. Stringari, World Scientific (Singapore) 1986.
6. O. Bohigas, A.M. Lane and J. Martorell, Phys. Rep. **51** (1979) 267
7. E. Lipparini and S. Stringari, to be published in Phys. Reports.
8. G.F. Bertsch, P.F. Bortignon and R.A. Broglia, Rev. Mod. Phys. **55** (1983) 287.
9. J. Speth and A. van der Woude, Rep. Prog. Phys. **44** (1981) 719.
10. see, e.g., Highly Excited States and Nuclear Structure, Editors N. Marty and Nguyen Van Giai, Journal de Physique **C4** (1984).
11. D. Vautherin and D.M. Brink, Phys. Rev. **C5** (1972) 626.
12. M. Beiner, H. Flocard, Nguyen Van Giai and P. Quentin, Nucl. Phys. **A238** (1975) 29.
13. P. Quentin and H. Flocard, Ann. Rev. Nucl. Part. Sci. **28** (1978) 523.
14. A.L. Fetter and J.D. Walecka, Quantum Theory of Many-Particle Systems, McGraw-Hill (New York) 1971.
15. P. Noziéres. Le Problème à N corps, Dunod (Paris) 1963.
16. A.M. Lane, Nuclear Theory, Benjamin (New York) 1964.
17. G.F. Bertsch and S.F. Tsai, Phys. Rep. **18C** (1975) 126.
18. J. W. Negele and D. Vautherin, Phys. Rev. **C5** (1972) 1472.
19. A.B. Migdal, Theory of Finite Fermi Systems and Applications to Finite Nuclei, Wiley (New York) 1967.
20. R. Courant and D. Hilbert, Methods of Mathematical Physics, Interscience Publishers, 1953.
21. K.F. Liu and Nguyen Van Giai, Phys. Lett. **65B** (1976) 23.
22. K.F. Liu and G.E. Brown, Nucl. Phys. **A265** (1976) 385.
23. S. Shlomo and G.F. Bertsch, Nucl. Phys. **A243** (1975) 507.
24. Nguyen Van Giai and H. Sagawa, Nucl. Phys. **A371** (1981) 1.
25. H. Sagawa and Nguyen Van Giai, Phys. Lett. **127B** (1983) 393.

26. N. Auerbach and Nguyen Van Giai, Phys. Lett. **72B** (1978) 289.

27. O. Bohigas, Nguyen Van Giai and D. Vautherin, Phys. Lett. **102B** (1981) 105.

28. Nguyen Van Giai, N. Auerbach and A.Z. Mekjian, Phys. Rev. Lett. **46** (1981) 1444.

29. N. Auerbach, A. Klein and Nguyen Van Giai, Phys. Lett. **106B** (1981) 347.

30. N. Auerbach and Amir Klein, Nucl. Phys. **A395** (1983) 77 ; Phys. Rev. **C28** (1983) 2075.

31. H. Sagawa and G.F. Bertsch, Phys. Lett. **146B** (1984) 138.

32. M. Barranco, M. Pi, J. Nemeth, C. Ngô and E. Tomasi, Nucl. Phys. **A464** (1987) 29.

33. Nguyen Van Giai, P.F. Bortignon, F. Zardi and R.A. Broglia, Phys. Lett. **199B** (1987) 155.

34. H. Feshbach, Ann. Phys. (N.Y.) **19** (1962) 287

35. S. Yoshida and S. Adachi, Z. Phys. **A325** (1986) 441.

36. Nguyen Van Giai, Ph. Chomaz, P.F. Bortignon, F. Zardi and R.A. Broglia, Nucl. Phys. **A482** (1988) 437c.

37. F. Zardi and P.F. Bortignon, Europhys. Lett. **1** (1986) 281.

38. F. Zardi, P.F. Bortignon, Nguyen Van Giai and R.A. Broglia, 5th Int. Conf. on Nuclear Reaction Mechanisms, Varenna, June 1988.

39. S. Adachi and S. Yoshida, Nucl. Phys. **A462** (1987) 61

40. W. Eyrich et al., Phys. Rev. **C29** (1984) 418 ;
S. Brandenburg et al., Nucl. Phys. **A466** (1987) 29

41. A. Bracco, Nucl. Phys. **A482** (1988) 421c.

42. A. Bracco et al., Phys. Rev. Lett. **60** (1988) 2603.

SUPERDEFORMATION

J.F. Sharpey-Schafer

Oliver Lodge Laboratory
University of Liverpool
Liverpool L69 3BX U.K.

1. INTRODUCTION

Due to the very strong interaction between nucleons at short distances, the nuclear shape giving the lowest energy for most light nuclei is spherical as it is the one that packs the nucleons as close together as possible. The stability of this spherical shape may be enhanced by quantum mechanics and the Pauli principle. The mean field acting quantum mechanically on a single nucleon allows only certain orbitals which may be filled with protons and neutrons according to the Pauli rule. For a spherical mean field the orbitals are grouped in degenerate energy levels characterised by the total angular momentum j of the single nucleon. In this shell model of the nucleus energy gaps arise as each of the orbitals is filled. Hence nuclei near closed shells are especially stable and are spherical in their lowest states.

In between closed shells quantum mechanics removes the stability imposed by sphericity. Any deformation of the nucleus removes the j degeneracy of the single particle nucleon energies. In particular a prolate quadrupole deformation causes the levels with small Ω, the projection of their angular momentum on the symmetry axis, to be lowered in energy and levels with large Ω to be raised in energy. This splitting gives rise to the well known Nilsson diagram where the shell structure is wiped out for moderate deformations. Thus for nuclei with nucleon numbers between shell closures it is energetically advantageous to fill the low Ω orbitals in a deformed mean field. The deformations reached in this manner are roughly egg shaped with major to minor axis ratios of about 1.3 to 1.

As nuclei become heavier the saturation of the nuclear force, at a binding energy of roughly 8MeV per nucleon, can no longer dominate the repulsive Coulomb forces between the protons. For the heaviest naturally occurring nuclei the nuclear and Coulomb forces are finely balanced indeed, allowing the shell effects of deformation to play a crucial role in determining the nuclear stability. Thus, as actinide nuclei are deformed the increase in surface energy due to the nuclear forces is almost compensated for by the decrease in Coulomb energy as the protons get further apart. Oscillations in the shell corrections [1] for actinide nuclei lead to the "double-humped" potential as a function of quadrupole deformation as shown in figure 1. The deformation of the

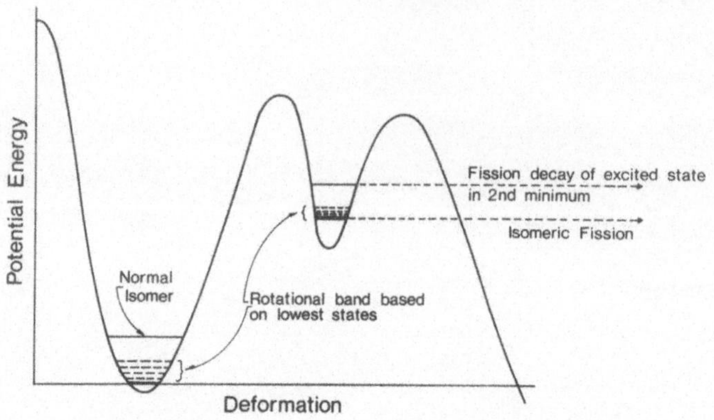

Fig. 1. The double-humped potential of Strutinski [1] giving rise to fissioning isomers in actinide nuclei. The second minimum has a major to minor axis ratio of 2 to 1.

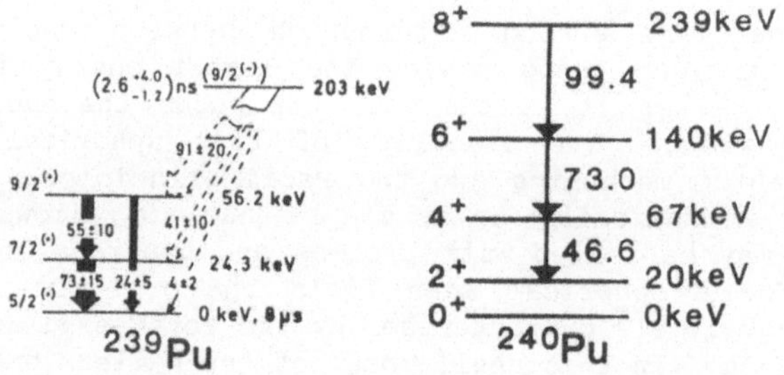

Fig. 2. Transitions observed by electron conversion studies in the second minima of ^{239}Pu [4] and ^{240}Pu [3]

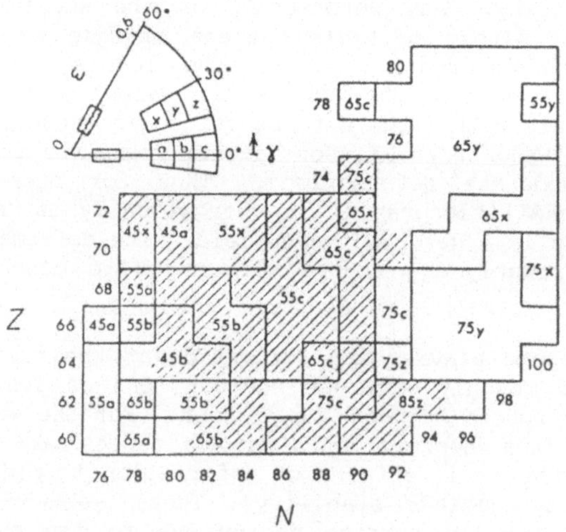

Fig. 3. Calculated [13] region of superdeformation near ^{152}Dy. The numbers give the spins at which the superdeformed states become yrast and the letters give the nuclear shape according to the labelling in the (ε,γ) plane shown in the top left hand corner.

second minimum in this potential is much larger than for normal nuclei and corresponds to a major to minor axis ratio of 2 to 1. States in this second minimum had been observed initially as spontaneously fissioning isomers by Polikanov et al [2].

As shown in figure 1, excited states must exist in both the first and second minimum of the double-humped potential. Indeed, due to the deformation at both minima, the nucleus is allowed to rotate about an axis perpendicular to the symmetry axis of the nucleus giving rise to rotational bands. These bands will have level separations governed by the moments of inertia $\mathcal{J}$ of the nucleus about the rotational axis. Clearly $\mathcal{J}$ increases with deformation and may be used as a measure of the shape at the second minimum if the levels in that minimum can be observed. The experimental difficulty with such observations is that in most reactions the second minimum is populated only very weakly, so that at best 1 in 10^5 fission events are delayed and from the decay of the fission isomer. In an experimental tour de force Specht and his co-workers in München observed [3] conversion electrons, from the decays in the second minimum, in coincidence with delayed fission events from the decay of the isomer of ^{240}Pu. The only other measurement on transitions in the second minimum is by Backe et al [4] in the odd nucleus ^{239}Pu. In both measurements 3 second minimum transitions were observed giving the decay schemes shown in figure 2. Lifetime measurements, which also confirmed the extreme deformation of the fissioning isomers, have been made for transitions in the second minimum [5,6,7].

In the mid 1970's, it was realised by theoretical groups from Copenhagen, Lund and Warsaw [8,9] that not only did the favoured shell corrections at the 2 to 1 axis ratio also occur for lighter nuclei, but in these cases the shape could be stabilised by nuclear rotation instead of the Coulomb interaction. Thus at very high spins the large moment of inertia $\mathcal{J}$ allowed states with the 2 to 1 axis ratio to be lowered below spherical or normally deformed states. The shell structure and shell energy correction at the 2 to 1 axis ratio are sensitive to proton and neutron numbers. A way of demonstrating this sensitivity is to consider the energy levels of a deformed quantum oscillator. Thus if one of the oscillator frequencies is allowed to change, in the Z-direction say, then

$$\omega_x = \omega_y = \omega_\perp \neq \omega_z \tag{1}$$

The z-axis then becomes the axis of symmetry and the total energy of the oscillator is

$$E = (n_x + n_y)\,\hbar\omega_\perp + n_z\,\hbar\,\omega_z \tag{2}$$

where n_x, n_y and n_z are the number of oscillator quanta in the x, y and z directions respectively. The energy E will have the largest degeneracy in situations where the ratio $\omega_\perp$ to ω_z is a simple fraction. Such a level diagram is to be found in Bohr and Mottleson's book [10] where it may be seen that there is a bunching of the oscillator levels and hence especially stable shapes at $\omega_\perp$: ω_z = 3:2, 2:1, 3:1 etc. for prolate deformations. If the potential depth below the Fermi surface is kept constant then as

$$V(z) = \tfrac{1}{2}\, m\, \omega_z^2\, z^2 \tag{3}$$

we have

$$\omega_z\, z_{RMS} = \text{constant} \tag{4}$$

as the nucleus is deformed and the minor to major axis ratios are inversely proportional to the oscillator frequencies. This also preserves the nuclear volume.

In more complex calculations [11,12] particular values of neutron number N and proton number Z are found to be extra stable at the 2 to 1 axis ratio. In particular the nucleus $^{152}_{66}Dy_{86}$ with N=86 and Z=66 was predicted [11] to be a good candidate for observing superdeformation. Superdeformed states were however predicted to be near the yrast line at high spin for all nuclei in a region close to the predicted "superdeformed magic numbers". In addition the deformation was predicted to change with proton and neutron number. The results of such a calculation by Åberg [13] are shown in figure 3 where both the superdeformed deformation parameter and the spin at which the superdeformed states were predicted to become yrast are shown as a function of (N, Z).

The problem with detecting the superdeformed states was that they were predicted to become yrast at spins between 50$\hbar$ and 60$\hbar$ in the most favourable cases. The record high spin states in 1982 were 38^+ in the prolate rotor ^{158}Er [14] and 38 in the oblate nucleus ^{152}Dy [15]. These high spin states were at about 15MeV excitation and were very untypical of the highest known spin in most other nuclei which seldom exceeded 30$\hbar$. The major development [16] in γ-ray spectroscopy that allowed discrete high spin level studies to be taken beyond 60$\hbar$ was the use of arrays of escape suppressed spectrometers (ESS). An ESS is a Ge γ-ray detector surrounded by scintillator, the escape suppression shield, which is operated in anti-coincidence with the Ge detector. This selects events in which all the γ-ray energy is absorbed in the Ge detector so that very good photo peak to total ratios are obtained. The operation of these devices and new physics that has resulted from their use has been discussed in a recent review article [17].

2. FIRST SIGHTINGS OF SUPERDEFORMATION

Attempts to find the predicted superdeformed states at high spin in ^{152}Dy using unsuppressed Ge detectors had insuperable difficulties due to the lack of signal compared to the background [18]. The first ESS array used on a major heavy ion accelerator was called TESSA2 [19] and consisted of 6 Ge detectors in NaI(Tℓ) suppression shields and a calorimeter of 50 BGO detectors to form a γ-ray calorimeter measuring the total γ-ray decay energy in an event and the number of γ-rays emitted. Using this spectrometer Nyakó et al [20] were able to establish for the first time the existence of a superdeformed band structure in ^{152}Dy using the $E\gamma_1$-$E\gamma_2$ correlation plot technique [21,22]. This technique uses the fact that classically the rotational energy E_R of a massive object rotating at an angular velocity ω about an axis for which its moment-of-inertia is $\mathcal{J}$ is given by

$$E_R = \tfrac{1}{2}\mathcal{J}\omega^2 = \underline{L}^2/2\mathcal{J} \qquad (5)$$

where $\underline{L}$ is the angular momentum. Hence quantum mechanically rotational energy levels are given by

$$E_R = I(I+1)\hbar^2/2\mathcal{J} \qquad (6)$$

where I is the rotational spin in units of $\hbar$. Because of the large electric quadrupole moments associated with a deformed rotating nucleus, the levels usually decay by E2 transitions with ΔI = 2 and with level separation given by the transitional γ-ray energy

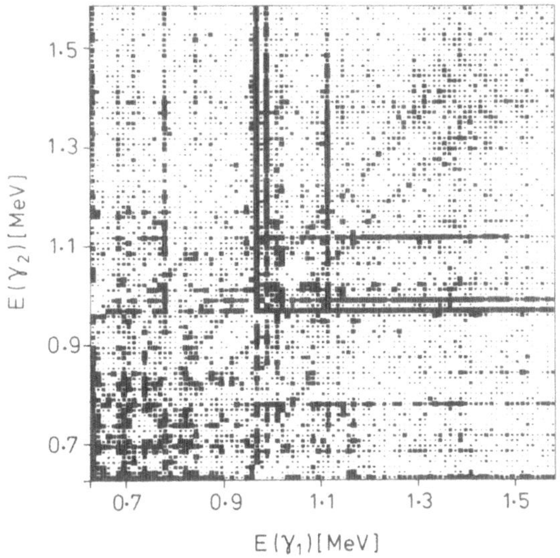

Fig. 4. Gamma-ray energy correlation contour plot for ^{152}Dy taken with TESSA2 using the ^{108}Pd(^{48}Ca,4n) reaction. The superdeformed structure is identified by two ridges parallel to the $E_{\gamma 1}=E_{\gamma 2}$ 45° diagonal.

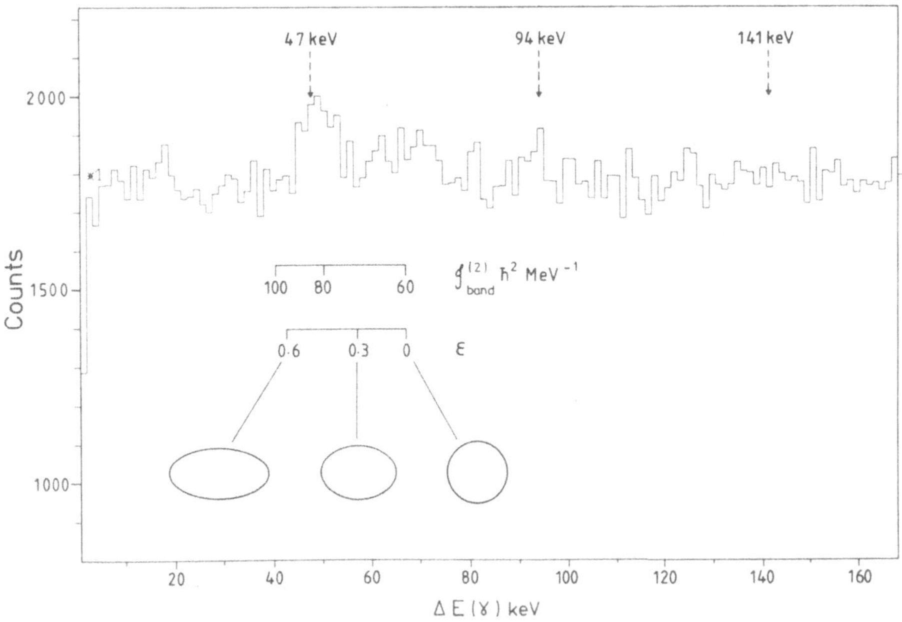

Fig. 5. Cut perpendicular to the $E_{\gamma 1}=E_{\gamma 2}$ 45° diagonal in figure 4 for mean γ-ray energies between 785 and 1330 keV in ^{152}Dy. The first ridge is clearly seen as a peak at ΔE=47 keV. The positions of possible second and third ridges are indicated.

$$E_\gamma = 2\hbar\omega = (2I + 1)\hbar^2/\mathcal{J}^{(1)} \tag{7}$$

so that $E_\gamma \propto I$. The separation of the γ-rays in an energy spectrum

$$\Delta E_\gamma = 4\hbar^2/\mathcal{J}^{(2)} = \text{constant} \tag{8}$$

Hence a spectrum of rotational γ-rays should have the evenly spaced structure of a picket fence. For a perfect classical rotor, the moments-of-inertia in equations (6), (7) and (8) should all be the same. As rotating nuclei are not so simple, the $\mathcal{J}^{(1)}$ and $\mathcal{J}^{(2)}$ of equations (7) and (8) respectively are not usually the same and are usually refered to as the "static" and "dynamic" moments-of-inertia. In a γ-γ coincidence experiment a plot of $E\gamma_1$ against $E\gamma_2$ for a single classical rotational band would produce an even raster of points [21,22] on a two dimensional contour plot. The square raster would be complete except for missing coincidences along the $E\gamma_1=E\gamma_2$ diagonal as an individual γ-ray would not be in coincidence with itself. Many such bands all with the same $\mathcal{J}^{(2)}$ and randomly displaced in energy with respect to each other would produce ridges parallel to the $E\gamma_1=E\gamma_2$ diagonal in our two dimensional contour plot. The moment-of-inertia $\mathcal{J}^{(2)}$ could be found from the separation of the first ridge from the diagonal which would be given by equation (8).

Figure 4 shows such an $E\gamma_1$-$E\gamma_2$ correlation plot for the $^{108}Pd(^{48}Ca,4n)^{152}Dy$ reaction at 205 MeV using data [20] taken with TESSA2. Thin stacked targets were used so that corrections to each E_γ had to be made for the full Doppler shift due to the recoil velocity of the residual nuclei. In order to see any structure the data has to be treated [21] to remove a large uncorrelated background. The first ridges are clearly seen parallel to the 45° diagonal. The vertical and horizontal stripes are caused by discrete γ-rays. The separation ΔE_γ of the first ridge from the diagonal is found to be very constant at $\Delta E_\gamma=(47\pm1)$keV giving $\mathcal{J}^{(2)}=(85\pm2)\hbar^2\text{MeV}^{-1}$. This value implies that the nucleus must be very deformed with quadrupole deformation parameter $\varepsilon\sim0.6$ implying a major to minor axis ratio of 2 to 1.

If a cut across the contour plot of figure 4 is made at right angles to the 45° diagonal the result shown in figure 5 is obtained. This is done by forming the spectrum of $\Delta E_\gamma = |E\gamma_1-E\gamma_2|$ taken over values of $\bar{E}_\gamma=(E\gamma_1+E\gamma_2)/2$ from 785 to 1330keV and subtracting some of the structure due to the strong discrete lines. Thus figure 5 looks along the diagonal at 45° in figure 4 and shows the first ridge at 47keV and perhaps a second ridge at 94keV. It should be noted that the first ridge is less than 10% of the height of the background illustrating the need for both very good peak to background performance of the detectors and the need for very good statistics. The first ridge was found to run down from $\bar{E}_\gamma=1.35$MeV to 0.80MeV where it disappeared in peaks due to coincidences between discrete γ-rays in ^{152}Dy. Assuming the rotation is classical so that $\mathcal{J}^{(1)}=\mathcal{J}^{(2)}$ and equation 7 holds, then the superdeformed rotation cascades from spin ~58ħ to 34ħ and maybe lower.

Prior to the experiment of Nyakó et al [20] described above an experiment [23] using the $^{100}Mo(^{34}S,4n)^{130}$ reaction had shown that similar ridge structures in ^{130}Ce were characteristic of almost as deformed nuclei as in ^{152}Dy. An experiment [24] to look for superdeformed $E\gamma_1$-$E\gamma_2$ correlations in the nucleus $^{154}_{66}Dy_{88}$ using the TESSA2 spectrometer and the $^{110}Pd(^{48}Ca,4n)$ reaction had found very weak ridges with a separation ΔE_γ between 42 and 55keV. Using the HERA spectrometer at Berkeley and beams of ^{40}Ar, de Voigt et al [25] confirmed the existence of superdeformed $E\gamma_1$-$E\gamma_2$ correlations in ^{152}Dy and suggested that such correlations may be seen very weakly in $^{154}_{68}Er_{86}$ and $^{150}_{66}Dy_{84}$ but not in $^{156}_{68}Er_{88}$. At one time the nucleus $^{144}_{64}Gd_{80}$ was the

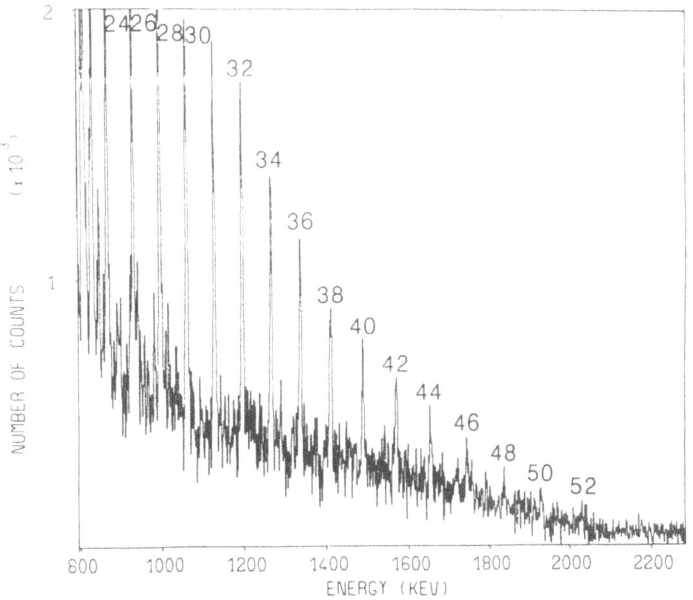

Fig. 6. Spectrum of the superdeformed discrete band in ^{132}Ce obtained using TESSA3.

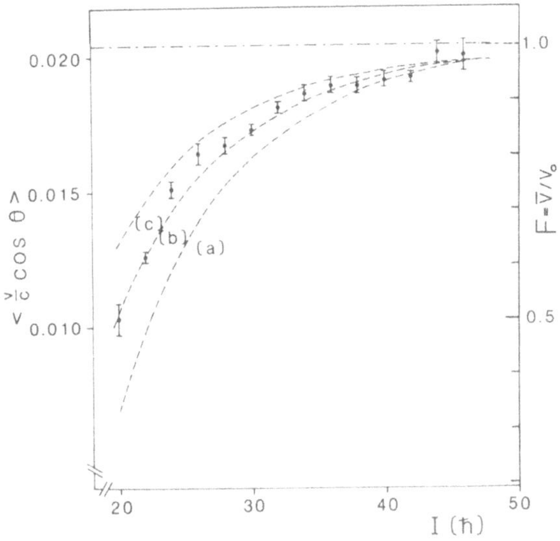

Fig. 7. The fractional Doppler shift F measured at θ=35° and 145° for the superdeformed band in ^{152}Dy. The curve (b) assumes a constant quadrupole moment Q_o=8.8eb for the band. Curves (a) and (c) indicate ±20% changes in Q_o.

most favoured candidate [26] for superdeformed structure, but searches in this nucleus have so far proved negative.

3. DISCRETE SUPERDEFORMED BANDS

The first evidence of discrete line rotational structure with extreme deformation was found by Nolan et al [27] in the ^{132}Ce nucleus. A very regular series of discrete γ-rays was seen from an estimated spin of 18 up to about spin 40 using the spectrometer TESSA2 and the ^{100}Mo(^{36}S,4n) reaction. A recent spectrum [16] of this band taken with the spectrometer TESSA3 is shown in figure 6. Seventeen discrete lines can be seen up to an estimated spin of 52 from a γ-ray energy of 809 to 2030keV. The spins have to be estimated as the γ-rays joining the bottom of the band to known levels have not been identified although very good statistics (4.10^8 triples events) have been obtained [28]. Indeed these data show that the decay from the extremely deformed band is fragmented and populated most of the known normal rotational bands at lower spins. The significance of the discovery of this band was not initially widely recognised. Firstly, the $\mathcal{J}^{(2)}$ for the band gave a deformation characteristic of 3 to 2 axis ratio rather than the "glamorous" 2 to 1 ratio. Secondly, very regular bands with apparent $\mathcal{J}^{(2)}$ that were characteristic of extreme deformation could be produced as an artifact where there was a strong interaction between crossing bands at a back-bend or quasi-particle alignment. Examples of such artifacts are to be found [29] in the nucleus ^{156}Dy. Thirdly, the inability to give a definite connection to the known decay scheme left potentially interested parties feeling nonplussed and encouraged judgements to wait until firm spins and excitation energies had been established. The highly deformed nature of this band has more recently [30] been established by very elegant lifetime measurements which are illustrated in figure 7. These data show that the feeding time for the levels is less than 15fs and that the measurements are consistent with a constant quadrupole moment Q_o=8.8eb throughout the length of the band. These lifetime data show that the large moment of inertia is not an artifact caused by progressive alignment, but is characteristic of an extreme prolate deformation with $\varepsilon \sim 0.4$ and a 3 to 2 axis ratio.

The most spectacular breakthrough in the study of superdeformation came with the discovery [31] that most of the intensity in the superdeformed structure in ^{152}Dy was concentrated into a single band. This remarkable and unpredicted observation was made using the improved spectrometer TESSA3 [16]. The spectrometer had 12 (now increased to 16) Ge detectors in compact shields [32] made of the very dense scintillator BGO as well as the same 50 detector BGO calorimeter used with TESSA2. This spectrometer gave an improvement of a factor greater than 10 in statistics allowing much weaker structures to be investigated in the spectra. The same ^{108}Cd(^{48}Ca,4n)^{152}Dy reaction as before was used, but decays from the 60ns 17^+ isomer were detected in delayed coincidence. A single superdeformed band of 19 discrete γ-rays (figure 8) with energies between 602 and 1449keV was discovered which populated the ^{152}Dy yrast line between the 1.5ns 27^- and the 60ns 17^+ isomers. The energy separation of the superdeformed transitions is extremely constant at ΔE_γ=47keV which is of course just the separation of the ridge from the diagonal seen in figures 4 and 5. As in ^{132}Ce it was not possible to find a connection from the end of the superdeformed band to the yrast state. Using intensity arguments regarding the feeding distribution along the yrast line it was estimated that the superdeformed γ-rays connected levels from spin 22^+ to $60^+\hbar$. The assumptions of even spin and positive parity rest entirely on the prediction of Åberg [33] that one such superdeformed band lies about 1MeV lower than other bands with the

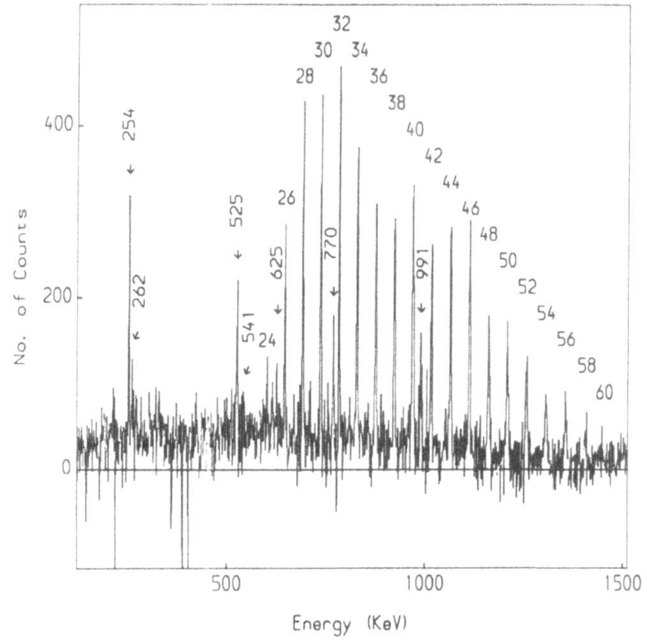

Fig. 8. Spectrum of the superdeformed band in ^{152}Dy using TESSA3 and gating on the 17^+ 60ns isomer. The γ-rays in the band are labelled by spin and those that are oblate yrast and near yrast γ-rays are labelled by their energies.

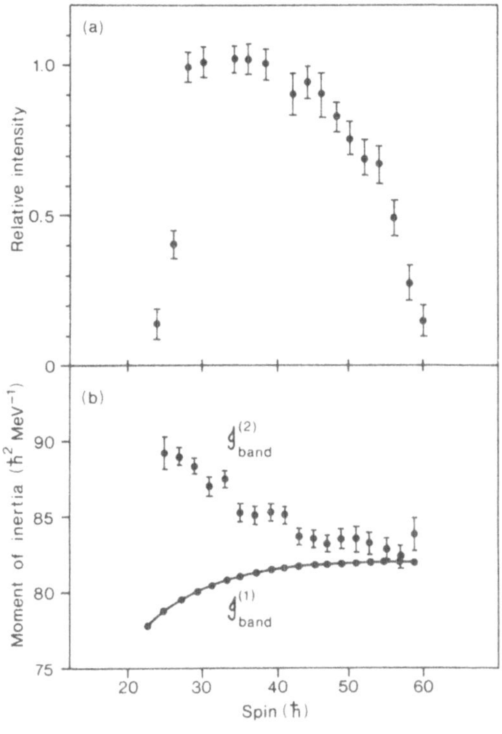

Fig. 9. (a) Relative intensities of the superdeformed γ-rays in ^{152}Dy as a function of spin (b) Moments of inertia $\mathcal{J}^{(1)}$ and $\mathcal{J}^{(2)}$ of the superdeformed band as a function of spin.

same deformation. The observation of a discrete γ-ray transition from spin 60ħ marked a dramatic advance in the study of high spin states. Previously the highest spin observed [34] was 46^+ in ^{158}Er and, after the initial extension of spins using TESSA2, progress to higher spins had been in steps of one or two ħ. The superdeformed band is populated mostly above spin 50ħ which can be seen from figure 9(a) where the relative γ-ray intensity is plotted against spin. From spin 50ħ down to the 693keV transition from the 28^+ level, the relative intensity is almost constant. The absolute maximum intensity is about 1% of the total to ^{152}Dy. The transitions from the levels assumed to have $J^\pi=26^+$ and 24^+ are weaker compared to the transitions above. This shows that the feeding out of the band is mainly from the 26^+ and the 24^+ levels. In figure 9(b) the static and dynamic moments of inertia $\mathcal{J}^{(1)}$ and $\mathcal{J}^{(2)}$ are plotted. The quantity $\mathcal{J}^{(1)}$ is affected by the spin assumptions and the curve would, for instance, be moved up if the superdeformed spins were too low. The quantity $\mathcal{J}^{(2)}$ is independent of the spin assumptions and is seen to fall slowly from 89 to 82 h^2 MeV^{-1}.

The decay path out of the bottom of the superdeformed band is not known which leaves the excitation energy and exact spins of the superdeformed states uncertain. Attempts have been made to establish the connection between the superdeformed and normal states, including the use of the fast sidefeeding into the states between the yrast isomers to isolate the feeding decays in the manner suggested by Sharpey-Schafer [35]. The data show that the decay path is highly fragmented and that exceptional statistics and signal to noise will be required to join the end of the superdeformed band to the yrast line. Recently the lifetimes of the levels in the superdeformed band have been measured [36] by repeating the experiment with a gold backing on the ^{108}Pd target and using the DSAM. The superdeformed γ-rays from levels with 50ħ and above have Doppler shifts that are not measurably different from the full shift. The lowest γ-ray observed in these data, from the 28^+ superdeformed state, has an attenuation factor F = 0.73 giving an effective lifetime for the feeding plus decay time of 190±10fs. The data are shown in figure 10 and an intrinsic quadrupole moment for the band can be derived assuming constant deformation at all spins. The best fit is given by Q_o=18±3 e.b which gives a B(E2) decay strength for the inband transitions of 2400W.u.! This should be compared with Q_o~5eb and B(E2)~200W.u. for rotational bands with normal deformation (ε_o = 0.2).

Because of the fast electronic stopping time α (calculated to be ~500fs for both the target and backing) only states with a very short effective lifetime will show a measurable centroid shift in the γ-ray energy. All the major intensity γ-rays in ^{152}Dy, including those of the lower deformation band, would appear as stopped transitions. Thus a subtraction of a total γ-ray projection at forward angles to the beam direction from a similar projection at backward angles, should show only the superdeformed transitions with all the other γ-rays cancelling out. Figure 11 shows the 35° projection subtracted from the 145° projection after normalisation on the 221keV γ-ray. Although there are no coincidence requirements, the resulting spectrum clearly shows the superdeformed band. It can also be seen from figure 11 that there are no other highly deformed rotational bands of significant intensity as these should also appear. This technique also enables a reliable measurement of (1.0±0.1)% for the total intensity of the superdeformed band relative to the total ^{152}Dy intensity to be made.

One of the most interesting aspects of the spectrum shown in figure 11 is the apparent lack of line shape effects for the superdeformed γ-ray transitions, resulting in a very narrow spectral line-width. This feature has been shown to be characteristic [37] of cascade feeding down

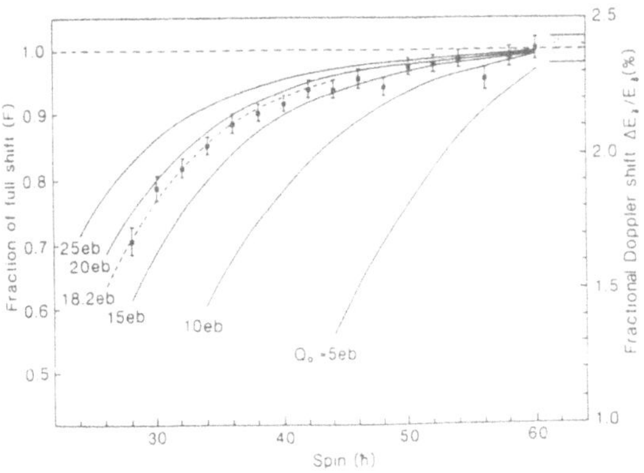

Fig. 10. The fractional Doppler shift for the ^{152}Dy superdeformed band. Calculated curves are for different values of the intrinsic quadrupole moment Q_o.

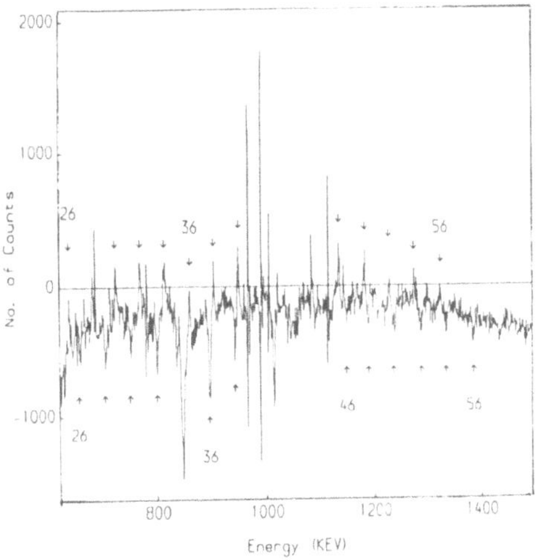

Fig. 11. Spectrum obtained by subtracting the θ=35° ^{152}Dy Doppler shift data of fig. 10 from the θ=145° data. Fast superdeformed γ-rays are indicated by arrows. Stopped γ-rays from oblate states cancel out.

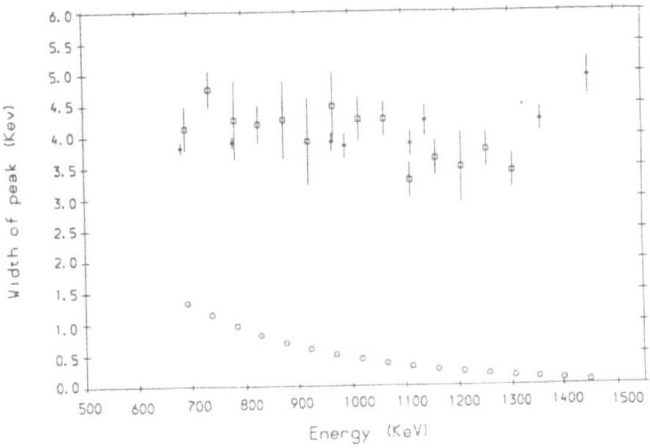

Fig. 12. Widths of γ-ray peaks for superdeformed (open points) and stopped (closed points) transitions. The calculated contribution to the line width from level lifetime effects is shown by the open circles at the bottom of the figure.

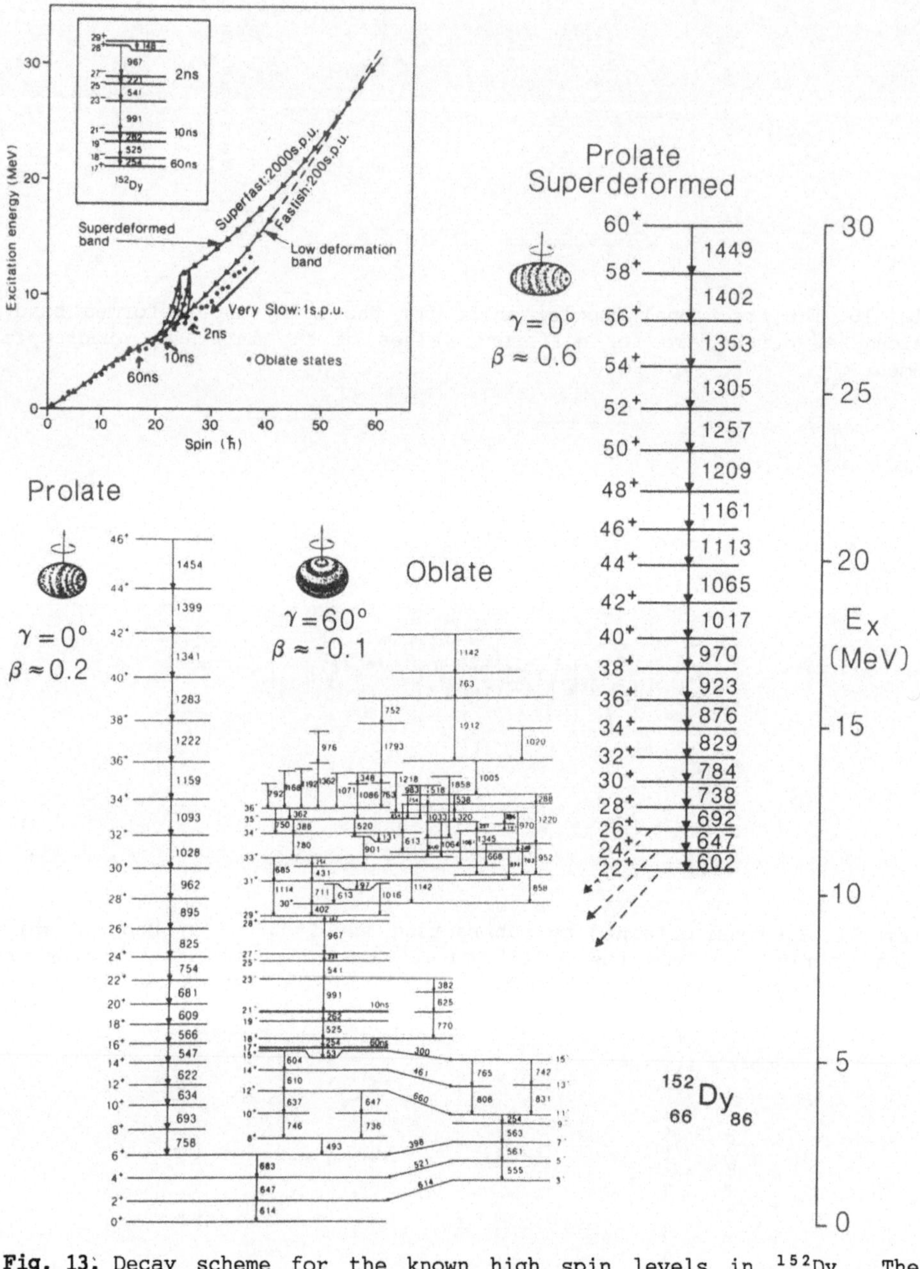

Fig. 13: Decay scheme for the known high spin levels in ^{152}Dy. The superdeformed band, reaching to spin 60ħ and excitation energy E_x~30MeV, is not attached to the other levels, but is known to decay to the yrast line between isomers at 27^- and 17^+. The inset plot of E_x versus spin shows schematically the relative positions of the superdeformed, the prolate (low deformation) and the oblate states.

a rotational band with negligible sidefeeding. Figure 12 shows the measured line-widths as a function of γ-ray energy, compared with those of the stopped transitions. Using a simple decay model [38] we calculate the recoil velocity distributions for the decays from each state in order to estimate the contributions to the line-widths from lifetime effects, assuming fast direct feeding. As the lifetimes of the states are now known to be extremely short, it is assumed that the recoils are attenuated only by electronic stopping of the form $v(t)=v_o e^{-t/\alpha}$ where v is the recoil velocity, after time t. Using the measured lifetimes, the r.m.s. deviation in the velocity distribution, and hence the spread in γ-ray energy, is calculated for each transition, and plotted in figure 12. It can be seen from this that lifetime effects will not make a measurable contribution to the line-widths as these are calculated to be much smaller than the experimental resolution of the germanium detectors.

The decay scheme of ^{152}Dy shown in figure 13 is one of the most remarkable for any nucleus: three different shapes of the nucleus co-exist between spins 22 and 40 and discrete line spectroscopy has been extended to spin 60ħ and 30MeV excitation energy. The oblate yrast states are known to about spin 40 and a prolate spin band of normal deformation, which bypasses the yrast isomers, has been observed to spin 40^+ [39] and has recently been extended to 46^+ [40]. Assuming that the superdeformed states become yrast when they cross a smoothly increasing projection of the low deformation band at about 52ħ (see insert to figure 13) then the highest discrete superdeformed state at spin 60ħ is at an excitation energy of about 30MeV.

4. SYSTEMATICS

The phenomenon of superdeformed states at high spin was predicted to be favoured in certain regions of the nuclear chart, but not to be confined to a single nucleus in that region. Such predictions were illustrated in figure 3 above. However the concentration of much of the superdeformed decay strength into a single band had not been predicted theoretically. The question arose as to whether the nuclei ^{132}Ce and ^{152}Dy had unique superdeformed properties, or whether similar bands could be found in neighbours of these initial superdeformed nuclei.

The matter was resolved by the discovery [41] of a superdeformed band in ^{135}Nd by the Berkeley group using the ^{100}Mo(^{40}Ar,5n) reaction. Thirteen superdeformed transitions are seen between 546 and 1362 keV from states estimated to be in the spin range 29/2 to 77/2. Additional superdeformed bands have been found [42] in the neighbouring even-even isotopes of ^{135}Nd. In ^{134}Nd a band is observed from spin 12 to spin 38 and in ^{136}Nd the band is from spin 16 to 40, In both these cases the connecting transitions from the super to the normal deformation are not observed. The Liverpool-York-Daresbury collaboration, using several versions of the TESSA spectrometers, have also observed superdeformed bands in ^{133}Nd and ^{137}Nd [43] and in ^{131}Ce [44]. In these three nuclei 16, 12 and 16 superdeformed transitions respectively have been observed, but in none of these cases have the connecting transitions been found. Perhaps the most remarkable of the Nd superdeformed bands is in ^{133}Nd where the band has up to 20% of the channel intensity. Indeed the superdeformed band dominates the γ-ray spectrum of ^{133}Nd above E_γ ~ 600keV. In figure 14, the $\mathcal{J}^{(2)}$ moments of inertia and the relative intensities are plotted against rotational frequency for the superdeformed bands observed in the Ce and Nd isotopes except for ^{136}Nd. It can be seen that most of the $\mathcal{J}^{(2)}$ moments of inertia peak at rotational frequencies between 0.5 and 0.6MeV and fall away at the upper and lower parts of the bands. Sudden increases are seen in $\mathcal{J}^{(2)}$ for the

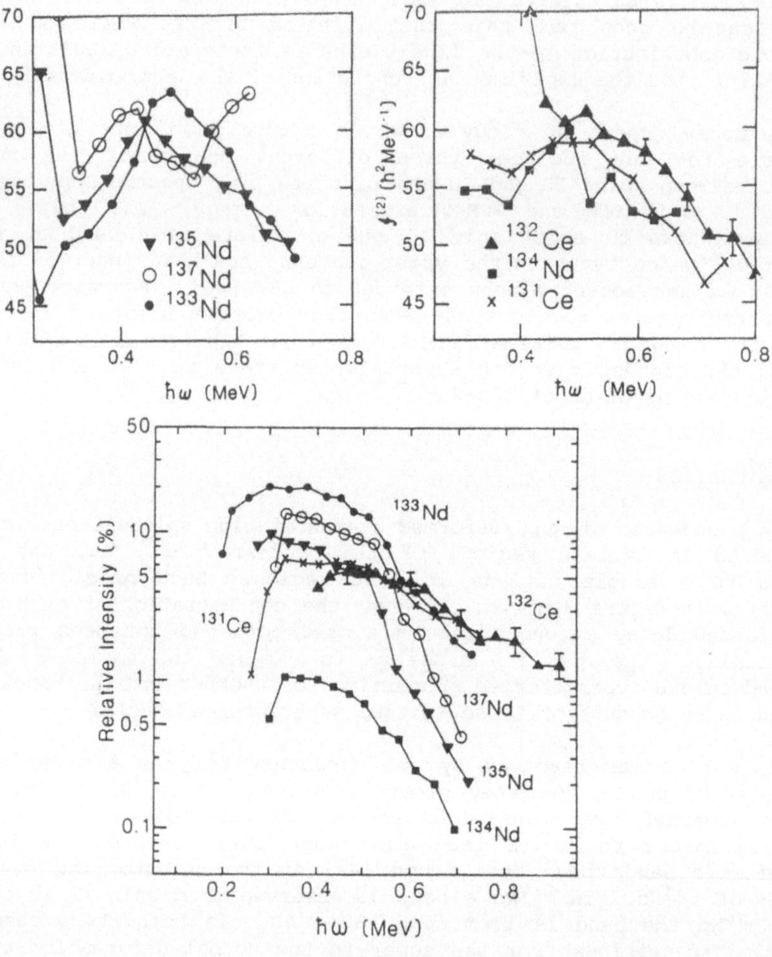

Fig. 14 The dynamic moment of inertia $^{(2)}$ and the relative intensity as a function of rotational frequency (ħω) for the superdeformed bands in the Ce and Nd nuclei. These data were measured with TESSA3 at the Daresbury Laboratory [28, 43, 44].

final transitions at the bottom of the bands in the odd Nd isotopes.

In the still more deformed region of nuclei near ^{152}Dy the consensus of recent calculations [13, 26, 45] was that the most favoured nucleus, in which the superdeformed minimum is lowest, would be $^{150}_{64}Gd_{86}$. Lighter gadolinium nuclei should also show signs of superdeformation as should nuclei with N=86 and even fewer protons than Gd. The nucleus ^{152}Dy is predicted to be on the upper edge of the region of superdeformation produced by the N=86 shell gap at a 2:1 axis ratio. The problem with carrying out experiments on the nuclei below ^{152}Dy is that they are very difficult to produce in standard heavy ion compound nucleus reactions while ensuring that sufficient angular momentum is put into the residual nucleus. It had initially been thought that it was essential in populating superdeformed states that the reaction must involve as high angular momentum as possible together with as cold a reaction as possible. Indeed it has been conjectured [46, 47] that the entrance channel could have strong effects on the population of superdeformed states. However, a second discrete superdeformed band in the N ~ 86 region was found in the nucleus $^{149}_{64}Gd_{85}$ by Haas et. al. [48]. They used the 8π spectrometer at Chalk River and the reaction ^{124}Sn(^{30}Si,5n) at 150MeV. The spectrum they obtain is very similar to that seen for ^{152}Dy. Again 19 γ-rays are observed from an energy of 617 to 1559 keV which the authors identify as decays from states with spins extending from about 51/2 to 127/2. Again the decays out of the band to the yrast line are not determined. The yield at a given spin is very similar to ^{152}Dy and lifetime measurements give Q_o = 17±2eb confirming the 2:1 axis ratio for the band in ^{149}Gd. The dynamic moment of inertia $\mathfrak{J}^{(2)}$ is found to be slightly smaller than for ^{152}Dy and to decrease more quickly with increasing spin.

The success of Haas et. al. [48] showed that the evaporation of neutrons could be used to cool the nucleus to sufficiently near the yrast line at high spin so that superdeformed states could be populated. Confirmation that this was the case was provided by the Berkeley group who observed [49] a discrete superdeformed band in $^{148}_{64}Gd_{84}$ both in the (^{48}Ca, 4n) reaction and in the (^{29}Si,5n) reaction. The spacing of the superdeformed γ-rays in both ^{148}Gd and ^{149}Gd is still very even, but in both cases the dynamic moment-of-inertia $\mathfrak{J}^{(2)}$ decreases rather more rapidly with spin than it does for ^{152}Dy. In contrast, the $\mathfrak{J}^{(2)}$ of a superdeformed band discovered in ^{151}Dy by the Argonne group [50] using the (^{34}S,5n) reaction actually increases with spin. These data demonstrate that the details of the microscopic configurations of the particles making up the superdeformed shapes are affecting the macroscopic dynamical behaviour.

At Daresbury we have recently used the (^{26}Mg,6n) and (^{27}Al,6n) reactions on ^{130}Te to observe [51] superdeformed bands in $^{150}_{64}Gd_{86}$ and $^{151}_{65}Tb_{86}$ respectively. Spectra showing γ-rays from the decay of these superdeformed states are shown in figure 15. The average spin at which the ^{150}Gd superdeformed band feeds into the yrast states is well established allowing the superdeformed spins to be estimated. These spins, as shown in figure 15, run from 34^+ up to 64^+. The point at which the superdeformed states in ^{151}Tb feed the yrast line is much more difficult to establish so that only the γ-ray energies of the transitions are given in figure 15. In figure 16 the relative intensities of superdeformed γ-rays in ^{150}Gd and ^{151}Tb are compared with those for ^{149}Gd and ^{152}Dy. It can be seen that for ^{150}Gd and ^{151}Tb the decay out of the bands occur at $\hbar\omega$ ~ 0.4MeV rather than ~0.3MeV for the original two nuclei. Additionally for ^{151}Tb the quantity $\mathfrak{J}^{(2)}$ is found to decrease more rapidly with increasing rotational frequency $\hbar\omega$ than even for ^{148}Gd. For ^{150}Gd the decrease is even more spectacular. These effects can be

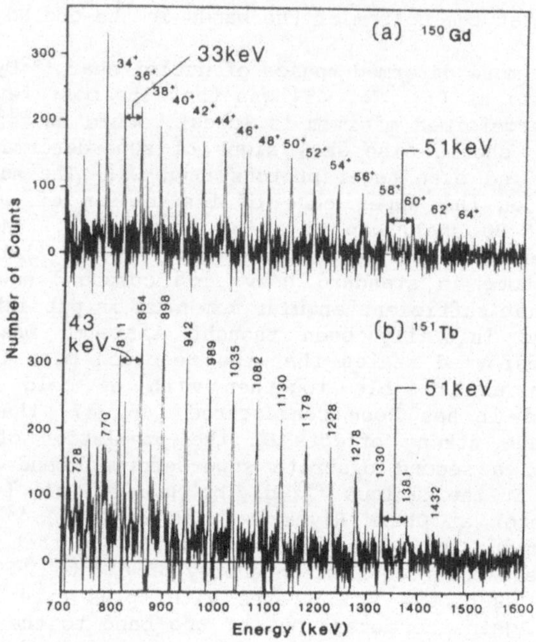

Fig. 15. Superdeformed bands in (a) ^{150}Gd and (b) ^{151}Tb measured [51] using the (^{26}Mg,6n) and (^{27}Al,6n) reactions on ^{130}Te and the spectrometer TESSA3.

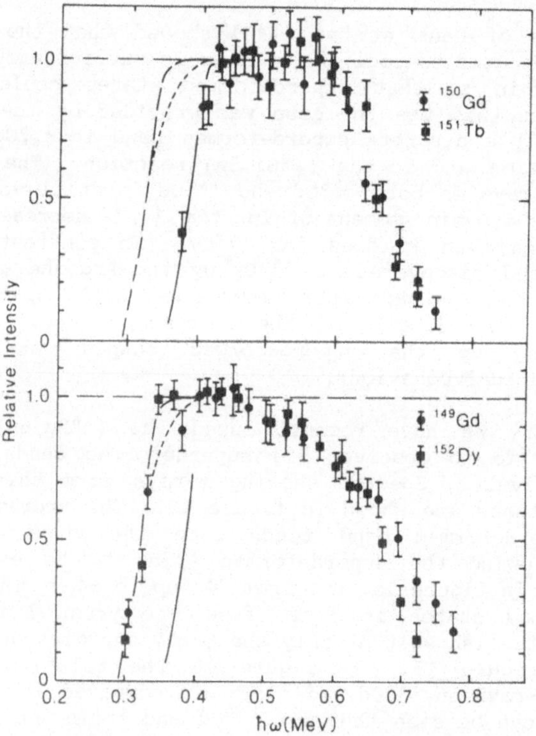

Fig. 16. Comparison of the relative intensities of superdeformed bands in ^{150}Gd, ^{151}Tb and ^{149}Gd, ^{152}Dy. The difference in the frequencies at which the bands exit from superdeformation is indicated.

seen from the spectra in figure 15. At low energies in ^{151}Tb the γ-ray separation is ~43keV in contrast to ~51keV at the highest energies. In ^{150}Gd the difference is even more spectacular with 33keV contrasted with 51keV. The microscopic causes of these changes in $\mathcal{J}^{(2)}$ will be discussed in the section below.

In addition to the regions of (N, Z) near ^{132}Ce and ^{152}Dy states of extreme deformation have been observed in Os nuclei and Pd nuclei. In ^{180}Os ridges in E_{γ_1}-E_{γ_2} correlations show evidence [52] of structures with $\varepsilon \sim 0.5$. Additionally discrete lines at very high spin on the yrast line in ^{178}Os give [53] an $\mathcal{J}^{(2)}$ characteristic of extreme deformation. In lighter nuclei similar states have been observed [54] in ^{104} ^{105}Pd.

5. MICROSCOPIC CONFIGURATIONS

It has been discussed in the introduction to these lectures how especially stable superdeformed configurations can arise in the simplest of simple harmonic oscillator models. In figure 17 the energies of single particle orbitals in a deformed Saxon-Woods potential [12] are plotted as a function of prolate quadrupole deformation β for both neutrons and protons. It can be seen that large energy gaps open up below areas of high level density. These gaps give rise to deformed "magic" numbers over a range of deformations. Such numbers are marked in figure 17. Extreme deformations will lie at low excitation energies where a nucleus has magic numbers for both protons and neutrons at the same deformation. Thus $^{132}_{58}Ce_{74}$ has magic numbers at a deformation of 0.45 and $^{152}_{68}Dy_{86}$ has magic numbers at $\beta \sim 0{,}7$. As the nucleus is rotated the orbitals in figure 17 will be split by the asymmetry introduced by the rotation. Orbitals with their angular momentum aligned with the axis of rotation, ie. with low Ω, will undergo considerable splitting as the rotation introduces a term $(-j_x\omega)$ into the Hamiltonian, where the rotation is about the x-axis. High Ω orbitals will suffer minimal splitting by the rotation. The energy of the nucleus may then be calculated [12] within the cranking approximation using the generalised Strutinski method as a function of spin I and nuclear shape. The Lund convention for the nuclear shape is illustrated [55] in figure 18 where the shape parameters are the quadrupole deformation β and the triaxility angle γ. The convention is such that the nucleus has γ=0° for prolate deformations rotating about an axis perpendicular to the symmetry axis. For oblate shapes, where the angular momentum is built up of the vector sum of individual particle spins aligned with the symmetry axis, the angle γ = 60°. Using this notation contour maps of the total energy of the nucleus may be calculated [55] as a function of total spin I. In figure 18 such contour plots are shown for the nucleus ^{152}Dy. It can be seen that as the spin increases the superdeformed minimum at $\beta \sim 0.6$ on the γ = 0°axis deepens and at the highest spins is below the energy for oblate deformations. In figure 20 the shapes of the energy surfaces are calculated at spin 60^+ and 40^+ for even-even nuclei with 86 neutrons. It can be seen that the superdeformed minimum is well formed and separated from other shapes by a significant barrier for proton number Z < 66, but becomes increasingly shallow for Z > 66. These impressive calculations reproduce the systematic behaviour of superdeformed structures very well at least in so far as present experimental data is concerned.

The way the underlying single particle configurations that go to make up the superdeformed bands in different nuclei affect the dynamical moment-of-inertia $\mathcal{J}^{(2)}$ of the bands has recently been calculated by the Lund group [56, 57, 58]. In figure 21(a) the proton single particle energies e^{ω}_{π} in the rotating frame have been calculated as a function of ω using deformation ε = 0.56 appropriate to ^{150}Gd. It can be seen that there is a suitable gap at Z = 64 for all ω which encourages the lowering

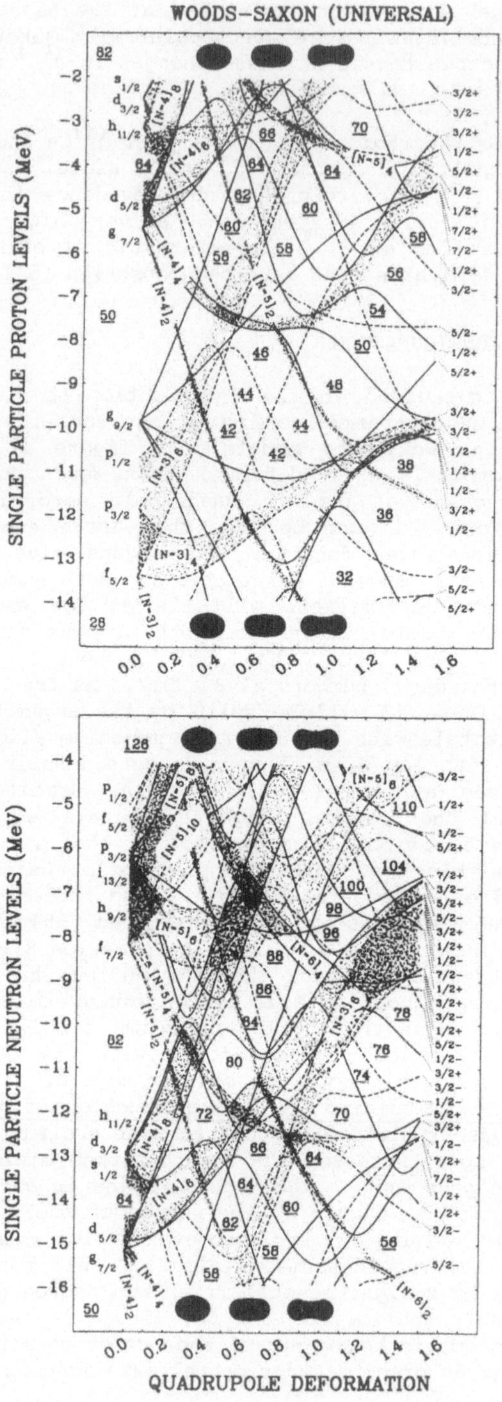

Fig. 17. Single particle levels for protons and neutrons as a function of the quadrupole deformation β_2. All non-intruder orbitals can be grouped into approximately degenerate multiplets which are marked by shaded areas. The chains of deformed shell closures are labelled with the number of occupied proton and neutron levels [55, 76].

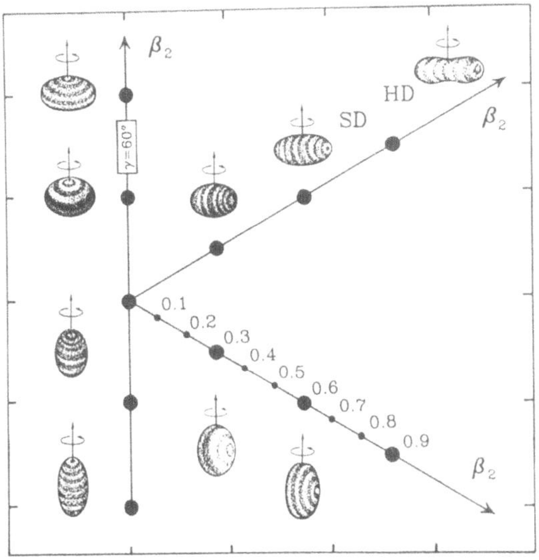

Fig. 18 The Lund convention for parameterising the nuclear shape. Shapes in the (β_2, γ) plane are illustrated where β_2 is the quadrupole deformation and γ is the triaxility parameter which increases anti-clockwise from -120° downwards, to 60° upwards.

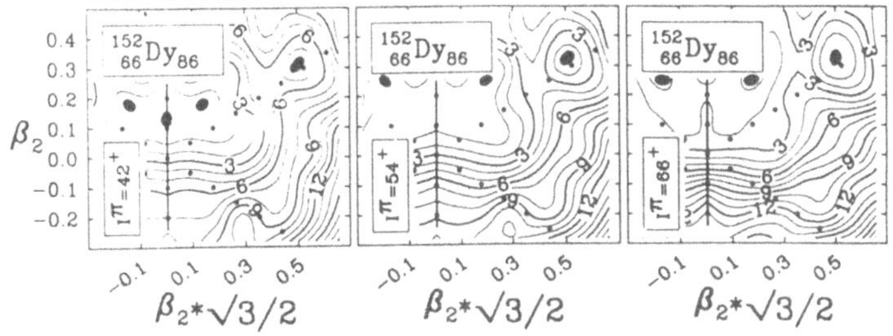

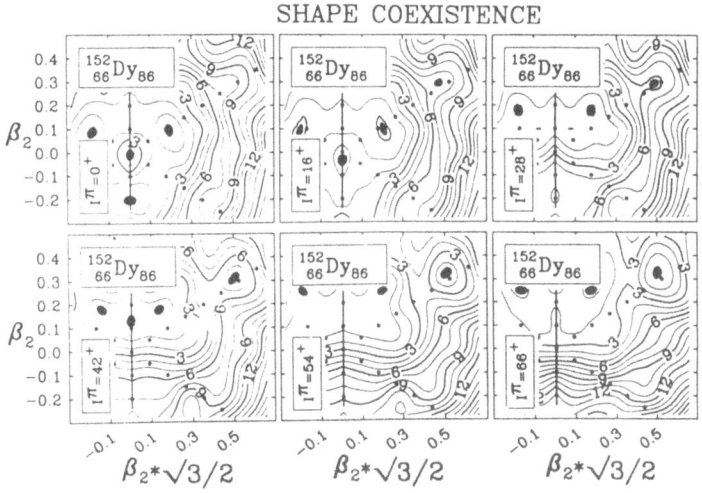

Fig. 19 Energy surfaces calculated [55] in the (β, γ) plane for ^{152}Dy for spins I^π up to 66^+. The development of the superdeformed minimum with increasing spin can be seen on the $\gamma=0$ axis near $\beta=0.6$.

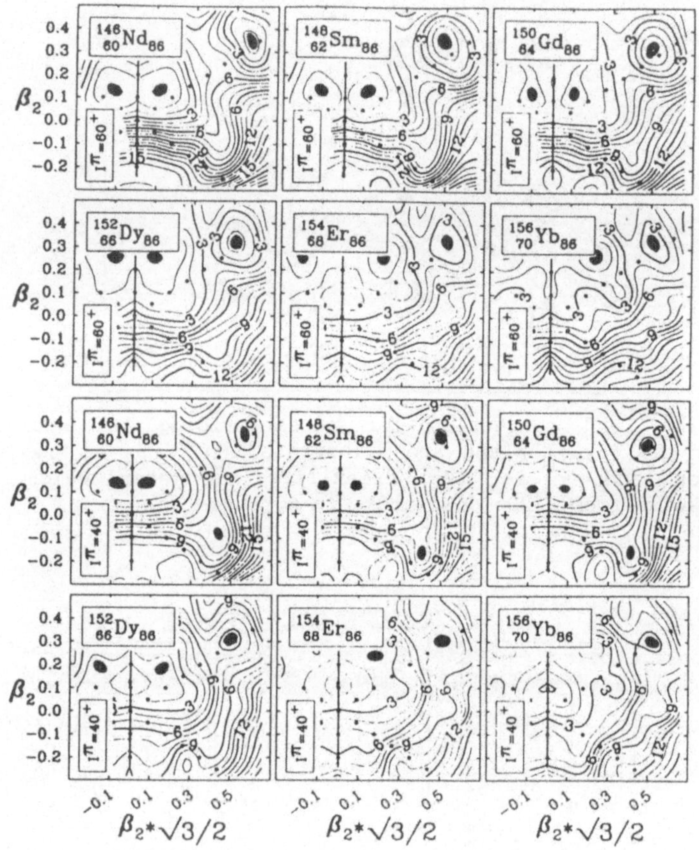

Fig. 20 Energy surfaces calculated [55] in the (β,γ) plane for even-even nuclei with 86 neutrons at spins 60^{+} and 40^{+}. For all these nuclei a superdeformed minimum exists on the γ=0° axis at about β=0.6. It can be seen that this minimum is best established for proton numbers less than 66.

and stability of a single positive parity superdeformed band. Changes in the deformation ε will mainly have the effect of altering the position of the high oscillator intruder orbitals with oscillator number N = 6 with respect to the N = 4 and 5 orbitals. It can be seen that the N=6 orbitals, which have Ω small, are split by the rotation. In contrast the N=4 and 5 orbitals, which have high Ω, are hardly affected. The contribution of a given orbital to the total angular momentum may be calculated from

$$i_{x,\pi} = \langle j_x \rangle \pi = -de_\pi^\omega/d\omega \qquad (9)$$

which is plotted for the four lowest N=6 proton orbitals in figure 21(b). The contribution of each orbital to the dynamic moment-of-inertia $\mathcal{J}^{(2)}$ is given by

$$\mathcal{J}^{(2)}_{orb,\pi} = di_{x,\pi}/d\omega = -d^2 e_\pi^\omega/d\omega^2 \qquad (10)$$

which are plotted as a function of ω in figure 21(c) for the same four orbitals. In figure 21(d) the contributions to $\mathcal{J}^{(2)}$ are summed for 1, 2, 3 and 4 protons in N=6 oscillator orbitals, again as a function of rotational frequency. It can be seen from figure 21(d) that the $\pi 6^4$ (Dy) contributions to $\mathcal{J}^{(2)}$ is roughly constant whereas this contribution decreases rapidly with increasing rotational frequency ω for $\pi 6^2$ (Gd) and $\pi 6^3$ (Tb).

In figure 22(a) the neutron routhians (single particle energy in the rotating frame) e_ν^ω are plotted as a function of ω, again for a deformation ε=0.56 which is appropriate for $^{150}_{64}Gd_{86}$. At the higher rotational frequencies there is a gap for 86 neutrons. In figure 22(b) the summed contributions of the N=7 neutrons to $\mathcal{J}^{(2)}$ is plotted as a function of Ω, together with the total contribution from eight N=6 neutrons plus the contribution from the N=76 core. It can be seen that apart from the N=7 valence neutrons, the contributions to $\mathcal{J}^{(2)}$ are rather constant with frequency. In figure 23 the experimental values of $\mathcal{J}^{(2)}$ and $\mathcal{J}^{(1)}$ are shown for the superdeformed bands in the nuclei ^{151}Tb, ^{152}Dy, ^{149} ^{150}Gd. The dotted lines are the sum of the calculations given in figure 21(d) and 22(b) for the appropriate number of protons and neutrons for each nucleus. It can be seen that the calculations reproduce very well the trend of the observed $\mathcal{J}^{(2)}$s with ω. Only in the case of ^{152}Dy do the calculations reproduce the absolute magnitude of $\mathcal{J}^{(2)}$ correctly. The calculations also give the correct slope of $\mathcal{J}^{(2)}$ versus ω for the superdeformed band in ^{148}Gd. In addition the observed small increase in $\mathcal{J}^{(2)}$ with ω in ^{151}Gd is reproduced.

The very large values of $\mathcal{J}^{(2)}$ for the lowest two frequency points of ^{150}Gd are not reproduced by the calculations as these values are too big to be due to the intrinsic nuclear shape. The pushing together of the γ-ray energies at the bottom of the ^{150}Gd superdeformed band to give this anomalous effect on the $\mathcal{J}^{(2)}$ must be due to a band crossing and will be discussed in a later section below.

The success of the Lund group's calculations [57,58] in reproducing the trends observed experimentally in $\mathcal{J}^{(2)}$ means that we should have confidence in these calculations in making spectroscopic predictions. In figure 24 their predictions [59] for the number of valence protons n_π in the N=6 and the number of neutrons n_ν in the N=7 intruder orbitals are given. It should be noticed that although these numbers increase, for the nuclei with 85 and 86 neutrons between proton number 64 and 66, instep with the neutron and proton numbers this is not the case for nucleon numbers outside this region. For example, the nucleus ^{148}Gd should have two N=6 protons $\pi 6^2$, but still has one N=7 neutron $\nu 7^1$. In

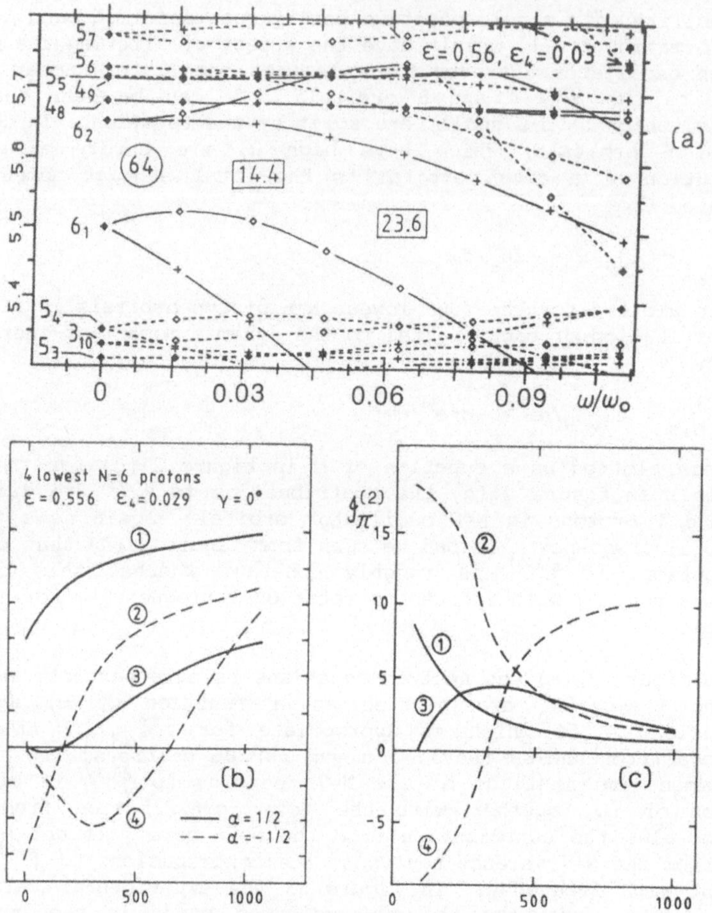

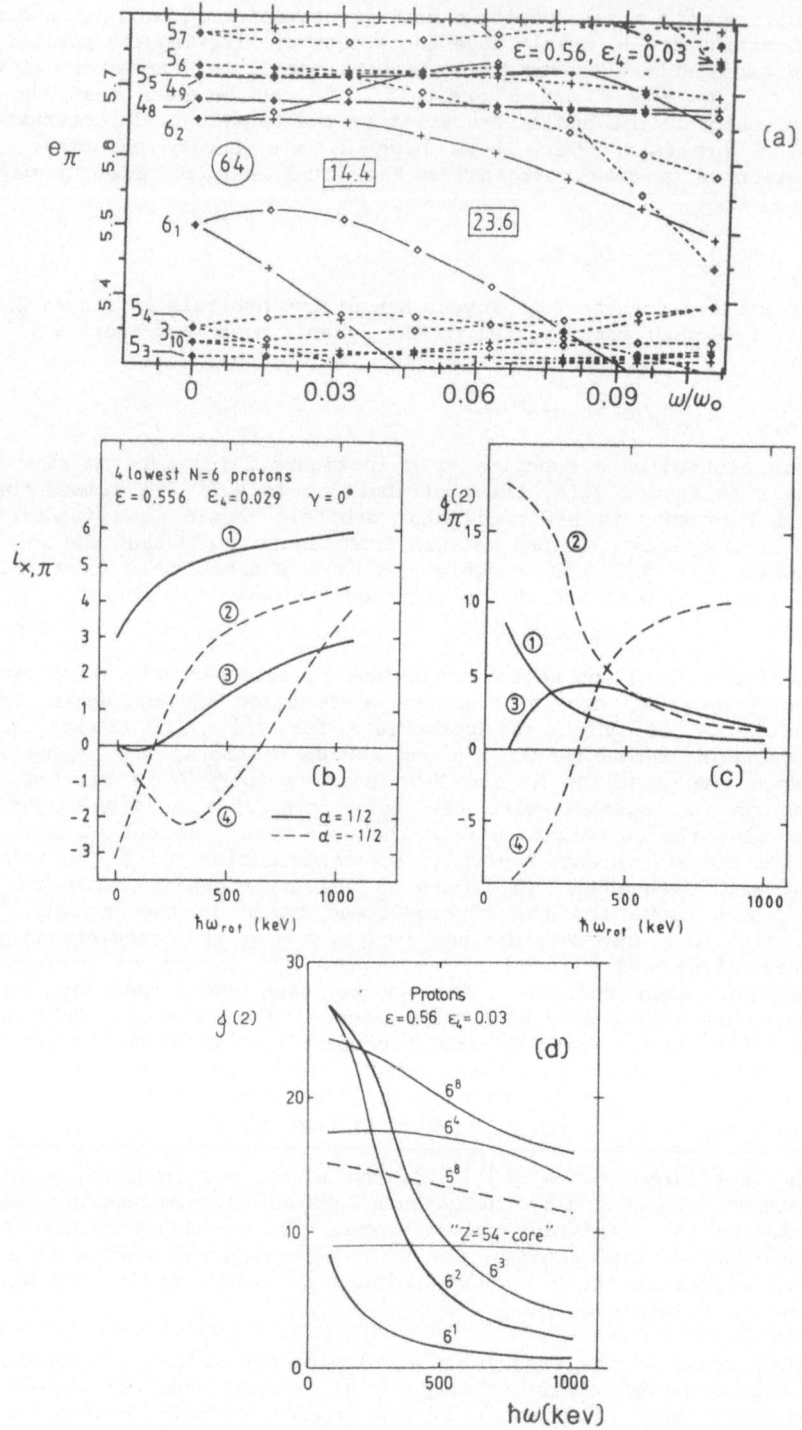

Fig. 21 Calculations of the Lund group [56,57,58] for a superdeformed potential appropriate for ^{150}Gd. (a) the energy e_π of protons in the rotating frame as a function of ω (b) the differential of (a) giving the aligned spin for the four lowest N=6 orbitals (c) the differential of (b) giving each orbitals contribution to $\mathcal{J}^{(2)}$ (d) the sum of (c) for N=6 protons giving their total contribution to $\mathcal{J}^{(2)}$.

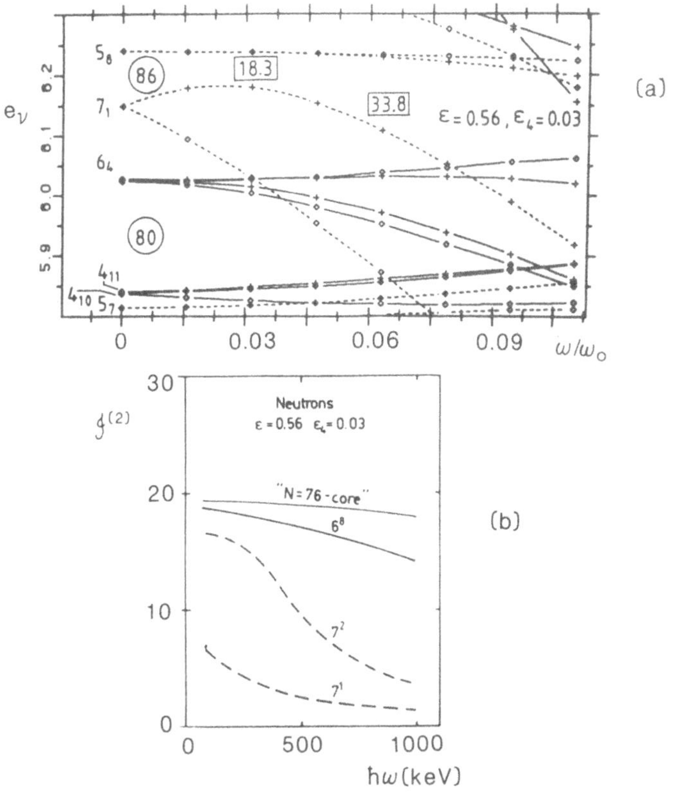

Fig. 22 Calculations of the Lund group [56,57,58] for a superdeformed potential appropriate for ^{150}Gd. (a) the energy e_ν of neutrons in the rotating frame as a function of ω showing the signature split N=7 intruder orbitals. (b) The neutron equivalent of fig. 21(d) showing the sum of contributions to $\mathcal{J}^{(2)}$ from the N=7 orbitals for occupation numbers n_ν=1 and 2.

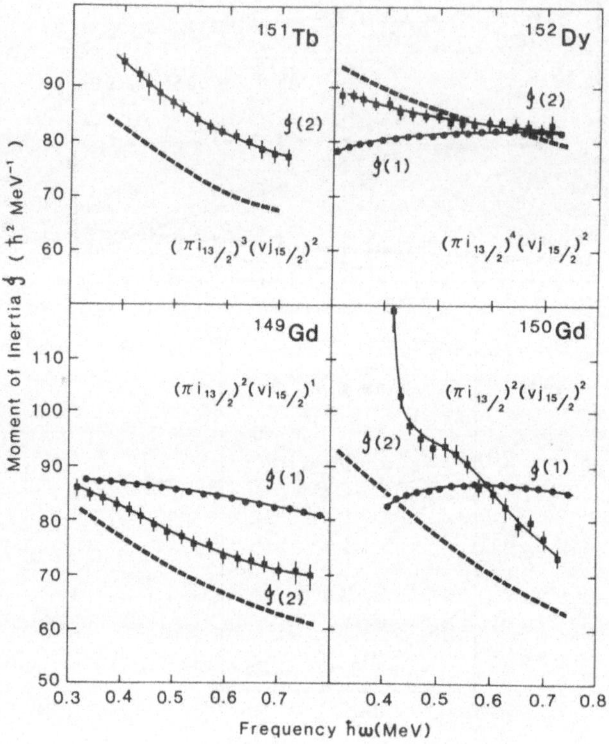

Fig. 23 Measured moments of inertia $\mathfrak{J}^{(1)}$ and $\mathfrak{J}^{(2)}$ for superdeformed bands in the nuclei ^{151}Tb, ^{152}Dy, ^{149} ^{150}Gd. The dotted lines are the calculated $\mathfrak{J}^{(2)}$ from the data given in figures 21 and 22 for the intruder orbital occupations given in the figure.

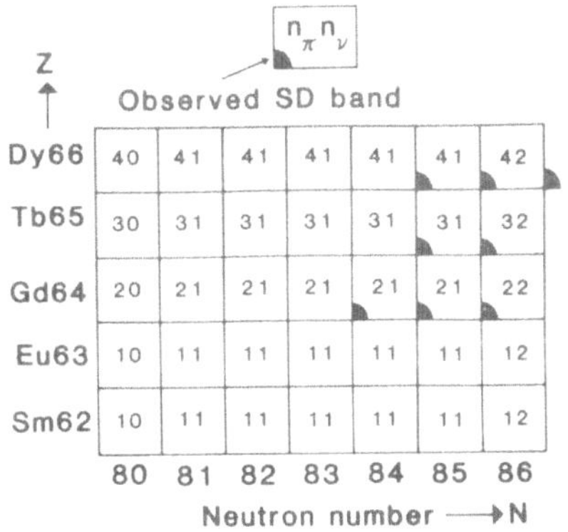

Fig. 24 Estimated [59] numbers of protons n_π in the N=6 and neutrons n_ν in the N=7 intruder orbitals for nuclei near A=150. It can be seen that holes in the lower oscillator shells must exit underneath the still occupied intruder orbits for lighter nuclei.

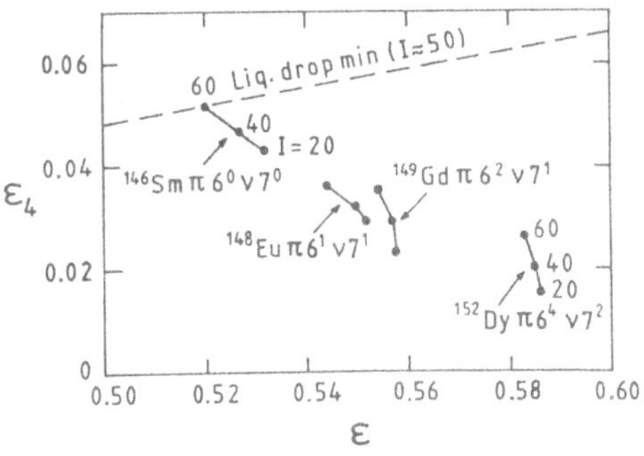

Fig. 25 Calculated [57] equilibrium shapes for superdeformed ^{146}Sm, ^{148}Eu, ^{149}Gd and ^{152}Dy as a function of spin for the intruder orbital configurations indicated. The dashed line shows for different quadrupole deformations ε the hexadecapole ε_4 deformation favoured by a rotating liquid drop at spin 50.

order to have the correct number of neutrons ^{148}Gd has to have in addition one hole in the deformation aligned neutron orbitals labelled 6_4 in figure 22(a). It can be seen that the higher pair of the $\nu 6_4$ orbitals have very little signature splitting. Hence these two unsplit orbitals should couple with the odd 7_1 rotational aligned orbital to produce a pair of superdeformed bands of either signature and no splitting. To date only one band has been observed [49] in this nucleus.

In figure 25, taken from [57], it can be seen that the calculations predict that the nuclear shape should be very stable throughout the length of any superdeformed band. For ^{152}Dy the quadrupole deformation ε hardly changes between spin 60 and spin 20 and the hexadecapole coefficient ε_4 decreases only slightly in this spin range. The predicted decrease in ε with decreasing proton and neutron numbers seen in figure 25 is consistent with the general trends anticipated by figure 17.

The data obtained in the first few 2 to 1 axis ratio superdeformed bands has given a most encouraging start to the spectroscopic study of the new superdeformed phase of nuclear matter.

6. FEEDING

The fact that discrete superdeformed states can be seen to spins of over $60\hbar$, which is very near the fission limit for these nuclei, asks the question: how do these bands get fed? The difference between the feeding intensities of discrete states in prolate normally deformed nuclei and the ^{152}Dy superdeformed band can be seen from figure 26. Whether any discrete state gets fed or not depends on the competition, for states above it, between "in-band" collective E2 decay and E1 "out-of-band" statistical decay probabilities to the fed states. The "in-band" E2 transitions loose angular momentum ($2\hbar$) but maintain the temperature of the nucleus; ie. maintain the energy above the yrast line. The E1 statistical decays cool the nucleus with little loss of angular momentum ($0\text{-}1\hbar$) and allow precipitation towards the yrast line. As the in-band E2 transition probabilities at ~2400W.u. are about ten times the normal speed of decay, the E1 precipitation from a non-yrast superdeformed state has to be even more enhanced if the lowest (yrast) superdeformed states are going to be populated. A combination of two effects has been proposed [60] to give this superdeformed E1 enhancement.

Firstly, due to the elongation of the superdeformed shape along the symmetry axis the Giant Dipole excitation in this direction is correspondingly lowered. The (GDR)s built on a superdeformed states is split into two components as illustrated in figure 27. The z-component is lowered to about 8MeV excitation while the x and y-components are pushed up in energy from the $(\text{GDR})_N$ normal excitation energy. This lowering of a third of the GDR strength increases, through its horizontal tail, the E1 dipole strength to be shared amongst the superdeformed states above the yrast line. This effect increases the E1 strength by about a factor 3 to 4.

Secondly, the lower density [33, 61] of superdeformed states amongst which to share the tail of the (GDR)s means that each state has to accept more strength. This gives another increase in the E1 strength of over a factor 3.

Using these assumptions Herskind and Schiffer [60,62] have been able to reproduce, in Monte-Carlo calculations, the population of a lowered [61] superdeformed band as seen in ^{152}Dy. A prediction of these calculations was that the statistical γ-rays feeding the superdeformed

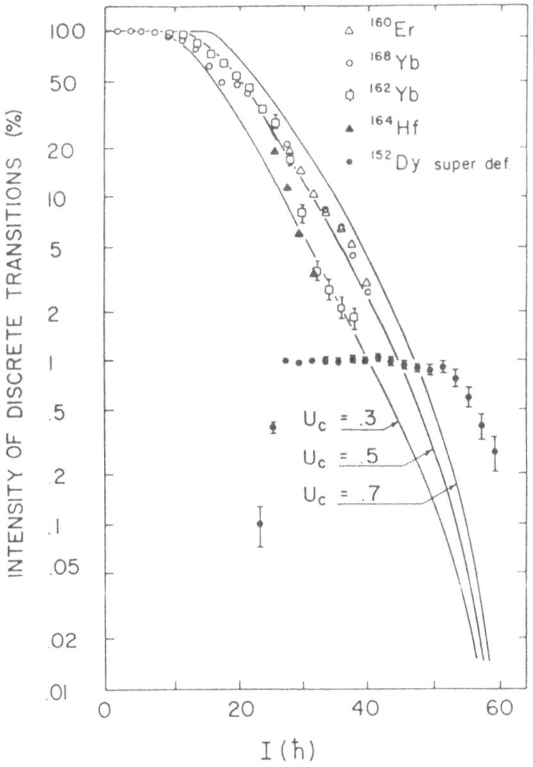

Fig. 26 Discrete line intensities as a function of spin normalised to that of the $2^+ \to 0^+$ transition for some normally deformed nuclei and compared to superdeformed intensities in ^{152}Dy. The intensities are the sum of all known discrete lines for a given spin. The lines are Monte Carlo calculations [62] for the intensities in ^{168}Yb using different values of the energy U_c (in MeV) above the yrast line in which the discrete intensity is included.

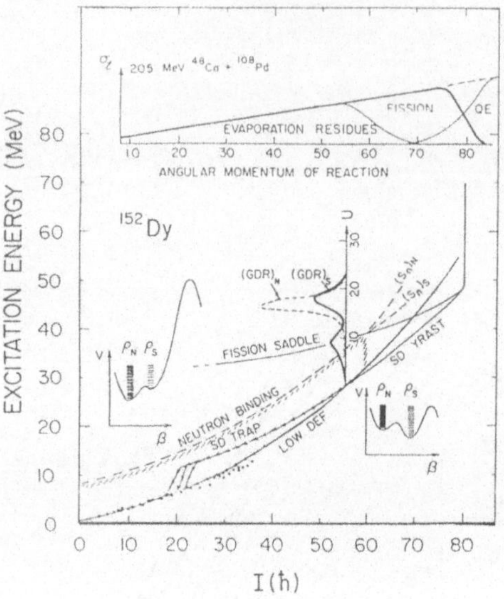

Fig. 27 Schematic yrast-diagram for ^{152}Dy. At I=54ħ the strength functions are shown for the Giant Dipole Resonances built on normal (GDR)n and super (GDR)s deformations. Level densities above and below spin 54 are also illustrated.

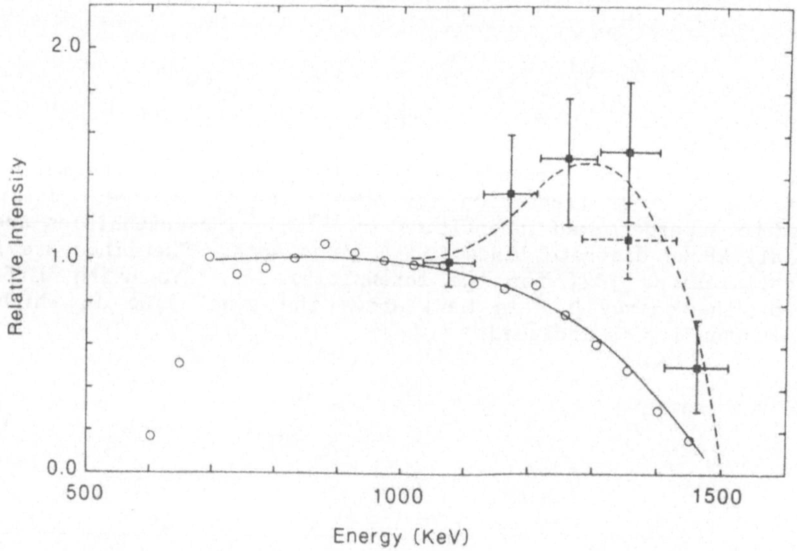

Fig. 28 Comparison of the intensities in the discrete line (open circles) in superdeformed ^{152}Dy with the total superdeformed intensity obtained from correlation ridges (closed squares with error bars).

states should be enhanced in intensity by a factor 3 for E1 transitions above 5MeV. Recent experiments [63,64] suggest that the intensity of the superdeformed states in fact decreases when gated by high energy γ-rays. These data favour an interpretation that the superdeformed discrete states are only populated when, after neutron evaporation, the residual excitation energy above the yrast line is very small.

The question then arises as to how much excited superdeformed bands are populated and how far do they extend before either decaying to the lowest superdeformed band or to normal deformed states. An attempt to answer this question has been made by measuring [64,65] the intensity of the first ridge in a $E_{\gamma 1}$-$E_{\gamma 2}$ correlation plot of ^{152}Dy data and comparing this with the intensity of the discrete superdeformed lines. These data are shown in figure 28 and imply that there is intensity in excited superdeformed states at rotational frequencies $\hbar\omega$>0.5MeV. The data also imply that any superdeformed band running parallel to the lowest band will be unlikely to have as much as 20% of the observed band's intensity.

The Monte-Carlo calculations [60,62] have several implications. The first is that at higher temperatures the nucleus can switch shapes between normal and superdeformation. This is illustrated for some decay paths in figure 29. A first consequence of this is that selecting discrete γ-rays at a low or even medium spin does NOT fix the shape at the initial entry point. Thus it is not possible to tag the decay of a split superdeformed (GDR)s by observing γ-rays in the discrete superdeformed bands. The initial state could have been either superdeformed <u>or</u> have normal deformation. However, there are possibilities to observe the effects of the switching of shapes. The lower transition rates associated with normally deformed states would delay at least a component of the feeding of the superdeformed band. This would be seen as a delayed fraction of the discrete γ-ray line shapes in lifetime measurements, an effect which is illustrated in figure 30. The line shapes shown are for the γ-rays from the 48^+ and 46^+ levels in ^{152}Dy assuming a 100Wu (slow) or 400Wu (fast) E2 decays of the normally deformed feeding states at high temperature. The measurements of Bentley et. al. [36] of the line shapes in ^{152}Dy do not give any hit of delayed components. Their data is compared with the Monte-Carlo calculations in figure 31, which shows that the normal B(E2) strength has to be of the order of 400Wu or more. Measurements of lifetimes of the main E2 component of the continuum radiation (E2 "bump") give [66,67] lifetimes for these decays that imply transition strengths in the region of 400Wu.

Calculations [55] of energy surfaces in the (β,γ) plane for nuclei near ^{152}Dy show that these shape parameters are not clearly defined at high temperatures. This has of course implications for the mean field description of these nuclei and the problem of usefully defining macroscopic quantities. However in the mass 130 region the calculations [55] show that for quite high temperature there is a single reasonably well defined minimum in the energy surface corresponding to the superdeformed shape. It is probably due to this effect that some superdeformed bands in this region have very strong, 20% in the case of ^{133}Nd [43], populations compared to the total population for that nucleus. It is therefore probable that some properties, such as $(GDR)_S$, of superdeformed shapes may best be investigated in the mass 130 region.

7. EXIT FROM SUPERDEFORMATION

A quite remarkable property of the superdeformed bands is their sudden demise at their lowest spins. This rapid exit is clearly seen for

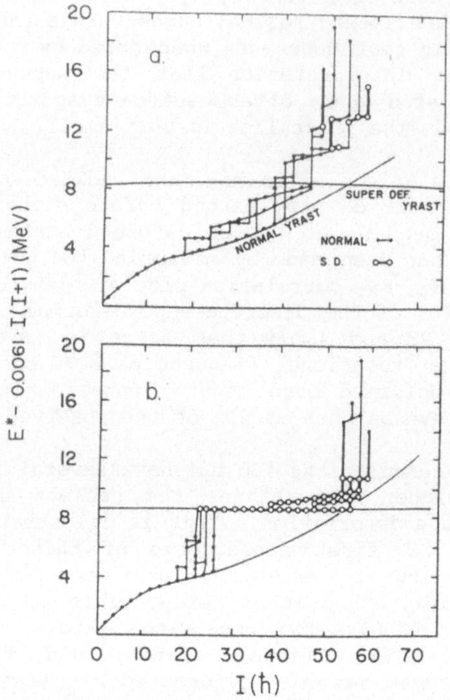

Fig. 29 Decay paths for some simulated [62] cascades in ^{152}Dy. (a) five simulated cascades selected so that at least one cascade is via a superdeformed state (b) five cascades which proceed via at least one superdeformed yrast state.

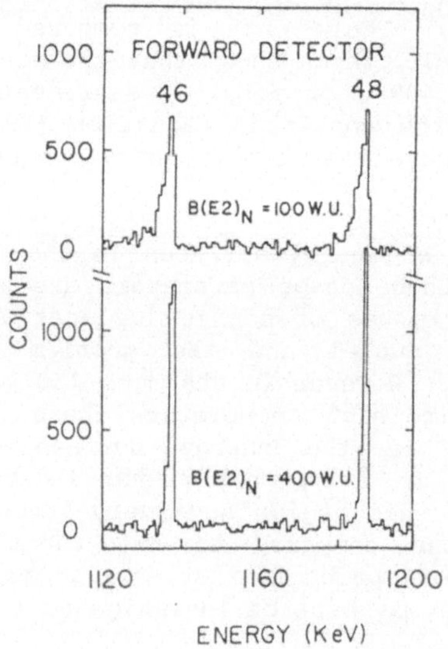

Fig. 30 Calculated [62] shapes for the 46^+ and 48^+ lines in superdeformed ^{152}Dy assuming $B(E2)_N$ values of 100 and 400W.u. for continuum states with normal deformation. The spectra have 0.8keV per channel and are for θ=35°

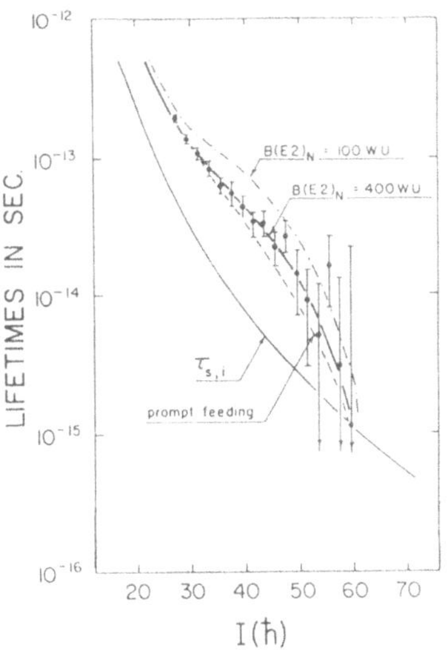

Fig. 31 Calculated effective lifetimes [62] using the assumptions of figure 30 and compared with the data of ref. [36]. The $\tau_{s,i}$ shows the intrinsic lifetimes of each individual superdeformed state.

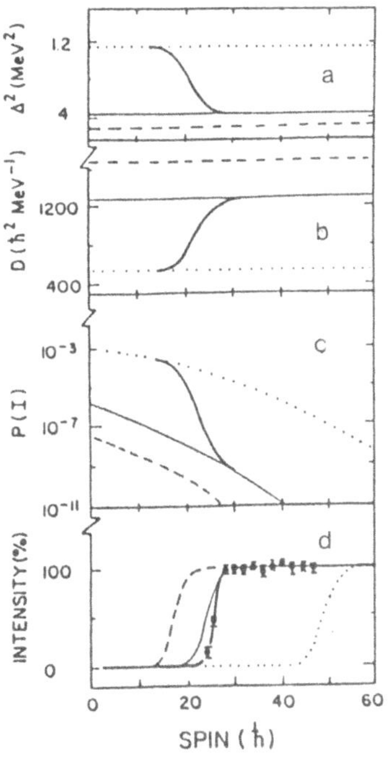

Fig. 32 Calculation [60] of how changes in the pairing energy Δ (a) affect the inertial mass D (b) the barrier penetrability P(I) (c) and the decay out of the ^{152}Dy superdeformed band (d).

152Dy in figure 9(a) where out-of-band decays occur for the two superdeformed levels with reduced intensity at the lowest γ-ray energies. Figure 16 shows that although the decays out of the first two 2 to 1 axis ratio superdeformed nuclei ^{152}Dy and ^{149}Gd occur at about the same frequency $\hbar\omega \sim 0.3$MeV, the decay out for ^{151}Tb and ^{150}Gd take place at a higher frequency $\hbar\omega \sim 0.4$MeV. All these decays take place very rapidly over one or two states. Straightforward barrier penetration calculations [61] do not manage to reproduce this sudden exit and require a steady decay of the band over 7 or 8 levels. That the decay out of the bands is due to the opening up of a new and even faster decay channel and not to the reduction of the in-band transition strengths can be seen for ^{132}Ce and ^{152}Dy in figures 7 and 10 respectively. These data show that at the bottom of the band there is no significant deviation from E2 decay dominated by the massive superdeformed quadrupole moment. Indeed, the lifetime data for ^{149}Gd show [68] that the lowest transition, which is reduced in intensity due to the exit channel, is actually faster than would be expected for constant Q_o and no other decay branch other than in-band E2.

The physical change that happens at the exit of the superdeformed bands has been conjectured [60] to be a sudden increase in the static pairing as the rotational frequency decreases. Now it is well known (see for instance the many references on the subject in [17]) that the major effect in decreasing pairing is the alignment of quasi-particles. In the superdeformed exit case a sudden increase in pairing would have to be caused by the dealignment and pairing off of two particles as the frequency decreases. As the lowest γ-ray energies in the superdeformed bands of nuclei such as ^{149}Gd, ^{151}Tb and ^{152}Dy (see figure 16) do not deviate systematically from the trend of the rest of the band, any band crossing must have a very weak interaction in these nuclei. In ^{150}Gd the last two transitions at the bottom of the band are squeezed together presumably by alignment effects as discussed in section 3 above, so that $\mathfrak{J}^{(2)}$ increases rapidly. This suggests that the interaction at the band crossing in superdeformed ^{150}Gd is longer than in the neighbouring superdeformed nuclei. The higher exit frequency for ^{151}Tb and ^{150}Gd also suggests that considerable pairing correlations survive to higher rotational frequencies than in ^{149}Gd and ^{152}Dy. In the mass 130 region the sudden increase in $\mathfrak{J}^{(2)}$ for the bottom one or two transitions for several nuclei (see figure 14) are probably due to effects similar to that in ^{150}Gd.

The reason that a change in pairing energies has such a dramatic effect on the barrier penetrability is that the penetrability depends on the Hamiltonian connecting the configurations in the superdeformed and normal wells in the potential. A large pairing interaction has the effect of mixing states within an energy range equal to the pairing energy Δ. This mixing increases the transition matrix elements connecting the two shapes and consequently to rapid decay out of the superdeformed band if a sudden increase in Δ occurs. This effect is illustrated in figure 32. It can be seen that in this model the frequency at which the exit out of the superdeformed band takes place will depend on the residual pairing energy for levels within the observed band. It has been pointed out [69,70] that the effect of dynamic pairing correlations within the observed bands is to bring the calculated angular momentum in the bands closer to the experimentally estimated values.

8. OPEN PROBLEMS

With the present generation of spectrometers [17] it is likely that the main thrust of research will be to delineate the limits of currently observable superdeformation in the A=130 and A=150 regions and to explore other newly found regions [52,53,54] of extreme deformation. Already detailed studies of the feeding and excitation of superdeformed states are being carried out [63,64]. In the mass 150 region an immediate task is to test the prediction [56,57] that superdeformed bands with neutron number N<85 and N>86 consist of pairs of bands of both signatures. It could be that there is more to be learnt from careful measurements of the lifetimes of superdeformed levels as discussed in section 6 above.

Major advances in our understanding of superdeformation probably require a new generation of spectrometers giving improvements in sensitivity of at least a factor ten. In the U.S.A. a proposal [71] has already been prepared for such a spectrometer. The proposal is to build a "GAMMASPHERE" consisting of 110 Ge detectors in a BGO honeycomb structure, operating in suppression mode. This Gammasphere has a 4π geometry, a price tag of M$\$_{US}$15 and would be scheduled to begin measurements in 1992. In Europe studies [72] are currently underway for a Ge shell subtending 4π structure at the target and consisting of about 500 detectors. A Ge shell of this kind requires developments to be made in the technology of large Ge detectors and hence a price tag is not available. The main advantage of such new generations of spectrometers is that multiple coincidences γ-γ-γ-....-γ (written γ^n where n>4) are detected with good efficiency. Such multiple coincidences can be used to define decay paths between the initial γ-ray decaying states, at high spin and excitation energy, all the way down to the ground state. The ability to do this while preserving good signal to noise is essential in picking out superdeformed structures and, at the same time, obtaining information on the feeding and exit transitions.

The problems of the superdeformed phase that clearly require study and will probably require the power of new generation spectrometers are:

(i) Unambiguous detection of the γ-rays feeding and exiting from the superdeformed bands. The importance of determining exact spins and excitation energies is augmented by the light this would throw on dynamical pairing [69,70] in the superdeformed phase.

(ii) Before pioneering work at Brookhaven [73] and Copenhagen [74] the study of high spin states was almost completely confined to the yrast line. So it is of similar interest to study the properties of p-h excitations in the superdeformed minimum. If figure 27 is a guide then excited superdeformed bands are likely to be at least a factor 5 to 10 less intense than the "yrast superdeformation" observed so far.

(iii) It is important in the study of the stability of different configurations at the fission limit to discover how high in spin the superdeformation can go before fission sets in. Because of the enormous E2 probabilities it would be ideal to Coulomb excite the nucleus up the superdeformed bands. At the time of writing this presents us with a few target problems!

(iv) There have been suggestions [75] that because the Coulomb barrier is lowered by the shape at the tips of a superdeformed nucleus that protons or alpha particles might escape preferentially from these locations in the nucleus. Any experiments involving particle-γ coincidences will be improved in sensitivity using very large arrays.

(v) There has been a recent calculation [76] showing that, at the highest spins, a minimum in the potential energy surfaces exists near the 3 to 1 major to minor axis ratio. The prediction is that this shape would lie lowest and be most observable for nuclei near ^{166}Er, ^{168}Yb and ^{170}Hf; nuclei with 98 neutrons. The calculated surfaces for ^{168}Yb for spins 20(10)70$\hbar$ are shown in figure 33. In-band E2 transition rates would be of the order of 10^4Wu and all

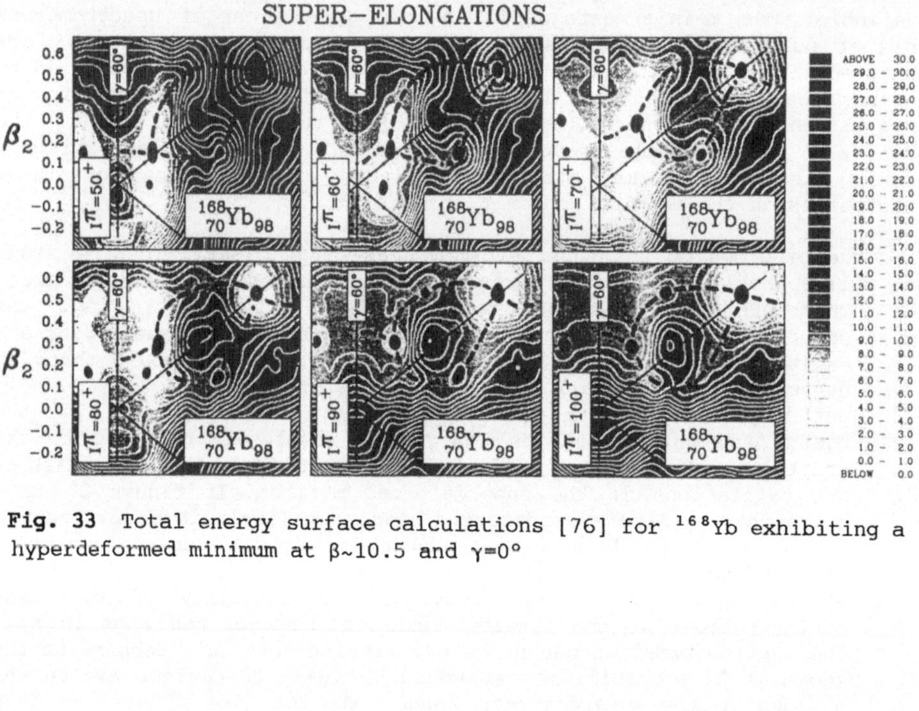

Fig. 33 Total energy surface calculations [76] for ^{168}Yb exhibiting a hyperdeformed minimum at $\beta \sim 10.5$ and $\gamma = 0°$

the nice physics that has been found for superdeformed 2 to 1 nuclei would be expected but more so! Hopefully it will turn out that hyperdeformed nuclei can exist and are not just the wrong side of the line of fission?

ACKNOWLEDGEMENTS

These lectures review the work of many people. I would like to thank numerous colleagues both in Europe and North America for many discussions over the exciting period of the last few years. My special thanks go to those experimentalists and theoretists who have worked directly with me at Liverpool, Daresbury, the Niels Bohr Institute and Lund; Sven Åberg, Andy Alderson, Tord Bengtsson, Mike Bentley, Alison Bruce, Howard Cranmer-Gordon, John Cresswell, Jerzy Dudek, Paul Fallon, Peter Forsyth, Bent Herskind, Debbie Howe, Andy Kirwan, Rahman Mokhtar, Dave Morrison, Andy Nelson, Paul Nolan, Barna Nyakó, Ingmar Ragnarsson, Mark Riley, John Roberts, Klaus Schiffer, John Simpson, Geirr Sletten, Peter Twin and Naomi Ward - to name but a few. Finally my deep gratitude to Judi Young for typing this at the eleventh hour and for the organisers of the Summer School for waiting so long for the manuscript.

This research has been supported by grants from the U.K. Science and Engineering Research Council, from the U.K. University Grants Committee and from the EEC, Directorate-General for Science, Research and Development "Stimulation Action" program.

REFERENCES

[1] V M Strutinski; Nucl. Phys. A95 420 (1967) and A122 1 (1968)
[2] S M Polikanov et al; Zh. Eksp. Teor. Fiz. 42 1464 (1962) and translated in Sov. Phys. JETP 15 1016
[3] H J Specht et al; Phys. Lett. 41B 43 (1972)
[4] H Backe et al; Phys. Rev. Lett. 41 490 (1979)
[5] G Ulfert et al; Nucl. Instr. Meth 148 369 (1978)
[6] V Metag et al; Hyperfine Interactions 1 405 (1976)
[7] D Habs et al; Phys. Rev. Lett. 38 387 (1977)
[8] R Bengtsson et al; Phys. Lett 57B 301 (1975)
[9] K Neergard and V V Pashkevich; Phys. Lett. 59B 218 (1975)
[10] Å Bohr and B Mottleson; Nucl. Structure Vol. 2 Benjamin, p592 (1975)
[11] I Ragnarsson et al; Nucl. Phys. A347 287 (1980)
[12] J Dudek et al; Phys. Rev. Lett. 59 405 (1987)
[13] S Åberg; Workshop in Nucl. Str. at High Spin, Risø, Denmark, p 5, May 1983
[14] J Burde et al; Phys. Rev. Lett. 48 (1982) 530
[15] T C Khoo et al; Phys. Rev. Lett. 41 1027 (1978)
[16] P J Nolan; Proc. Int. Nucl. Phys. Conf. Harrogate, U.K. eds J L Durell et al, IOP Conf. Series 86 Vol. 2 155 (1986)
[17] J F Sharpey-Schafer and J Simpson; Prog. in Part. and Nucl. Phys. 21 293 (1988)
[18] Y. Schutz et al; Phys. Rev. Lett. 48 1534 (1982)
[19] P J Twin et al; Nucl. Phys. A409 343c (1983)
[20] B M Nyakó et al; Phys. Rev. Lett. 52 507 (1984)
[21] O Andersen et al; Phys. Rev. Lett. 43 687 (1979)
[22] B Herskind; J. de. Phys. 41 C10-106 (1980)
[23] P J Nolan et al; Phys. Lett. 128B 285 (1983)
[24] J F Sharpey-Schafer et al; Proc. XXIV Winter Meeting on Nucl. Phys. Bormio, Italy, January 1986 Univ. degli studi di Milano, Supp. 49, p669
[25] M J A de Voigt et al; Phys. Rev. Lett. 59 270 (1987)

[26] J Dudek and W Nazarewicz; Phys. Rev. C31 298 (1985)
[27] P J Nolan et al; J. Phys. G11 L17 (1985)
[28] A J Kirwan et al; Daresbury Annual Report 1986/87, Nucl. Str. Appendix, p28
[29] M A Riley et al; Nucl. Phys. A486 456 (1988)
[30] A J Kirwan et al; Phys. Rev. Lett. 58 467 (1987)
[31] P J Twin et al; Phys. Rev. Lett. 57 811 (1986)
[32] P J Nolan et al; NIM A236 95 (1985)
[33] S Åberg; Proc. XXV Int. Winter Meeting on Nucl. Phys. Bormio, Italy January 1987; Univ. degli studi di Milano, Supp. 56 p661
[34] P O Tjøm et al; Phys. Rev.Lett. 55 2405 (1985)
[35] J F Sharpey-Schafer; Proc. Int. Conf. on Weak and Electromag. Interactions in Nuclei (Springer) ed. H V Klapdor, 88 (1986)
[36] M A Bentley et al; Phys. Rev. Lett. 59 2141 (1987)
[37] J C Bacelar et al; Phys. Rev. Lett. 57 3019 (1986)
[38] N. Rowley; private communication (1988)
[39] B M Nyakó et al; Phys. Rev. Lett. 56 2680 (1986)
[40] M A Bentley et al; submitted to J. Phys. G (1988)
[41] E M Beck et al; Phys. Rev. Lett. 58 2182 (1987)
[42] E M Beck et al; Phys. Lett. B195 531 (1987)
[43] R Wadsworth et al; J. Phys. G13 L207 (1987)
[44] Y-X Luo et al; Z. Phys. A329 125 (1988)
[45] R. Chasman; Phys. Lett. B187 219 (1987)
[46] A Ruckelshäusen et al; Phys. Rev. Lett. 56 2357 (1986)
[47] T L Khoo; Proc. Int. Conf. on Weak and Electromag. Interactions in Nuclei (Springer) ed. H V Klapdov 98 (1986)
[48] B Haas et al; Phys. Rev. Lett. 60 503 (1988)
[49] M A Deleplanque et al; Phys. Rev. Lett. 60 1626 (1988)
[50] G-E Rathke et al; to be published
[51] P Fallon et al; Phys. Lett. B. (in press)
[52] T Rzaca-Urban et al; Z. Phys. A328 379 (1987)
[53] J Burde et al; Proc. Conf. on High Spin Nucl. Str. and Novel Nuclear Shapes, Argonne, U.S.A.;p 36 April 1988
[54] A O Macchiavelli et al; Phys. Rev. C38 1088 (1988)
[55] J Dudek; JIHIR, Oak Ridge, Document 88-01
[56] T Bengtsson et al; Phys. Lett. B208 39 (1988)
[57] S. Åberg et al; XXVII Int. Winter Meeting on Nucl. Phys., Bormio. Italy; Univ. degli studi di Milano, Supp. 63 p 546 January 1988
[58] S Åberg et al; Proc. 3rd Int. Conf on Nucl-Nucl Collisions, St. Malo, France; Nucl. Phys. A488 147C (June 1988)
[59] S Åberg; private communication
[60] B Herskind et al; Phys. Rev. Lett. 59 2416 (1987)
[61] I Ragnarsson and S Åberg; Phys. Lett. B180 191 (1986)
[62] B Herskind and K Schiffer; Proc. Int. School "Enrico Fermi", Societa Italiana Di Fisica (Varenna, 1987)
[63] P Taras et al; Phys. Rev. Lett. 61 1348 (1988)
[64] P J Twin; Proc. Conf. on Contempt. Topics in Nucl. Str. Phys.; Cocoyoc, Mexico (June 1988)
[65] M A Bentley et al; to be published in J. Phys. G
[66] R Holtzmann et al; Phys. Lett. B195 321 (1987)
[67] A Nourreddine et al; Phys. Rev. C36 2687 (1987)
[68] J Gascon; private communication
[69] Y R Shimizu et al; Phys. Lett. B198 33 (1987)
[70] W Nazarewicz et al; Phys. Lett. B196 404 (1987)
[71] M A Deleplanque and R M Diamond Eds, Gammasphere, a proposal; Berkeley, U.S.A., March 1988
[72] R M Lieder Ed;, Euroball design study, KFA Jülich, BRD, May 1988
[73] O C Kistner et al; Phys. Rev. C17 17 (1978)
[74] L L Riedinger et al; Phys. Rev. Lett. 44 (1980) 568
[75] M Blann and T T Komoto; Physica Scripta 24 93 (1981)
[76] J Dudek et al; Phys. Lett. B211 (1988) 252

THE NUCLEAR EQUATION OF STATE

László P. Csernai

Physics Department, University of Bergen

Allégaten 55, N-5007 Bergen, Norway

1. Introduction

In these two lectures we will study two regions of the nuclear equation of state (EOS): the energy and density region which is reachable in intermediate energy heavy ion collisions up to a few GeV/nucl. energy, and some aspects of the Quark - Gluon Plasma (QGP) phase transition. In the intermediate energy region we will pay particular attention to the compressibility of nuclear matter and to the liquid - gas phase transition. Some basic facts about the nuclear multifragmentation will also be mentioned. Since the formation and signatures of QGP are discussed in the lectures of Bernd Müller at this summer school [Mü88], we will discuss the features of the phase transition to QGP only from the EOS view point, and the sensitivity of the phase transition to the nuclear compressibility. We will concentrate on the connections between experimental data and the EOS rather than on theoretical derivation of a particular EOS in the framework of a particular theoretical model.

The EOS provides only limited information about the nuclear matter: the static thermal equilibrium properties. Before we proceed it has to be mentioned that in heavy ion collisions non- equilibrium processes are very important, thus nuclear transport properties will play an equally important role. It is also possible to extract transport coefficients from the data. An example of this is given in [BC87, BC88] where scaling properties of the data were studied and this led to conclusions about the Reynolds number (i.e. viscosity).

2. Intermediate Energy EOS

2.1 Bulk Nuclear Matter

2.1.1 The Nuclear Compressibility

From conventional nuclear physics we know that there is a stable equilibrium state at the normal nuclear density $n_0 = 0.145 - 0.17 fm^{-3}$ [My76, Be71] with a compressibility which was earlier assumed to be in the range of $K = 180 - 240\ MeV$ [BG76] and a binding energy of 16 $MeV/nucleon$. If we want to learn about the EOS at high densities and high temperatures we have to rely mostly on theoretical estimates. The high density high temperature part of the equation of state is decisive in the first, compression stage of the collision. The low density behavior of nuclear matter determines the observables and the reaction mechanism of the final expansion stage in a collision before the breakup. In this first part of the lecture we will concentrate on the low density part of the nuclear equation of state, which is directly related to the final fragmentation, nuclear compressibility, momentum dependence, etc.

After an energetic nucleus-nucleus collision, many light nuclear fragments, a few heavy fragments and a few mesons (mainly pions) are observed in the 100 MeV – 4 $GeV/nucleon$ beam energy region. Thus the initial kinetic energy of the projectile leads to the destruction of the ground state nuclear matter and converts it into a dilute gas ($n << n_0$) of fragments, which then loses thermal contact during the breakup or freeze-out stage. These frozen-out fragments and their momentum distributions can be measured by the detectors. Some excited fragments can of course decay while reaching the detectors.

One of the most standard methods to calculate the nuclear EOS is in the mean field theory. At this school the nuclear mean field theory will be introduced in Prof. Tjon's lectures [Tj88]. We start out with a Lagrangian including the nucleon field, ψ, a scalar meson field, ϕ and a vector meson field, V_μ. Customarily the contribution of the scalar field is described by a quartic polynomial. The coefficients and the coupling constants determine the behaviour of the calculated EOS. Not all the parameters free are obviously, since basic nuclear parameters like the binding energy and the saturation density should be reproduced by the model. Also the compressibility, K, and the effective nucleon mass, m^*, are sometimes considered as known parameters.

Waldhauser, *et al.*, based on a mean field theoretical calculation, however, pointed out recently that the characterization of the EOS with the ground state compressibility is sometimes very misleading [WM88]. For example at $T = 100\ MeV$, and if the effective mass is $m^* = 0.55m$ the EOS at $n = 2 - 3n_0$ is practically the same for different compressibilities like $K = 210,\ 300,\ 400\ MeV$. On the other hand the EOS is very sensitive to the effective mass at high densities. This finding explains the earlier experience that if some phenomenon, which is sensitive to the EOS at high densities, is satisfactorily described in a theoretical model with one given $K(n_0, T = 0)$, it is still possible that other models have to use a different constant value for the ground state K. So to debate about the nuclear compressibility is meaningful only if apart of the value of K also the particular modell or parametrization is also discussed.

The nuclear compressibility is in the focus of an international debate recently. With the advancement of the relativistic heavy ion physics we reached the stage where *quantitative* conclusions about the high temperature high density EOS became possible. The compressibility

$$K_\sigma = 9\frac{\partial p(\sigma, n)}{\partial n},$$

influences a great number of experimental observables. These were summarized recently by Glendenning [Gl88]. Following his work we can briefly summarize the different phenomena leading to some conclusions about the EOS.

Landau Sum Rule. In the Landau theory of Fermi liquids the compressibility is given by $K = 3\hbar^2 k_F^2(1 + F_0)/m^*$, where F_0 is one of the Landau parameters caracterizing the liquid. Brown and Osnes [BO85] determined F_0, and thus K, from the Landau sum rule which connects the Landau parameters. Collecting the information available for them the authors concluded that the compressibility is $K = 106\ MeV$. Glendenning, on the other hand analysing the accuracy of this estimate found that since the Landau parameters are not known really well the compressibility can be in the range of $K = 74 - 371\ MeV$.

Pion Multiplicities in Relativistic Heavy Ion Collisions. One of the first attempts to determine the EOS from high energy experiment was done by Stock it et al. [SB82]. The idea was that there are less pions observed than one would expect based on a cascade calculation or on a (noninteracting) ideal gas model. So, some kinetic energy should be missing during the collision, and this causes the smaller pion production rate. This missing energy should then be the compressional energy. In several subsequent works this effect was studied in more sophisticated models. First the compression was calculated by using the EOS from the Rankine-Hugoniot relations for shock compression. Then it turned out that the final expansion should also be taken into account because pion reabsorption is also important. These calculations are quite involved finally but the in most of them a large compressibility, $K > 200\ MeV$ was needed to reproduce the pion multiplicity data. A basic problem was pointed out recently by Maruhn and Stöcker [MS87]. The pion multiplicities were measured at high energies only, and there is a sizeable energy gap between the ground state and the lowest energy data. This leads to an essential uncertainty if we want to calculate the EOS directly from the data using the Rankine-Hugoniot relations. Most authors do not realize this because they assume some given parametrization of the EOS which connects the two regions in an arbitrary way. To avoid this problem the measurement of K around the ground state would be needed, or in other words the first and second derivative of K (versus n and T) at the ground state.

Sidewards Flow in High Energy Nuclear Collisions. The existence of shock waves and the collective "bounce off" of nuclei of each other was predicted [SM74,CJ73] long before the first really convincing experinents [GG84]. By now the flow analysis is one of the well established methods to extract information about the EOS, and even about the transport properties of the hot nuclear matter. Earlier it was described satisfactorily in the fluid dynamical model but the more recent transport theoretical models (VUU-BUU-LV) [GB87,AR87] have the advantage of being able to incorporate finite particle number and non-equilibrium effects. The nuclear mean field potential is an organic constituent of these models, so the nuclear compressibility can be explicitely read off from the calculations. The most recent model calculations include also momentum dependent interactions which are especially important in the initial not completely equilibrated stage of the collision. These calculations indicate that the compressibility should be in the range of $k = 200 - 400\ MeV$ to fit the flow data. The momentum dependence of the potential allows for the lower compressibility values in this range while non momentum dependent interactions lead to stiffer EOS.

Supernova Explosions. A very interesting contribution to the nuclear EOS has been provided by theoretical calculations of Supernova explosions. At late stages of star evolution a star of about $10 M_\odot$ may explode if its iron core is in the range of $1.3 - 1.35 M_\odot$. Baron *et al.* foud that if the EOS is sufficiently soft at high densities a successful prompt supernova explosion may occur due to the shock wave which develops after the gravitational collapse of the core [BC85]. The compression modulus depends on the proton fraction Z/A, which is smaller in the supernovae than in nuclei. The EOS which led to the explosion had $K(Z/A = 1/3) = 138\ MeV$ and this corresponds to a $K(1/2) = 180\ MeV$.

Neutron Stars. Glendenning [Gl88] used the same EOS [BC85] to calculate the maximum mass of a neutron star by solving the Tollman - Oppenheimer - Volkov equation. The stiffer the EOS the heavier neutron star can be supported by it. He found that with $Z/A = 1/3$ the maximum neutron star mass would be $1.25 M_{\odot}$. However, the neutron stars are more neutron rich, so $Z/A = 1/5$ might be more appropriate value. In this case the maximum neutron star mass would be only $1 M_{\odot}$. Since there is a neuron star with $M = 1.451 \pm 0.007 M_{\odot}$ (PSR1913+16), and another where the mass is less accurately measured with $M = 1.85^{+0.35}_{-0.30} M_{\odot}$. These indicate that the EOS may be more stiff than the supernova calculations predicted. According to Glendenning's calculations at least $K = 200\ MeV$ is necessary to account for the observed neutron star masses.

Giant Monopole Resonance. New results for K have been reported by the Groningen group who made precision measurements of the breathing mode of 5 Sn and 4 Sm isotopes [SB88, WB87]. These data were analysed in conjunction with the already existing data on ^{208}Pb and ^{24}Mg nuclei. They determined the compressibility of infinite nuclear matter, the surface, the isospin and the Coulomb contribution to the data:

$$K_A = K_{\infty} + K_s A^{-1/3} + K_{\tau}(\frac{N-Z}{A})^2 + K_C Z^2 A^{-4/3}.$$

The resulting value for K_{∞} was $299 \pm 25\ MeV$, much more than the value extracted from the earlier data.

The above mentioned cases are not complete, ther are still other ways to gain information about the EOS and the compressibility. The most accurate measurements of course are still apply to the ground state nuclear matter (Giant Monopoles) or to the cold matter (Neutron Stars). The other data deal with more dynamic situations and with hot and compressed matter so it is not surprising that there is still room for improving the present estimates.

2.1.2 A Simplified Equation of State

Considering the most essential properties of the nuclear equation of state for densities below n_0 the theoretically a liquid gas phase transition is clearly predicted with $T = 15 - 20\ MeV$ and $n_c = 0.3 - 0.5 n_0$. More accurate information and further details can be obtained only from thorough experimental research and by comparing experimental and theoretical results. Before we discuss the properties of the nuclear equation of state let us introduce the general notation of thermodynamic variables (Table 1). If we have defined one of the "state functions" or "thermodynamical potentials" in terms of its proper variables like $e(s,n)$, $F(T,V,N)$ or $\mu(T,p)$ all others thermodynamical variables can be obtained by differentiating the thermodynamical potential. For example: The equation of state $p = p(T,n)$ can be obtained from the Helmholtz free energy density as $p(T,n) = n\ f_{,n} - f$. (The comma denotes the partial derivative: $a_{,x} = \partial a/\partial x$.)

As an example which is used widely in the literature [SB83, SN80, CB80,CS83, Da79, GK84, Ka84, Ni79, MS83], let us define an analytic parametrization for the

Table 1

THERMODYNAMICAL VARIABLES

S = *entropy*	N = *particle number* $\sigma = S/N$	V = *volume* $s = S/V$
Extensives	Specific Extensives $(1/N)$	Extensive densities $(1/V)$
$E(S,V,N) = TS - pV + \mu N$ $dE = TdS - pdV + \mu dN$	$\epsilon(\sigma,\nu) = T\sigma - p\nu + \mu$ $d\epsilon = Td\sigma - pd\mu$	$e(s,n) = Ts + \mu n - p$ $de = Tds + \mu dn$ eg.: $p = -e + se_{,s} + ne_{,n}$
One intensive:		
Enthalpy: $H(S,p,N) = E + pV = TS + \mu N$ $dH = TdS + Vdp + \mu dN$	$\chi(\sigma,p) = \epsilon + p\nu \quad = T\sigma + \mu$ $d\chi = Td\sigma + \nu dp$	$w(s,n) = e + p = Ts + \mu n$ $dw = Tds + \mu dn$ (redundant)
Helmholtz free energy: $F(T,V,N) = E - TS = \mu N - pV$ $dF = -SdT - pdV + \mu dN$	$\Phi(T,\nu) = \epsilon - T\sigma = \mu - p\nu$ $d\Phi = -\sigma dT - pd\nu$	$f(T,n) = e - Ts = \mu n - p$ $df = -sdT + \mu dn$
$X(S,V,\mu) = E - \mu N = TS - pV$ $dX = TdS - pdV$	–	$x(s,\mu) = e - \mu n = Ts - p$ $dx = Tds - nd\mu$
Two intensives:		
Gibbs free energy: $G(T,p,N) = E + pV - TS = \mu N$ $dG = -SdT + Vdp + \mu dN$	$\mu(T,p) = -T\sigma + p\nu$ $d\mu = -\sigma dT + \nu dp$	–
$\Omega(T,V,\mu) = -pV = E - TS - \mu N$ $d\Omega = -SdT - pdV - Nd\mu$	–	$z(\mu,T) = -p = e - Ts - \mu n$ $dz = -sdT - nd\mu$
$Y(S,p,\mu) = TS = E + pV - \mu N$ $dY = TdS + Vdp - Nd\mu$		
Gibbs-Duhem relation:		
$E + PV - TS - \mu N = O$ $-SdT + Vdp - Nd\mu = O$	$d\mu = -\sigma dT + \nu dp$	$dp = sdT + nd\mu$

nuclear equation of state. The thermodynamical potential $e = e(n,s)$ as a function of baryon density n, and entropy density s is given by:

$$e(n,s) = e_c(n) + e_F^*(n,s) - e_F^*(n,0),$$

where $e_c(n)$ is the ground state energy density, and $e_F^*(n,s)$ is the energy density of an ideal Fermi-gas. We can parametrize the ground state energy density as [Ka84]

$$e_c(n) = n_0 \sum_{i=2}^{5} a_i \left(\frac{n}{n_0}\right)^{\frac{i}{3}+1},$$

where $a_i = +21.1, -38.3, -26.7, +35.9\ MeV$ for $i = 2, ..., 5$ respectively. This parametrization yields a binding energy $\epsilon_0(n_0) = e_0(n_0)/n_0 = -8\ MeV$ (instead of -16 to simulate finite size effects) and a nuclear compressibility $K = 210\ MeV$ at $n_0 =$

$0.15 fm^{-3}$. Note that this parametrization is used for small nuclear densities $n < 2n_0$. At high densities the sound speed exceeds the speed of light. For the thermal part of the energy density we use the non-relativistic ideal Fermi-gas approximation because for the low density and temperature at the breakup relativistic corrections are negligible. Then the energy density e depends on the density n and specific entropy $\sigma = s/n$ as [LL54]:

$$e_F^*(n,s) = (\frac{n^{5/3}}{m})y(\sigma),$$

where y is a dimensionless quantity and it depends on the dimensionless specific entropy σ (or μ/T). $y(\sigma)$ can be given in integral form [LL54], but in actual calculations usually practical analytic parametrizations are used [Ka84, CK86].

Other thermodynamical quantities can then be calculated from standard thermodynamic relations:

$$T(n,s) = e_{,s} = \frac{n^{2/3}}{m} y'(\sigma),$$

$$\mu(n,s) = e_{,n} = \frac{1}{3}\sum_{i=2}^{5}(i+3)a_i(\frac{n}{n_0}) + \frac{5}{3n}e_F^*(n,s) - T(n,s)\sigma,$$

$$p(n,s) = p_c(n) + \frac{2}{3}e_F^*(n,s),$$

where $p_c(n) = \frac{n_0}{3}\sum_{i=2}^{5} i a_i(\frac{n}{n_0})^{i/3+1}$. The equation of state represents a stable equilibrium configuration only if the energy has a minimum. This condition is satisfied if the matrix $M_{ik} = e_{,ik}$ (where $k, i = n, s$) is positive definite. This requirement leads to two independent constraints on the derivatives of the thermodynamical parameters [LL54, Section 21]:

$$c_\nu = Ts(T,\nu)_{,T} > 0, \quad \text{and} \quad \kappa_T = -\frac{1}{\nu}\nu(p,T)_{,p} > 0,$$

where κ_T is the isothermal compressibility, and c_ν is the isochoric specific heat. In nuclear physics the compressibility is customarily characterized by another positive quantity:

$$K_\sigma = 9p(\sigma,n)_{,n}\,, \quad \text{and} \quad K_T = 9p(T,n)_{,n}\,.$$

If these requirements are satisfied then the adiabatic sound speed is positive and larger than the isotherm sound speed.

There are regions in the $[T, n]$ plane where these stability conditions are not satisfied. That is, our equation of state does not represent a stable equilibrium. The region where $u_T^2 < 0$ is contained within the unstable region. There are speculations [SB83, LS84] that the matter in a relativistic heavy ion collision might penetrate into the unstable region because of rapid expansion during the collision.

2.1.3 Phase Coexistence between Liquid and Gas Phases

If the temperature and density of our system falls into the unstable region, or even close to this region, it may split up into two phases. Theoretically this is also a consequence of the stability requirements. If we allow for two co-existing phases we have one more free parameter in our thermodynamical problem, the volume fraction of the phases $i = L, G$:

$$\lambda = V_i/V,$$

or equivalently the particle number fractions:

$$\alpha_i = N_i/N.$$

The sum of both is normalized to 1, $\alpha_L + \alpha_G = 1$, $\lambda_L + \lambda_G = 1$ and there is a relation among α and λ:

$$\lambda_i = \frac{n}{n_i}\alpha_i, \quad \text{and} \quad \lambda_L = \frac{n - n_G}{n_L - n_G}.$$

Now the requirement of the energy minimum, leads to Gibb's criteria of phase equilibrium: $p_L = p_G = p$, $T_L = T_G = T$, and $\mu_L = \mu_G = \mu$. For a two phase system these requirements restrict the region of stability on the $[n, s]$ plane to a line! This is the Maxwell construction line, and it lies in the stable region of the previous stability study.

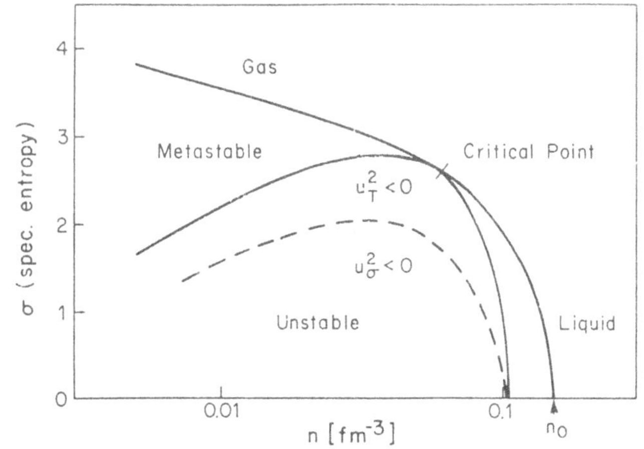

Fig. 1 Phase diagram on the entropy density plane. Phase equilibrium is possible above the critical entropy too!

Outside the region confined by this line the matter is stable in one single phase. Within this line but outside the $u_T^2 < 0$ region the matter is mechanically stable if formation of the other phase is hindered or delayed. The region between the Maxwell construction line and the boundary of instability $u_T^2 < 0$ is metastable, matter can be stable in this region if the other phase is not present. These are the phenomena of superheating and supercooling which are quite common in relatively slow thermodynamic processes, so we expect these phenomena to occur in relativistic heavy ion collisions. If we solve the Gibb's criteria for our equation of state the extensive thermodynamic quantities are given along the Maxwell construction line as functions of one intensive parameter, say T. In a heavy ion reaction in principle we might reach the phase mixture region with arbitrarily high energy collisions in the subsequent quasi-adiabatic expansion [CB80] if the breakup density is sufficiently low.

2.1.4 Critical Exponents

It will be imperative to mention a few results about critical phenomena. The critical opalescence in liquid gas phase transition was observed more than a century ago and in the 1940's Guggenheim [Gu45] realized that several fluids behave similarly around the critical point of the liquid-gas phase transition. This lead to the extended study of the critical exponents which started in the 1960's. (see ref.[St71]). Let us introduce the "order parameter" $n_L^{eq}(T) - n_G^{eq}(T)$, $(= n_L - n_G)$ and the relative deviation from the critical temperature

$$\varepsilon = (T - T_c)/T_c.$$

Guggenheim's observation was that just below the critical point

$$n_L - n_G \propto (-\varepsilon)^\beta,$$

where β is a *critical exponent*, which was found to be universally $\beta = 1/3$ for the liquids he studied. Similarly another critical exponent δ is defined at $T = T_c$ by

$$p - p_c \propto (n - n_c)^\delta \text{sign}(n - n_c).$$

At the critical point the isotherm compressibility, κ_T, diverges or K_T tends to zero. This divergence can be parametrized by a critical exponent too:

$$\kappa_T \propto (-\varepsilon)^{-\gamma'}, \quad \text{if: } \varepsilon < 0,$$

$$\kappa_T \propto (\varepsilon)^{-\gamma}, \quad \text{if: } \varepsilon > 0,$$

below and above the critical point respectively. Similarly the specific heat can be parameterized around the critical point as:

$$c_\nu \propto (-\varepsilon)^{-\alpha'}, \quad \text{if: } \varepsilon < 0,$$

$$c_\nu \propto (\varepsilon)^{-\alpha}, \quad \text{if: } \varepsilon > 0.$$

The critical exponents can be calculated for a given equation of state. So far in nuclear physics applications, however, the critical exponents were seldom evaluated. In Table 2 some critical exponents are listed for different models and systems:

Table 2

Values of critical-point exponents for selected systems. From [St71].

	α $T > T_c$	α' $T < T_c$	β $T < T_c$	γ $T > T_c$	γ' $T < T_c$	δ $T = T_c$
Fluids	~ 0.1	~ 0.1	~ 0.34	1.35	~ 1	4.2
3 dim Ising model	$\sim 1/8$	$\sim 1/8$	$\sim 5/16$	$\sim 5/4$	$\sim 5/4$	~ 5
Classical mean field (Van der Waals)	0	0	1/2	1	1	3

In [GK84] for a simple analytic equation of state the above mentioned critical exponents were evaluated and the same values were obtained as in the Van der Waals theory.

2.1.5 Fragment Mass Distributions

There are numerous models describing fragment mass distributions. A concise review is given in ref. [CK86]. The overwhelming majority of the models describe a static situation at the "freeze-out moment". It is possible that at this moment some excited nuclear fragments exist and their final decay by particle emission is also considered in the most sophisticated calculations [SB83,FR83,BB86,CK86b]. Most models are of statistical origin and in principle they would yield an equation of state. (This is not so in some percolation models where the connection between the bond-breaking probability and physical quantities like energy and density is not defined.) The evaluation of the equation of state is, however, not a trivial task and in practice it is very seldom performed [CF86b]. Thus it is not always clear whether a statistical model which satisfactorily describes the experimental data exhibits a liquid- gas phase transition or not. Here only some very basic facts will be mentioned about the fragment distributions and a few of the recent works not mentioned in [CK86] will be discussed.

At high beam energies the system breaks up after the collision with considerable excitation energy, and so that the system is rather dilute at freeze out. In this case the description of fragment mass distribution is simpler because we are close to an ideal gas behaviour. This situation will be discussed in the next section. At lower accelerator energies the situation might get more involved, due to the influence of the liquid gas phase transition. Both in equilibrium and in non-equilibrium expansion if finally two phases exist, they are very different. The gas phase is very dilute and has a large entropy $\sigma = 3.5-4$, while the liquid phase has low entropy $\sigma = 1-2$ and density close to n_0. What is the fragment distribution in such a phase mixture? The gas phase, having large entropy, consists of very light fragments with an exponentially decreasing mass spectrum. In this limit there is not much difference in the model estimates. From the experimentally observed light fragment (proton to alpha) abundances all previously discussed models extract an entropy value on the order of $3-4$, down to a few 100 MeV beam energy or even lower [Ka84, JS84].

The prediction of the mass distribution of heavier fragments representing the liquid phase is a more involved problem. The thermodynamical limit does not yield a definite prediction. Surface effects, nuclear size, reaction geometry, fission, final state decays and even the collective flow pattern may influence the intermediate and heavy fragment mass distribution. The light fragment distributions are not independent of the liquid phase. The final decay or fission of the heavier fragments can change the light fragment distributions too. While for the light fragments the grand canonical treatment is acceptable, the behavior of intermediate mass fragments is already strongly influenced by the limited nucleon number. These finite size and surface effects will be discussed later in sect. 2.2.

2.1.6 Law of Mass Action

The law of mass action as applied to ideal gases is the most basic law describing the fragment distributions. Ignoring relativistic, quantum and isospin effects the number density of ground state nuclei of mass number A is

$$n_g(A) = g_A\left(\frac{mTA}{2\pi}\right)^{3/2} e^{A(\mu+W_0)/T} \tag{1}$$

where g_A is the spin degeneracy, m is the nucleon mass, and $W_0 > 0$ is the binding energy per nucleon. The non-relativistic chemical potential per nucleon, μ is related to the relativistic chemical potential by $\mu = \mu_{rel.} - m$. If $\mu < -W_0$ then the number density is an exponentially decreasing function of A. Once $\mu = -W_0$ the nuclei would like to coalesce, to form uniform liquid nuclear matter.

Using Eq.(1) for p and d, and neglecting the binding energy difference the deuteron to proton ratio is: $x \equiv n_d/n_p = \frac{3}{2}\, 2^{3/2} e^{\mu/T}$. It follows that $\mu/T = lnx - 1.445$. Now from $e = Ts + \mu n - p$ by inserting the Boltzmann ideal gas expressions $e = n\frac{3}{2}T$ and $p = nT$ we get $\sigma = s/n = -\mu/T + 2.5$. Using the expression of μ/T in terms of x we can express the entropy by the d/p ratio:

$$\sigma = 3.945 - \ln x.$$

This result was first obtained by Siemens and Kapusta [SK79], and it served as the basis for experimental measurements of entropy later.

At the freeze out, however, not only nuclei in their ground states but also nuclei in various excited states will be present. To explicitly count them we should additively include

$$n_i(A) = \frac{g_i}{g_A} n(A)_g e^{-E_i^*/T},$$

where g_i is the degeneracy of the excited state and E_i^* is its excitation energy above the ground state. If the total baryon density is known as usual, μ can be obtained from the total nucleon density of the system at break-up

$$n = \sum_A \sum_{g,i} A n_i(A).$$

There are several large numerical models which calculate the nuclear fragment mass distribution based on the law of mass action for ideal gases. In [RK81, FR82, FR83, RF82] all known nuclear states with $A < 16$ having a width $\Gamma < 1\ MeV$ were included explicitly, and these levels for $A > 4$ were supplemented by an effective level density formula for the higher lying states which are not known experimentally [FR83, FR86]. Since this model includes an excluded volume approximation, the equation of state belonging to this is somewhat different from the ideal gas equation of state, the pressure increases sharper at higher densities as $n \to n_0$. It does not show a first order phase transition because only repulsive interactions are included, long-range attraction is not. This code has recently been named FREESCO [FR86]. It is an approximate microcanonical event generator where the exact microcanonical fragment distribution is calculated recursively by approximating the one- fragment inclusive distributions in each step by the grand canonical distribution. Another fragmentation model is the Quantum Statistical Model (QSM) [SC81,SB83] which calculates the grand canonical one-fragment inclusive distribution functions, but it includes as a special feature quantum statistics. The known particle-stable and metastable nuclear states with $A < 20$ are included in this model, and the repulsive interactions are simulated by the excluded volume approximation also.

Both models are based on the same physical picture: namely a first fast explosion creating light and medium mass fragment according to the law of mass action followed by sequential evaporation from these products in a final decay step. These two models, which can be regarded as different implementations of a general statistical model for nuclear disassembly, were compared to each other and to experimental results recently [CK86b]. It was found that in the breakup temperature range of $T = 30 - 90\ MeV$ there is an essentially unique relationship between the "d- like/p-like" fragment ratio, X, and the specific entropy of the ideal gas mixture σ. The lower temperature isotherms begin to deviate from the universal curve at low entropies. At high entropies and low X the "Siemens-Kapusta" formula [SK79] $\sigma = 3.945 - \ln X$ is a good approximation to the results of the more sophisticated statistical models. The experimentally determined values of X at the maximum charged particle multiplicity for different experiments ranging from 400 to 1050 $MeV/nucleon$ beam energy [DG85] are between 0.48 and 0.68. According to both above mentioned models this corresponds to entropy values of $\sigma = 3.45 - 3.9$ at the break- up.

Temperatures extracted from the energy spectra of different fragments with a moving source fit from intermediate energy heavy ion reactions. The temperatures are impressively constant independently of the particle [JW87]! This might suggest thermal and phase equilibrium. The above-mentioned experiments [DG85] are of relatively high energy and we do not expect the system to reach the nuclear liquid-gas phase transition before breakup. Therefore the above theoretical models which neglect attractive interactions yield satisfactory results. At lower energies the same is not true anymore. While the light fragments show a relatively high entropy according to the analysis, the intermediate fragments have an entropy value by almost one unit smaller [CF87]. This indicates that the above model cannot yield satisfactory results at lower energies, and other effects like the nuclear liquid-gas phase transition [Cs85], microcanonical statistics, attractive and Coulomb interactions should be considered.

2.2 Finite Systems and Fragment Abundances

2.2.1 Phase Transition in Finite Systems

For a system with a finite number of particles in a very strict sense no phase transitions exist and fluctuations can be important. Could it be that nuclear systems are so small that these fluctuations completely wash out the first order liquid-gas phase transition below T_c? This question was first addressed in the context of heavy ion reactions in [GK84]. Consider a system held at fixed temperature and pressure. We are interested in density fluctuations of this system. Instead of a nuclear system it may be helpful to think of a finite number of particles placed in a cylinder which is maintained at a fixed temperature T, with a movable piston at one end which exerts a constant pressure p on the gas particles. Only a finite number of particles per unit time collide with the piston, so the position of the piston will fluctuate with time about some mean position. Thus the density of the gas will also fluctuate.

The ratio of probabilities for a system to be at density n_1 or n_2 is

$$P(n_2)/P(n_1) = \exp[-(G(n_2) - G(n_1))/T]$$

where $G(n)$ is the Gibbs free energy at p and T. For an infinite system in equilibrium the density n is determined by the EOS once p and T are specified. It is necessary therefore to know $G(n)$ for densities not permitted by the equation of state. This is provided by the Landau theory [LL54] in which n is treated as an independent variable not restricted by p and T. Such an analysis was carried out in [GK84]. A simple form for the nuclear EOS was chosen

$$p = -a_0 n^2 + 2a_3 n^3 + nT, \tag{2}$$

$(a_0 = 293\ MeV fm^3,\ a_3 = 666\ MeV fm^6,\ n_0 = 0.15 fm^{-3},\ W_0 = 8\ MeV)$ which has a critical point at $n_c = a_0/(6a_3),\ T_c = a_0 n_c\ ,\ p_c = \frac{1}{3} T_c n_c$. One can expand the EOS (2) around the critical point by introducing $t = T - T_c$ and $\eta = n - n_c$ so that,

$$p - p_c = n_c t + t\eta + 2a_3\eta^3 \,. \tag{3}$$

This equation of state behaves similarly to the Van der Waals EOS, for negative t the phase equilibrium points can be found by the Maxwell construction [GK84]:

$$\eta_L = -\eta_G = \sqrt{-t/2a_3}.$$

The essential feature of the Landau approach is the construction of the free energy in terms of a power series in the order parameter η. Thus $G(p, T, \eta)$ will be defined at nonequilibrium values of η too, for a fixed p and T. In the neighborhood of the critical point the Gibbs free energy is then:

$$G(p,T,\eta) = G_0(p,T,\eta) + \alpha(p,T)\eta + A(p,T)\eta^2 + C(p,T)\eta^3 + B(p,T)\eta^4 + \ldots \tag{4}$$

The EOS (3) can be used to obtain the coefficients in (4) since the equilibrium value of η can be obtained from the requirement that G has an extremum in equilibrium:

$$\frac{\partial G}{\partial \eta} = \alpha + 2A\eta + 3C\eta^2 + 4B\eta^3 = 0. \tag{5}$$

This should be the EOS (3). Comparing (3) and (5) we obtain for the coefficients: $\alpha = -(p - p_c - n_c t)D,\ A = \frac{1}{2}tD,\ B = \frac{a_3}{2}D,\ C = 0$, where $D = N/n_c^2$ and N is the total number of nucleons in the system. This choice of D gives the correct G for equilibrium states. So the G in the order parameter expansion is

$$G = G_0(p,T) + \frac{N}{n_c^2}[-(p - p_c - n_c t)\eta + \frac{1}{2}t\eta^2 + \frac{a_3}{2}\eta^4].$$

The density or η values at the phase equilibrium η_L and η_G are the solutions of the EOS (3) if $p = p_c + n_c t$. At this pressure $p = p_c + n_c t$ the probability distribution of the density of the system is given by

$$R(n) = \frac{P(n)}{P(n_L)} = \exp[-(G(p,T,\eta) - G(p,T,\eta_L))/T]. \tag{6}$$

This probability is plotted in Fig. 2.

For T not too close to T_c there are two well defined peaks corresponding to a separation of liquid and gas phases, thus exhibiting a reasonably sharp first order phase transition. As Tapproaches T_c from below the valley separating the two peaks gets filled in and the distinction between liquid and gas gets washed out. At T_c the distribution is flat at the top. These large density fluctuations at the critical point give rise to the phenomenon of critical opalescence in atomic systems.

To find the relative probability for a system composed of N nucleons, N not necessarily 100, one simply scales the results of Fig. 2 to the power $N/100$, $R^{N/100}$, because in Eq. (6) the Gibbs free energy was taken to be proportional to the total

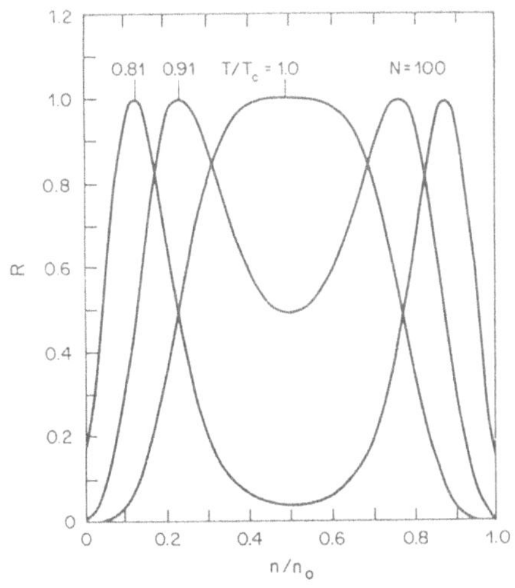

Fig. 2 The relative probability for the system to be at density n compared to the thermodynamically favored values n_L or n_G. The number of nucleons is $N = 100$. The pressure is the equilibrium pressure. From [GK84].

number of particles. For the density midway between n_L and n_G the relative probability assumes the simple form $R(\frac{1}{2}(n_L + n_G)) = \exp(-0.75(T - T_c)^2 N/(TT_c))$. Thus a larger number of nucleons sharpens the distinction between liquid and gas phases.

2.2.2 Droplet and Bubble Formation

Let us now consider the surface effects. Suppose that in a central collision between heavy nuclei an intermediate state of high temperature and density is reached and that subsequently it undergoes an adiabatic expansion. Then, no matter what the entropy per baryon is, it will eventually intersect the Maxwell curve separating liquid and gas phases if it does not break up before. (See Fig. 1). What happens next depends on whether the system hits the Maxwell curve from the liquid side ($n > n_c$) or from the gas side ($n < n_c$). If from the liquid side, bubbles begin to form, and if from the gas side, droplets begin to form [Si83]. For definiteness we shall consider the formation of droplets in a gas.

The probability of droplet formation is estimated by calculating the change in the Gibbs free energy of the system when a droplet appears in the gas [LL54,Re65]. Suppose that a spherical droplet containing A nucleons spontaneously forms in a gas consisting originally of a total number $A + B$ nucleons.

$$G_{no\ drop} = \mu_G(A + B), \tag{7}$$

$$G_{drop} = \mu_L A + \mu_G B + 4\pi R^2 \sigma_s + T\tau \ln A. \tag{8}$$

Here μ_G and μ_L are the nucleon chemical potentials in the gas and liquid phase respectively at pressure p and temperature T. The third term in Eq. (8) is the surface free energy for a droplet of radius R and with surface tension $\sigma_s = \sigma_s(T)$. The last term in Eq. (8) was introduced by Fisher [Fi67] in his droplet model. It takes into account the fact that the droplet surface closes on itself which reduces the total entropy associated with surface fluctuations. He introduced the critical exponent $\tau = 2 + 1/\delta$, and since in mean field theories $\delta = 3$, thus $\tau \equiv 2 + 1/\delta = 7/3$.

The probability of formation of the droplet is proportional to $\exp(-\Delta G/T)$, where ΔG is the difference between Eqs. (8) and (7). The yield of a fragment of mass A is

$$Y(A) = Y_0 \exp[\frac{\mu_G - \mu_L}{T} A - \frac{A\pi r_0^2 \sigma_s}{T} A^{2/3} - \tau \ln A]. \tag{9}$$

Here Y_0 is a normalization constant and r_0 is related to the droplet radius by $R = r_0 A^{1/3}$ and to the density by $n_L^{-1} = 4\pi r_0^3/3$. The importance of the surface effects was first observed by the Purdue-Fermilab group [FA82, MA82, HB84] and applied to high energy, $80 - 350$ GeV, proton-nucleus reactions. Mass and charge distributions for A up to 30 were measured with higher precision than ever before possible because of the use of an in beam gas jet target. Arguments based on emulsion experiments [Ta77] and on temperature measurements suggested that these fragments come from a common thermalized source. It was noticed that a power law $A^{-2.65}$ fits the data better than an exponential $e^{-\alpha A}$. The novel interpretation was that the target nucleus was almost instantaneously heated by the passage of the ultra-relativistic proton, and that subsequently the heated nucleus expanded in size until it passed through the critical point, $T = T_c$ and $n = n_c$, of the liquid-gas phase transition. At that point the distribution of droplets is $Y(A) = Y_0 A^{-\tau}$ because in Eq. (9) $\mu_G = \mu_L$ and $\sigma_s = 0$ at the critical point, so the volume and surface free energy terms vanish. There is no distinction between liquid and gas at the critical point, only long range fluctuations.

There are at least two difficulties with the above interpretation. First, why should one be so lucky to hit the critical point of nuclear matter accidentally with proton energies ranging from 80 to 350 GeV and with targets so different in size as krypton and xenon? Second, according to Fisher's version of the droplet model, $2 < \tau < 2.5$, whereas the data were outside this range.

The group recently remeasured the mass distributions depending on the proton energy in the range of $E_p = 1 - 20$ GeV [MB88]. Based on Eq. (9) they introduced a parametrization

$$Y(A) = Y_0 \, x^{A^{0.6386}} \, y^A \, A^{-\tau}.$$

Thus if the system would approach the critical point x and y should tend to 1, according to (9). They determined x, and y by fitting the experimental mass yields at different energies and found that x and y tend to 1 monotonically from below (above) respectively! At $E_p = 2$ GeV, $x = 0.2, y = 1.4$ and around 10 GeV both reach 1 already. At this fit τ was kept constant at 2.2. These data indicate that the path in the thermodynamical space is really energy dependent and it gets in the vicinity of the critical point only at higher proton energies. When τ was independently fitted to the data it showed a similar convergence to $\tau \approx 2.1$ from below.

These recent results of the group are consistent with the liquid gas phase transition picture. With increasing bombarding energy multifragmentation occurs first in the mechanical instability region, then in the supersaturated vapour region and finally at energies above 10 GeV in the critical region.

To draw a conclusive opinion about the nuclear fragmentation models would be too premature now. One remark, however, is probably important to make: The connection between the nuclear fragmentation models and the nuclear EOS should be firmly established before a final conclusion about the nuclear liquid- gas phase transition can be drawn. So far the EOS underlying the statistical models was seldom calculated (apart from some simple cases [FR83]). In statistical fragmentation models the evaluation of the EOS is in principle possible although it may be very cumbersome. We may be confident, however, that in the near future a consistent nuclear EOS and fragmentation theory will arise form the large scale theoretical effort.

On the experimental side the problems are to separate central heavy ion collisions and eliminate geometric effects arising in peripheral reactions. The most promising development in the near future will be provided by the 4π detector at MSU with good mass and energy resolution. This will lead to a major step in understanding the mechanism of heavy ion reactions in the nuclear liquid gas phase transition region.

3. The Nuclear EOS and the Quark Gluon Plasma

On QGP the equation of state side most of the theoretical work is invested in the study of pure SU(N) Yang-Mills theory on the lattice. These calculations, however, are restricted so far to zero net baryon density or zero chemical potential [Ka87]. To form such a low or "zero" baryon density matter in the deconfined phase one expectedly needs extremely high energy. Relatively simple "phenomenological" theories on hand, are able to provide us with an equation of state (EOS) in the phase transition region for cold matter [BC76,CN77,FM78], for zero baryon charge at finite temperature [CS79], or in the complete phase space for finite density and temperature [BC85, BK84,85, SS86, HS86, KL80,CG86]. These phenomenological equation of state studies can yield a good qualitative insight into the phase transition problem until a priori QCD calculations will be available in the complete density-temperature domain. There are even some advantages in the phenomenological approach: The results of these nuclear EOS studies can easily be incorporated into the phenomenological phase transition models.

3.1 Hadronic Equation of State

We discussed the nuclear equation of state extensively in these lectures. Similar phenomenological EOS can be used here too, however, more attention to high temperature and high density behavior is necessary.

In sect. 2.1.1 we introduced a simple parametrization of the nuclear EOS. In the literature several other parametrizations are also used. In one other paramet rization the energy density e in terms of density n and temperature T is parametrized as

$$e = n[m - W_0 + K(n/n_0 - 1)^2/18 + 3T/2], \tag{10}$$

where m is the nucleon rest mass, $W_0 > 0$ is the binding energy, the third term is the compressional energy e_c, usually called "quadratic", and the last term is the thermal energy described as that of a Boltzmann ideal gas. (This approximation must be sufficient at high temperatures). At high temperatures at least pion pairs should also be taken into account. Otherwise the energy density would be zero in baryon free matter. The simplest way to take this additive mesonic component into account, is by neglecting their rest mass:

$$e_m = g_1(\pi^2/30)T^4, \quad p_m = e_m/3, \quad s_m = \frac{4}{3}e_m/T,$$

where g_1 is the degeneracy of states. If we consider only pions, $g_1 = 3$ and so:

$$e_\pi = \pi^2 T^4/10, \quad p_\pi = \pi^2 T^4/30, \quad s_\pi = 4\pi^2 T^3/30.$$

At high temperatures some nucleons can be exited. The most important contribution is coming from delta resonances. Since the total baryon charge is conserved $n = n_N + n_\Delta$, in the Boltzmann approximation the delta to nucleon ratio is given by

$$n_\Delta/n_N = 4(m_\Delta/m_N)^{3/2}\exp(-[m_\Delta - m_N]/T).$$

This causes a change in the energy density where the rest mass term is now $n_\Delta m_\Delta + n_N m_N$, and also influences the other thermodynamical variables. The sum of two or more of the above mentioned combinations provides the total hadronic (h) EOS. In the simplest case $e_h = e_n + e_\pi$.

At high densities there is another constraint on the EOS, the requirement of causality. Eq. (10) yields a sound speed larger than the speed of light at large densities [GK85], and thus it is acausal. This can be remedied by using another functional form for the compressional energy, the "Sierk-Nix" parametrization

$$e_c = n\ 2K(\sqrt{n/n_0} - 1)^2/9,$$

or the so called "linear" form

$$e_c = Kn_0(n/n_0 - 1)^2/18.$$

These parametrizations provide almost identical behavior [GK85] at $n = 3-4\ n_0$ if the compressibility is chosen for the "Quadratic": $K = 275\ MeV$, for the "Sierk-Nix": $K = 550\ MeV$, and for the "Linear": $K = 1800\ MeV$.

It is important to emphasize that the nuclear EOS strongly influences the phase transition and the phase diagram. The compressional energy is particularly important. When it is neglected [CG86] the resulting phase diagram may lead to pathological behavior, the matter at n_0, and $T = 0$ being in the mixed phase. (Also the possibility of a first order phase transition is restricted to a very small range of bag constants: $\sqrt[4]{B} = 149 - 154\ MeV$ [CG86].) One way of including the compressional energy into the hadronic phases is the excluded volume approximation [SS86], which is a standard way of treating nuclear matter in relativistic nuclear collisions, first introduced in ref. [SC81]. This approximation leads to a phase diagram [SS86] similar to the nuclear EOS-s with explicit compressional energy.

3.2 QCD - Plasma Equation of State

The QCD Lagrangian leads to an equation of state which should in principle describe both the nuclear and quark-gluon plasma phase. Due to the nonlinear interactions it is not easy to find this EOS. At, high energy densities, however, the coupling tends to zero between quarks and gluons and an "asymptotic freedom" sets in. In this limit, i.e. at high enough temperatures and densities, the EOS of the quark world [Gy85] would be quite trivial. It would correspond to a non-interacting gas of N_f flavor quarks that come in N_c colors, and $(N_c^2 - 1)$ spin 1 gluons. In this case the EOS is given by the Stefan-Boltzmann expressions:

$$e_{SB}(T,\mu) = \frac{\pi^2}{15}(N_c^2 - 1 + \frac{7N_cN_f}{4})T^4 \ + \ \frac{N_cN_f}{2}(T^2\mu^2 + \frac{\mu^4}{2\pi^2}),$$

$$p_{SB}(T,\mu) = \frac{1}{3}e_{SB}(T,m),$$

$$n_{SB}(T,\mu) = \frac{N_c N_f}{9\pi^2}(\mu^3 + \pi^2 T^2 \mu),$$

where T and $\mu = \mu_q$ are the quark temperature and chemical potential ($\mu_b = 3\mu_q$), and $n_{SB} = n_b$ is the *baryon charge* density in the quark phase.

It is plausible that the vacuum in which the ideal gas of quarks and gluons exist differs from our everyday vacuum. Since we do not see the quarks and gluons in our nonperturbative physical vacuum [Sh80] , this vacuum should have an energy lower than the QCD perturbative vacuum where they can exist. Phenomenologically, we can try to take this effect into account by adding a constant $Bg^{\mu\nu}$ to the energy momentum tensor of the "quark world". This leads to the EOS :

$$e_q(T,\mu) = e_{SB}(T,\mu) + B,$$

$$p_q(T,\mu) = p_{SB}(T,\mu) - B,$$

where B is called the bag constant and this EOS is the "Bag Model" EOS. Usually for applications in heavy ion physics we can restrict ourselves to two flavors (u and d) in the quark- gluon phases, so $N_f = 2$ and $N_c = 3$ (for u, d, s quarks $N_f = 3$). In zeroth order of perturbation theory then the pressure p_q in terms of T and μ_b is

$$p_q = 37\pi^2 T^4/30 + \mu_b^2 T^2/9 + \mu_b^4/162\pi^2 - B,$$

where μ_b is the chemical potential associated with the baryon charge. For phase transition studies this simple form is frequently used. In some cases 1-loop [SS86,HS86] or 2-loop [KL80,Ch78] perturbative corrections are also included. The introduction of these perturbative terms leads to a 10-20% increase of the critical temperature and to a similar decrease of the critical densities n_{cq} and n_{ch}.

3.3 Phase Mixture

Having defined both the Hadronic and QCD plasma EOS one can create a complete EOS by Maxwell construction, containing pure phases and a region where the above two phases coexist. In this region if the plasma has zero baryon charge 2 of Gibb's criteria $p_q = p_h$, $T_q = T_h$, and in baryon-rich plasma an additional one: $3\mu_q = \mu_h$ should be satisfied. For baryon free plasma $p_q = 37\pi^2 T^4/90 - B$ and for a pionic gas $p_h = 3\pi^2 T^4/90$, thus from the requirement that $p_q(T_c) = p_h(T_c)$ we can get the critical temperature T_c :

$$T_c^4 = 90B/(34\pi^2)$$

The phase transition is first order. At T_c the coexisting hadronic and quark phase have different energy and entropy densities. For example if $B = \Lambda^4/(\hbar c)^3 = 0.397\ GeV/fm^3$, then the critical temperature and pressure are $T_c = 169\ MeV$, $p_c = 35\ MeV/fm^3$, and the critical energies at T_c are $e_h(T_c) = 106\ MeV/fm^3$, and $e_q(T_c) = 1.695\ GeV/fm^3$.

For baryon-rich matter in this approach the Maxwell construction can be done relatively easily since $p_q(\mu, T)$ is given and the chemical potential of the hadronic phase is also well known. For the EOS (10) in the Boltzmann approximation

$$\mu_b = T\ln(\frac{n_b C}{dT^{3/2}}) + m_N + W_0 + K(n_b - n_0)(3n_b - n_0)/(18n_0^2),$$

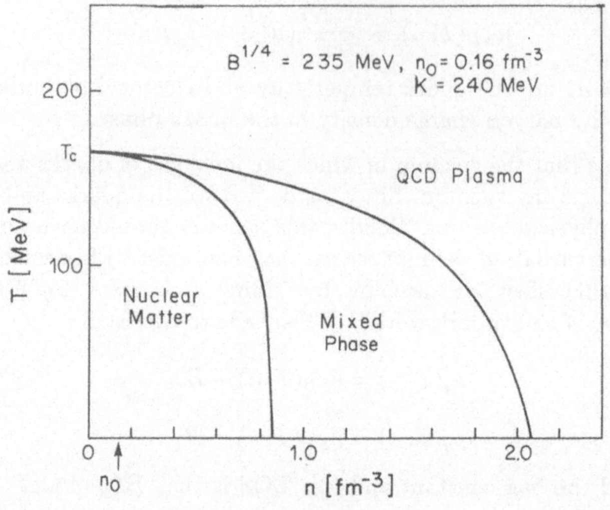

Fig. 3 Phase diagram of the nuclear matter quark matter phase transition from a simplified phenomenological model. From [CK86].

where $C = (2\pi(\hbar c)^2/(mc^2))^{3/2}$, and d is the degeneracy of the nucleon gas, $d = 4$. Now the phase equilibrium at a give temperature T_c can be found from the Gibbs criteria, i.e. by solving a single equation (numerically) for n_b. A typical phase diagram arising from this construction is shown on Fig. 3.

3.4 QGP Phase Transition and Nuclear Compressibility

The phase diagram of the first order phase transition is sensitive on both the nuclear and plasma parameters. The increase of compressibility K leads to a decrease of both critical densities, n_{cq} and n_{ch} while increase of the bag constant B leads to the increase of the critical temperature, and densities. The inclusion of hadronic resonances has negligible effect on the phase diagram at $T = 0$ or $\mu = 0$ but it pushes the phase boundaries to higher n and T values in the intermediate region, leading to an increase of the pure nuclear matter domain on the $[\mu, T]$ plane. The equilibrium pressure at fixed intermediate chemical potentials also increases due to the inclusion of hadronic resonances. The equilibrium pressure is higher at $T = 0$ than at T_c which is an interesting feature first observed in ref. [KL80].

The energy density where the mixed phase formation becomes possible is about $1-2\ GeV/fm^3$ at finite densities, and it decreases below $1\ GeV/fm^3$ when the density tends to zero. To form pure QCD plasma one should, however, reach $2-6\ GeV/fm^3$ energy density at finite densities and $1-4\ GeV/fm^3$ at $n = 0$. This of course does not mean that $n = 0$ QCD plasma can be formed with less beam energy! For comparison the energy density of the normal nuclear matter is $0.134\ GeV/fm^3$.

Acknowledgements

I would like to thank Miklos Gyulassy, Joseph Kapusta, Horst Stöcker, and Dan Strottman for discussions and fruitful collaboration.

4. References

AS86 J. Aichelin and H. Stöcker, Phys. Lett., 176B (1986) 14.

AR87 J. Aichelin, A. Rosenhauer, G. Peilert, H. Stöcker, and W. Greiner, Phys. Rev. Lett. 58 (1987) 1926.

BC76 G. Baym, S.A.Chin; Phys.Lett. 62B, 241 (1076)

BC85 H.W. Barz, L. P. Csernai, B. Kampfer and B. Lukács, Phys. Rev. D 32 (1985) 115.

BK84 H.W. Barz, B. Kampfer, L.P. Csernai and B.Lukács, Phys. Lett. 143B (1984) 334.

BB86 H.W. Barz, J.P. Bondorf, R. Donangelo, and H. Schulz, Phys. Lett. 169b (1986) 318.

Be71 H.A. Bethe, Ann. Rev. Nucl. Sci., 21 (1971) 93.

BG76 J.P. Blaizot, D. Gogny and B. Grammaticos, Nucl. Phys. A265 (1976) 315.

BO85 G.E. Brown, and E. Osnes, Phys. Rev. Lett. 159B (1985) 223.

BC85 E. Baron, J. Cooperstein, and S. Kahana, Phys. Rev. Lett. 55 (1985) 126.

CS79 T. Celik and H. Satz, Z. Phys. C1 (1979) 163.

CJ73 G.F. Chapline,M.H.Johnson, E.Teller and M.S.Weiss,Phys. Rev.D8 (1973) 4302.

CN77 G.Chapline, M.Nauenberg; Phys.Rev. D16, 456 (1977) CR86 M. E. Carrington and M. J. Rhoades-Brown State University of New York Report.

Ch78 S.A.Chin; Phys.Lett. 78B, 552 (1978).

CG86 J.Cleymans, R.Gavai, E.Suhonen; Phys.Rep. 130, 217 (1986).

CB80 L.P. Csernai and H.W. Barz, Z. Phys. A296 (1980) 173.

CG81 L.P. Csernai and W. Greiner, Phys. Lett. 99B (1981) 85.

CS83 L.P. Csernai,H. Stöcker, P.R. Subramanian, G. Graebner, A. Rosenhauer, G. Buchwald, J.A. Maruhn and W. Greiner, Phys. Rev. C28 (1983) 2001.

Cs85 L.P. Csernai, Phys. Rev. Lett. 54 (1985) 639.

CK86 L.P. Csernai, and J. Kapusta, Phys. Rep. 131 (1986) 223.

CK86b L.P. Csernai, J.I. Kapusta, G. Fai, D. Hahn, J. Randrup, and H. Stöcker, Phys. Rev. C submitted (1986) LBL-22183.

CF86b L.P. Csernai, and G. Fai, Acta Phys. Hung. in press (1986).

Da79 P. Danielewicz, Nucl. Phys. A314 (1979) 465.

DG85 P. Danielewicz and M. Gyulassy, Phys. Rev. D31 (1985) 53.

DG85 K. G. R. Doss, A. A. Gustafsson, H. H. Gutbrod, B. Kolb, H. Lohner, B. Ludewigt, A. M. Poskanzer, T. Renner, H. Riedesel, H. G. Ritter, A. Warwick, and H. Wieman, Phys. Rev. C32 (1985) 116.

FR82 G. Fai and J. Randrup, Nucl. Phys. A381 (1982) 557.

FR83 G. Fai and J. Randrup, Nucl. Phys. A404 (1983) 551.

FR86 G. Fai and J. Randrup, Comp. Phys. Comm. subm., LBL-21537.

FC85 G. Fai, L.P. Csernai, J. Randrup, and H. Stöcker, Phys. Lett. 164B (1985) 265.

FA82 J. E. Finn, S. Agarval, A. Bujak, J. Chuang, L. J. Gutay, A. S. Hirsch, R. W. Minich, N.T. Porile, R.P. Scharenberg, B. C. Stringfellow, and F. Turkot, Phys. Rev. Lett. 49 (1982) 1321.

Fi67 M.E. Fisher, Physics (N.Y.) 3 (1967) 255.

FM78 B. Freedman, L.McLerran; Phys.Rev. D17, 1109 (1978).

GB86 C.Gale, G. Bertsch, and S. Das Gupta, Phys. Rev. (1986) subm.

Gl88 N.K. Glendenning, Phys. Rev. C (1988) in press.

GC86 N.K. Glendenning, L.P. Csernai, and J.I. Kapusta, Phys. Rev. C33 (1986) 1299.

GK84 A.L.Goodman, J.I. Kapusta and A.Z. Mekjian, Phys. Rev. C30 (1984) 851.

GK85 C. Grant and J. Kapusta, Phys. Rev. C32 (1985) 663.

Gu45 E. A. Guggenheim; J. Chem. Phys. 12 (1945) 253.

GG84 H.A. Gustafsson, H. H. Gutbrod, B. Kolb, H. Lohner, B. Ludewigt, A. M. Poskanzer, T. Renner, H. Riedesel, H.G. Ritter, A. Warwick, F. Weik and H. Wieman, Phys. Rev. Lett. 52 (1984) 1590.

GG84b H.A. Gustafsson, H. H. Gutbrod, B. Kolb, H. Lohner, B. Ludewigt, A.M. Poskanzer, T. Renner, H. Riedesel, H. G. Ritter, A. Warwick, F. Weik and H. Wieman, Phys. Rev. Lett. 53 (1984) 544.

HS86 U. Heinz, P. R. Subramanian, H. Stöcker, and W. Greiner J. Phys. G: Nucl. Phys. 12 (1986) 1237.

HB84 A.S. Hirsch, A. Bujak, J. E. Finn, L. J. Gutay, R. W. Minich, N. T. Porile, R. P. Scharenberg, and B. Stringfellow, Phys. Rev. C29 (1984) 508.

IM85 Y. Ivanov, I. Mishustin, L. Satarov, Nucl. Phys. A433 (1985) 619.

JS84 B.V. Jacak, H. Stöcker and G.D. Westfall, Phys. Rev. C29 (1984) 1744.

JW87 B.V. Jacak, G.D. Westfall, G. Crawley, D. Fox, C.K. Gelbke, L.H. Harwood, B. E. Hasselquist, W.G. Lynch, D.K. Scott, H. Stöcker, M.B. Tsang, G.Buchwald, and T.J.M. Symons, Subm. to Phys. Rev. C.

Ka84 J.I. Kapusta, Phys. Rev. C29 (1984) 1735.

KL80 J. Kuti, B. Lukács, J. Polonyi, and K. Szlachanyi Phys. Lett. B95 (1980) 75.

LL54 L.D. Landau and E.M. Lifshitz, Statistical Physics (Nauka, Moscow, 1954).

LS84 J.A. Lopez and P.J. Siemens, Nucl. Phys. A431 (1984) 728.

MB88 M. Mahi, A.T. Bujak, D.D. Charmony, Y.H. Chung, L.J. Gutay A.S. Hirsch, G.L. Paderewski, N.T. Porile, T.C. Sangster, R.P. Scharenberg, and B. C. Stringfellow, Phys. Rev. Lett. 60 (1988) 1936.

MA82 R.W. Minich, S. Agarval, A. Bujak, J. Chuang, J.E. Finn, L.J. Gutay, A.S. Hirsch, N.T. Porile, R.P. Scharenberg, B.C. Stringfellow and F. Turkot, Phys. Lett. 118B (1982) 458.

MS83 I.N. Mishustin and L.M. Satarov, Yad. Fiz. 37 (1983) 894.

MS86 J.Maruhn, and H. Stöcker, UFTP preprint 186/1986, and,

Mü85 B. Müller, The Physics of the Quark-Gluon Plasma, Lecture Notes in Phys. 225 (1985), Springer-Verlag.

Mü88 B. Müller, Lectures at this school.

My76 W.D. Myers, Atomic Data Nucl. Data Tables 17 (1976) 411.

Ni79 J.R. Nix, Prog. in Part. and Nucl. Phys., 2 (1979) 237.

OS86 E. Osnes, and D. Strottman, Phys. Lett. 166B (1986) 5.

PR87 G. Peilert, A. Rosenhauer, B. Waldhauser, J.A. Maruhn, H. Stöcker, and W. Greiner, Inv. talk at Int. Symp. on Nucl. Phys., Madras, India, January 22-25, 1987. in press.

RK81 J. Randrup and S.E. Koonin, Nucl. Phys. A356 (1981) 223.

RF82 J. Randrup and G. Fai, Phys. Lett. 115B (1982) 281.

Re65 F. Reif: Fundamentals of statistical and thermal physics (McGraw-Hill, 1965).

SM74 W. Scheid, H. Müller and W. Greiner, Phys. Rev. Lett. 32 (1974) 741.

SK79 P.J. Siemens and J.I. Kapusta, Phys. Rev. Lett. 43 (1979) 1486.

SN80 A.J. Sierk and J.R. Nix, Phys. Rev. C22 (1980) 1920.

St71 H.E. Stanley: Introduction to phase transitions and critical phenomena (Oxford University Press 1971).

SB82 R. Stock, R. Bock, R. Brockmann, J.W. Harris, A. Sandoval, H.Strobele, K.L. Wolf, H.G. Pugh, L.S. Schroeder, M. Maier, R.E. Renfordt, A. Daca and M.E. Oritz, Phys. Rev. Lett. 49 (1982) 1236.

SB82b H. Stöcker, G. Buchwald. L.P. Csernai,G. Graebner, J.A.Maruhn and W.Greiner, Nucl. Phys. A387 (1982) 205c.

SB83 H. Stöcker, G. Buchwald, G. Graebner, P. Subramanian, J.A. Maruhn, W. Greiner, B.V. Jacak and G.D. Westfall, Nucl. Phys. A400 (1983) 63c.

SB88 M.M Sharma, W.T.A. Borghols, S. Brandenburg, S. Crona, A. van der Woude, and M.N. Harakeh, Phys. Rev. C (1988) in press.

SC81 P.R.Subramanian, L.P. Csernai, H.Stöcker, J.Maruhn, W.Greiner and H.Kruse, J. Phys. G7 (1981) L241.

Tj88 J.A. Tjon, Lectures at this school.

WM88 B. Waldhauser, J. Maruhn, H. Stöcker, and W. Greiner, Rhys. Rev. C38 (1988) in press.

WB87 A. van der Woude, W.T.A. Borghols, S. Brandenburg, and M.M. Sharma, Phys. Rev. Lett. 58 (1987) 2383.

RELATIVISTIC HEAVY ION COLLISIONS

Berndt Müller

Institut für Theoretische Physik
Johann Wolfgang Goethe-Universität
Frankfurt am Main, West Germany

INTRODUCTION

Collisions between heavy nuclei at "relativistic" energies are tremendously complicated processes, evolving from a simple initial state (two nuclei in their ground states) to highly complex final states involving hundreds of free particles. Nobody in his or her right mind would voluntarily investigate such processes were it not for the hope to study the properties of hadronic matter at high density and high excitation energy (the term "high temperature" is customarily used to express this condition). The theory of strong interactions, QCD, predicts that a phase transition occurs under such conditions, in which hadronic matter, i.e. matter composed of baryons and mesons, is converted into a quark-gluon plasma consisting of quarks and gluons that are no longer confined into clusters of the size of about 1 fm.

This phase change is expected to require an energy density of about 1-2 GeV/fm^3, corresponding to a baryon density of more than $8\rho_0$(ρ_0 = 0.16/fm^3 being the saturation density of nuclear matter) or a temperature T greater than 160-200 MeV. Although the new state of hadronic matter is often simply called "quark matter", the term "quark-gluon plasma" is more appropriate since about half the excitation energy is predicted to reside in gluonic depress of freedom.

Various signatures have been suggested to allow for an experimental detection of this phase transition, most notably involving measurements of transverse particle momenta, strangeness and charm production. These will be discussed, together with some current ideas about the space-time evolution of hadronic matter in a nuclear collision. We will then turn to the first results from the experiments at Brookhaven and CERN, which show some very interesting features. Finally, we will briefly consider a different approach to hadronic matter at high energy and density, namely through the dynamics of a gas of relativistic (hadronic) strings.

One other remark may be appropriate here: We will understand the term "relativistic collisions" as implying that the kinetic energy in the center-of-mass-system exceeds the nuclear rest mass. This occurs at a laboratory beam energy

$$(E/A)_{beam} \gtrsim 6 \text{ GeV} \quad .$$

Lower energies will not be considered here; I refer to Laszlo Csernai's lectures. A brief list of suggested literature for our subject is given at the end.

THE QUARK-GLUON PLASMA

Our present picture of the structure of the nucleon, i.e. of the building block of strongly interacting matter, is roughly as follows: The three valence quarks are confined to a core region of size $R_c \sim 0.6$fm by the action of the color force between them. In the context of bag models this is expressed by saying that the normal color vacuum does not support the propagation of states that are not color singlets. The quarks therefore must "dig" a hole into this normal vacuum, replacing it by a state often called the "perturbative" vacuum of quantum chromodynamics (QCD). This costs energy BV, where V is the volume of the quark bag and B, the bag constant, is the pressure that the normal QCD vacuum exerts on the bag. A crude estimate gives

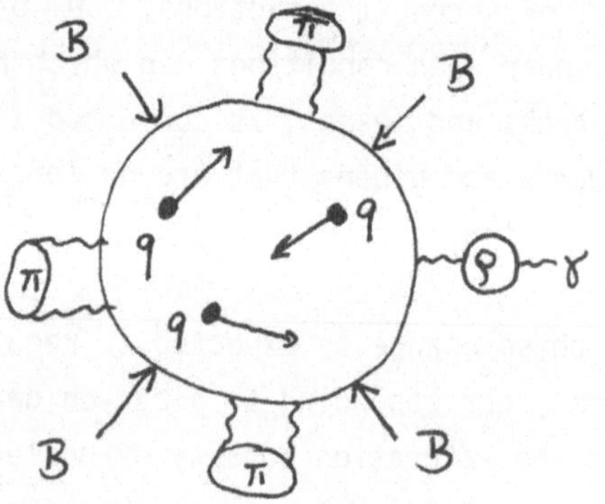

$$B \sim (200 \text{ MeV})^4 \sim 200 \text{ MeV/fm}^3 \quad .$$

Around the quark core there extends a cloud of virtual mesons, mainly π- and ρ-mesons, which increases the size of the nucleon to the value $R_N \sim 0.8$fm measured as charge radius in electron scattering.

In a nucleus, the nucleons are separated by an average distance $2r_o$ with $r_o \sim 1.2\text{fm} \sim 2R_C$. In other words; only about 1/8 of the nuclear volume is filled by the quark cores of its nucleons. However, the separation between the quark bags shrinks when nuclear matter is compressed, until all "empty space" between them is squeezed out at a nuclear density $\rho_C \sim 8\rho_o$. Beyond that density, the nucleons may be expected to dissolve into one continuous region occupied by quarks, i.e. quark matter. (An alternative outcome would be that the nucleon bags shrink under pressure, but there are strong general arguments in QCD against this scenario.) This may actually occur in the interior of neutron stars, where densities up to $10\rho_o$ are predicted in the center, but it is not clearhow the transition to quark matter can be observed in that case.

The second way of getting rid of the void between the nucleons is by filling it with other hadrons, i.e. pions, kaons, etc. Since these are unstable particles this procedure corresponds to putting nuclear matter into a highly excited state, which can be characterized by a temperature T in case the excitations are in thermodynamic equilibrium. Under these conditions the new phase of hadronic matter would be expected to contain, besides quarks, an almost equal number of antiquarks originating from the

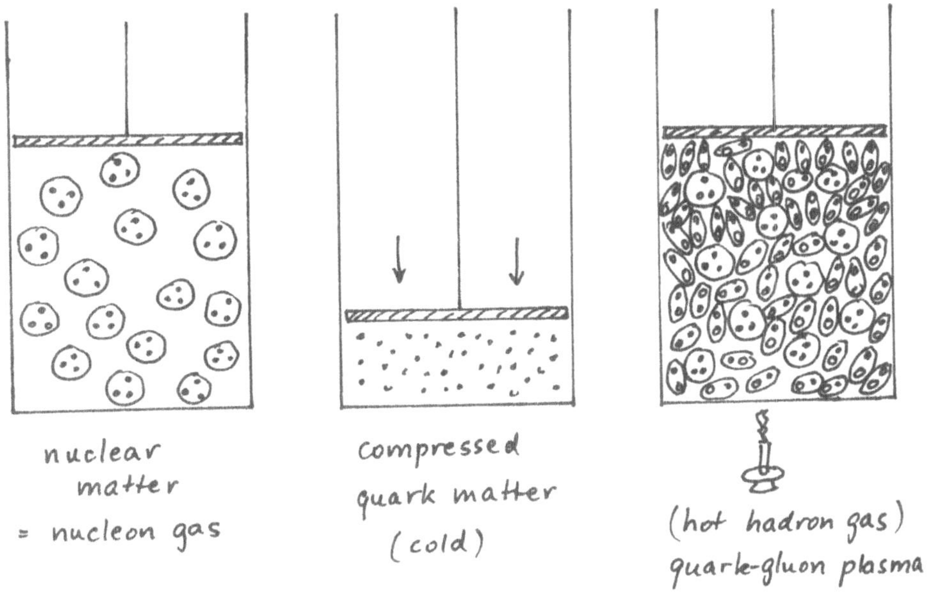

mesons and, because a quark-antiquark pair can annihilate to form a gluon, also a large number of gluons. For this reason the new state is usually called a "quark-gluon plasma". To obtain a crude estimate of the critical temperature T_c, let us estimate what temperature we need to fill space completely with pions. Neglecting the pion rest mass (we shall soon see that $T_c > m_\pi$) and setting the Boltzmann constant $k_B=1$, the number density of pions is

$$n_\pi = 3\int\frac{d^3k}{(2\pi)^3}\left(e^{-k/T}-1\right)^{-1} = \frac{3}{\pi^2}\zeta(3)\,T^3$$

Taking a pion radius $R_\pi \sim 0.6$fm, space is filled with pions if

$$n_\pi V_\pi = \frac{3}{\pi^2}\zeta(3)\,T_c^3\cdot\frac{4\pi}{3}R_\pi^3 = \frac{4}{\pi}\zeta(3)\left(T_c R_\pi\right)^3 = 1$$

This gives

$$T_c \sim 0.85\; R_\pi^{-1} \sim 280\ \text{MeV},$$

where we have used $(\hbar c) \approx 200$ MeVfm to convert inverse length into energy. This value of T_c is an overestimate, because other mesons are excited as well leading to a much higher hadron density near T_c, which is thus reduced to about 200 MeV.

At $T>T_c$, quarks and gluons are predicted to move essentially freely all over the region of high energy density. As (u,d) quarks and gluons are practically massless particles then, the energy density per degree of freedom is given by the general Stefan-Boltzmann law

$$\varepsilon/d = \frac{\pi^2}{30}T^4 .$$

All that remains is to count the available number of degrees of freedom d. For gluons we have

$$d_G = 2(\text{spin}) \times 8(\text{colour}) = 16 ,$$

and for quarks (u,d) we find

$$d_Q = 2(\text{spin}) \times 3(\text{colour}) \times 2(\text{isospin}) \times \frac{7}{4}(\text{Fermions}) = 21 .$$

So, altogether, we have effectively 37 degrees of freedom in the quark-gluon plasma. Including a finite quark chemical potential μ (Fermi energy) to account for a baryon surplus, the equation of state becomes:

$$\varepsilon = \frac{37}{30}\pi^2 T^4 + \pi^2 T^2 + \frac{1}{2\pi^2}\mu^4 \quad ,$$

$$\varepsilon \quad \sim (T/160\ \mathrm{MeV})^4\ [\mathrm{GeV/fm}^3] \quad . \quad (\mu = o) \quad .$$

With $T_c \sim 200$ MeV we thus need an energy density $\varepsilon > 2$ GeV/fm³ to achieve the transition to quark gluon plasma.

There are three circumstances under which such conditions may (have) prevail(ed) in nature:

(a) in the core of neutron stars, here would be $\mu > \mu_c$, $T \sim o$;

(b) in the very early big bang of the universe, with $T > T_c$, $\mu \sim o$;

(c) and relativistic heavy ion collisions (RHIC), where both T and μ are generally large.

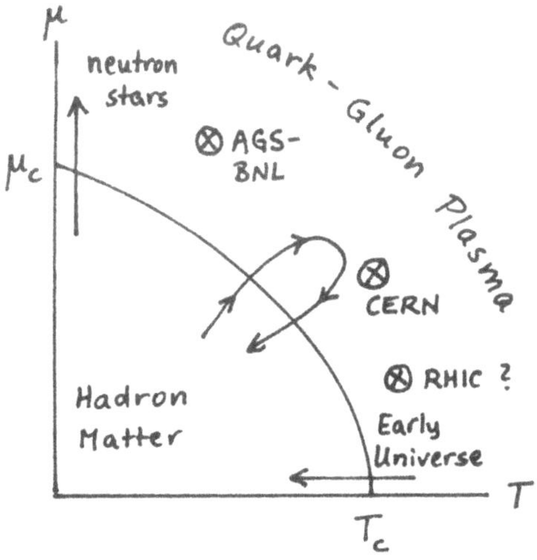

Here we are concerned with the last of these cases. Two quite extreme scenarios have been presented how a high energy density could develop in nuclear collisions. In the first, the "low-energy" or stopping scenario one assumes that a large target nucleus is able to stop an approaching projectile even at rather high energy. In this case a "fireball" is formed out of the colliding parts of the nuclei, containing a large fraction of baryons. In the second, "ultra-high energy" scenario one assumes that nuclei are essentially transparent and that high energy density is formed out of hadronizing strings between the nuclei after they have passed through each other.

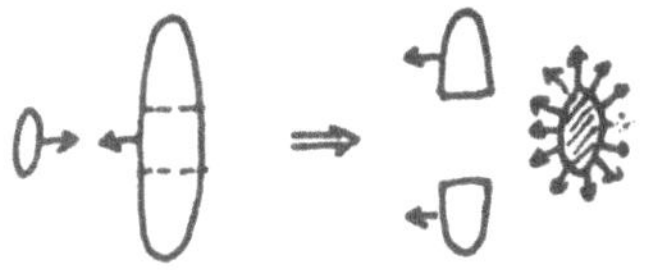

stopping & fireball formation

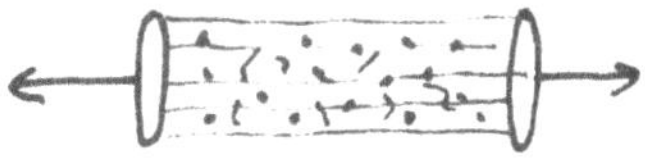

transparency

Today we know that the stopping hypothesis is satisfied to rather good degree up to the highest available energies (200 GeV/n. beam energy at CERN). At this energy, in a central ^{16}O and ^{208}Pb collision, there are about 16+56 = 72 participants, with an effective c.m. energy of about 500 GeV. This corresponds to a fireball rapidity

$$Y_{cm} = \text{artanh}\sqrt{\gamma^2-1}/(\gamma_p+A_T^{eff}/A_p) \sim 2.37 ;$$

and assuming a fireball radius of 3 fm, the energy density ε and baryon density ρ_B are

$$\varepsilon \sim 5.4 \text{ GeV/fm}^3 , \quad \rho_B \sim 0.7\text{fm}^{-3} .$$

Using the previously given expression for ε in the quark-gluon phase, one find that this corresponds to the values

$$T \sim 235 \text{ MeV} , \quad \mu_B = 3_\mu \sim 400 \text{ MeV},$$

indicated in the sketch of the phase diagram.

A crude estimate of the attained energy density has been extracted from the experimental data by means of a formula suggested by Bjorken

$$\varepsilon \sim \frac{dE_T/dy}{\pi R^2 \ \tau_o} ,$$

where E_T is the transverse energy, R is the projectile radius, and τ_o is the time required for thermalization. This formula is based on the "high-energy", transparency model, and thus should not really be applied at today's energies. Nonetheless, values of 2-4 GeV/fm³ were deduced from the experiments in this way.

CURRENT R.H.I.C. EXPERIMENTS

Experiments with highly relativistic heavy ions are presently carried out at CERN and Brookhaven (AGS), with energies of 60 and 200 GeV/n. and 15 GeV/n., respectively. At CERN, where ^{16}O and ^{32}S beam have been available, there are three large general-purpose experiments:

- NA35 (Stock et al.) "Streamer chamber"

  measuring dN/dy, E_T, π^-, K_s^o, Λ, etc.

- WA80 (Gutbrod et al.) "Plastic Ball, Lead Glass", measuring E_T, π^o, η, γ, target fragmentation;
- NA34 (Specht, Willis, et al.) "Helios", measuring E_T, dN/dy, e^+e^-, γ, etc.

Moreover, there exist three large dedicated experiments:

- NA38: $\mu^+\mu^-$ spectrometer (Kluberg et al.)
- NA36: Time-projection chamber (Gruhn et al.)
- WA85: Omega-spectrometer (K_S^o, Λ, $\bar{\Lambda}$) (Quercigh et al.)

At Brookhaven, 15 GeV/n ^{16}O and ^{28}Si beam were available at the AGS with two large experiments running:

E802 (Nagamiya, Hansen, et al.) with a particle spectrometer and a Lead glass array;

E814 (Braun-Munzinger, et al.) with Calorimeters, etc., and a third experiment (E810, TPC) is being set up.

The experiments carried out so far have clearly shown that nuclei are not transparent even at energies of 200 GeV/u. In the most central collisions a detector at zero degrees see no paaticle at all. The rapidity distribution of negative pions has a peak right at the rapidity of the centre of mass of the projectile and the tube of matter of the target nuclei lying geometrically in its way. The π-transverse momentum distribution looks like that emitted by a fireball of temperature 180-200 MeV. Pion-pion interferometry has indicate a final fireball size of about 8fm at central rapidity. Finally, energy densities well above 2 GeV/fm^3 have been deduced with help of the Bjorken formula; other evaluations on the basis of Landau's hydrodynamic model even yield values of 5 GeV/fm^3 at AGS energies (15 GeV/n.).

SIGNATURES OF QUARK MATTER

A long list of possible signals for the formation of a quark-gluon plasma has been suggested. Presently, the most promising signals are probably:

1) Plateau and further increase of $\langle P_T \rangle$ versus dN/dy;
2) Depletion of J/ψ formation;
3) Enhanced production of strange hadrons (k,Λ,$\bar{\Lambda}$,...).

Let us discuss these three signals in some detail.

1) According to an argument of Shuryak and van Hove, the imminent presence of a phase transition with large latent heat shows up as a plateau in the rise of fireball temperature with increasing energy density.

Identifying temperature T with transverse momentum $<P_T>$ and energy density ε with transverse energy per unit rapidity dE_T/dy, an experimentally observable signal is obtained.

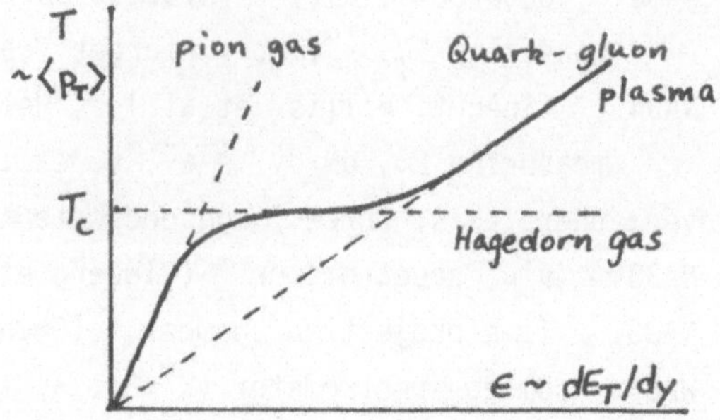

Put in simple words the idea is that, when the critical temperature T_c is reached, additional energy is required to convert the hadron phase into the quark phase. The temperature remains constant, and only continues to rise when the phase change has been completed. So far, no indication for this phenomenon has been observed in nuclear collisions.

2) As pointed out by Matsui and Satz, colour charges are screened in the deconfined quark-gluon phase. The linearly rising, confining potential that binds a $(c\bar{c})$ pair into charmonium states J/ψ, ψ', etc., is replaced by a short-range, screened potential in the new phase, which does not support a bound state if $T > 1.2\ T_c$. Therefore the formation of charmonium should be suppressed, if a quark-gluon plasma is formed. Since it takes a while (~1-2fm/c) until the J/ψ state is formed out of a newly created $(c\bar{c})$-pair, this suppression should be alleviated for fast moving states which can escape from the fireball before the (cc)-pair can dissociate. Thus the suppression should be most notable at small momenta. Precisely this effect seems to be observed at CERN by the NA38 experiment. New calculations have shown, however, that a very similar pattern of suppression can be caused by hadronic mechanisms even in the absence of deconfinement. The status of this effect as a valid signal for plasma formation is therefore in doubt.

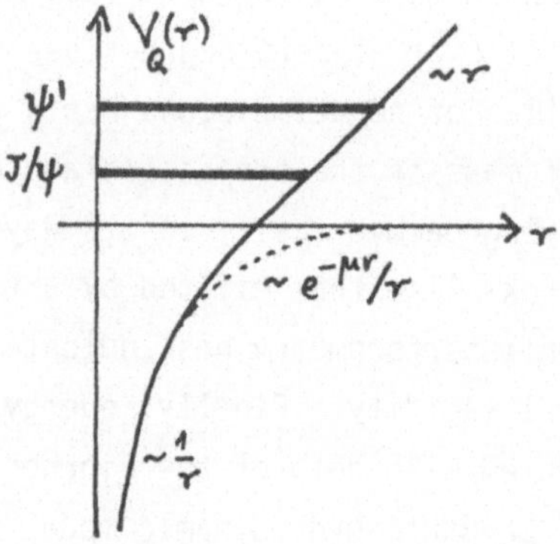

3) As was shown by Rafelski and Müller, strange quarks can be produced much more easily in the quark-gluon plasma. The

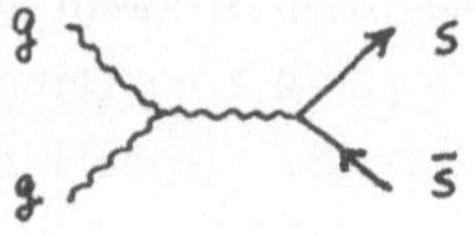

reasons for this effect include a much lower energy threshold (~ 350 MeV vs. ~ 700 MeV) and the much larger efficiency of strangeness production by gluons as opposed to light quarks. The large phase-space density of gluons in the deconfined phase, commanding 16 independent degrees of freedom, facilitates the reaction rate for the process $gg \to s\bar{s}$ being an order of magnitude larger [$A_s \sim 10^{23} s^{-1}$] than characteristic rates for strangeness production, e.g. $NN \to NK\Lambda$, $\pi N \to K\Lambda$, $\pi\pi \to K\bar{K}$, in the hadronic gas phase [$A_s \sim 10^{22} s^{-1}$]. Considerably enhanced production of strange hadrons in AA, as compared to pp, collisions would therefore signal the intermediate existence of a dense quark-gluon phase; strange antibaryons are probably the most sensitive signal in view of their difficult production in secondary reactions involving nucleons or pions.

Considerable enhancement in K^+ and Λ production has been observed in the AGS (E802) and CERN (NA35) experiments, and a $\bar{\Lambda}/\Lambda$ ratio as high as 0.3 has been seen in the WA85 data. At present, these results appear to lack an explanation in the context of a reaction model involving only hadrons, and no deconfined phase. However, scientific caution requires to wait for better data and more refined calculations before a claim to the observation of a quark-gluon plasma can be made. Part of the difficulty lies in the multitude of final state interactions that can alter the abundance of any species of strange hadrons, combined with our rather rudimentary understanding of the hadronization of a quark-gluon plasma. Although much insight has been gained in the past few years, more systematic studies are required, especially when abundant data on particle distributions in AA collisions become available.

In order to distinguish between a quark-gluon plasma and colour-confined hadronic matter, one needs a realistic model for the hadron gas. Assuming a pion gas at T = 300 MeV, as many authors have done, is not adequate, since we know from experiment that many excited hadron states (rho-meson, delta-resonance, etc.) are excited when the temperature exceeds 100-150 MeV. Probably the most realistic model, originally proposed by Hagedorn, assumes an excitation spectrum that increases in density exponentially with hadron mass: $\rho(m) \simeq \rho_o \exp(+ m/m_o)$. One can show that this leads to a limiting temperature $T_c = m_o$, at which all thermodynamic quantities (energy, entropy, etc.) diverge. A dynamical model that yields precisely this mass spectrum is the relativistic string model. Here the hadrons are viewed as strings of colour flux, with a quark Q, antiquark $\bar{Q}$ or a diquark (QQ) at the ends. Except for the quark masses, the single parameter of this model is the string tension K, which is known from experiment (Regge slope) to be of order 1 GeV/fm ~ 15 tons. The critical temperature can be expressed in terms of the string constant:

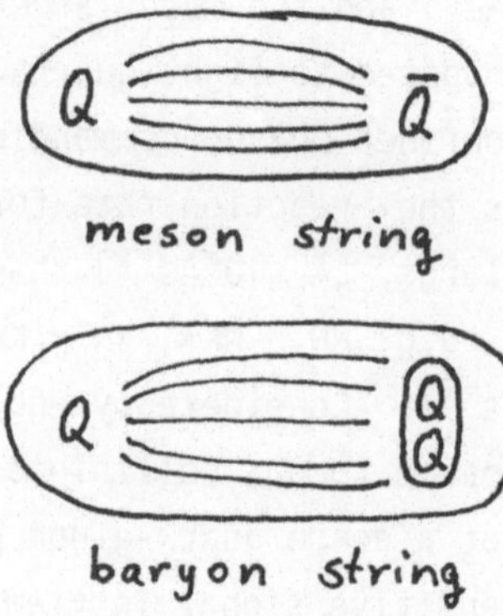

$$T_C \sim \frac{1}{2}\pi^{1/6} K^{1/2} \sim 250 \text{ MeV},$$

not far from the expected transition to the deconfined phase.

Mathematically, a string is described by its world-sheet $x^\mu(\tau,\sigma)$, where τ measures the proper time and σ parametrizes the points on the string. The whole string is determined by the motion of its endpoint $y^\mu(\tau) = x^\mu(\tau,\sigma = o)$; this world-line is called the directrix. Choosing the time gauge $x^o \equiv \tau$, the directrix gradient vector has unit length, $|d\vec{y}/dt| = 1$, and is semiperiodic:

$$\vec{y}(t + \frac{2E}{K}) = \vec{y}(t) + \frac{2\vec{P}}{K} ,$$

where $E,\vec{P}$ are total energy and momentum of the string. An ensemble of strings can then be modelled on the computer by choosing a set of directrices $\vec{y}_\alpha(t)$, e.g. by a stochastic polygon construction.

Sailer, Greiner and myself have recently performed such numerical simulations of a (non-interacting) string gas. Our results show that the mass spectrum is, indeed, rising exponentially, and that pressure, energy and entropy density all diverge at T_C. Simulations of colliding nuclei require the addition of interactions among the strings, i.e. cross-over of ends and string breaking. First results with interacting strings look promising, e.g. the equilibration of the mass distribution starting from nucleons is quite fast. Whether and how the interactions modify the Hagedorn equation of state, is an interesting question which is presently studied.

CONCLUSIONS

In collisions of nuclei at very high energy one hopes to observe the predicted transition from a colour-confined hadron phase to a deconfined quark-gluon plasma. Serious experiments, which began about two years ago, have clearly shown that a very high energy density is reached in such collisions. Proposed signals, such as strangeness enhancement and charmonium suppression, are being observed. However, more theoretical work is needed to study whether these or other possible signals are unambiguous signatures of quark matter.

REFERENCES

E.V. Shuryak, QCD and the Theory of Superdense Matter, Phys. Rep. 61:71 (1980).

B. Müller, The Physics of the Quark-gluon Plasma, Lecture Notes in Physics, vol. 225, Springer-Verlag, Heidelberg (1985).

L. McLerran, The Physics of the Quark-Gluon Plasma, Rev. Mod. Phys. 58:1021 (1986).

J. Cleymans, R.V. Gavai, and E. Suhonen, Quarks and Gluons at High Temperatures and Densities, Phys. Rep. 130:217 (1986).

P. Koch, B. Müller, and J. Rafelski, Strangeness Production in Relativistic Heavy Ion Collisions, Phys. Rep. 142:167 (1986).

K. Kajantie and L. McLerran, Probes of the Quark-Gluon Plasma in High Energy Collisions, Ann. Rev. Nucl. Part. Science 37:293 (1987).

PARTICIPANTS

ANGULO, P.C.	Departamento di Fisica Nuclear Faculdad de Ciencias Universidad de Granada E-18071Granada/Spain
ARIAS, F	Departamento de Fisica Moderna Faculdad de Ciencias cl Fuentenueva sin E-18071Granada/Spain
BOERSMA, H.F.	K.V.I. Zernikelaan 25 9747AA Groningen/TheNetherlands
BOOTEN, J.G.L.	R.J. van de Graaff Lab. Rijksuniversiteit Utrecht Postbus 80.000 3508 TA Utrecht/The Netherlands
BUDA, A.J.	Institute of Nuclear Research, Dept. P2 05-400 Swierk/Poland
BULTEN, H.J.	NIKHEF-K Postbus 41882 1009 DB Amsterdam/The Netherlands
CABALLERO, J.A.	Instituto de Estructura de la Materie Consejo Superior de Investigaciones Cientificas Serrano 119-123 E-28006 Madrid/Spain
CHOWDHURY, S.K.	Dept. of Theoretical Physics Indian Association for the Cultivation of Science Jadavpur Calcutta-700032/India
COSTER, C.J.A. DE	Institute for Nuclear Physics Proeftuinstraat 86 B-9000 Gent/Belgium
DAMAN, M.A.	NIKHEF-K Postbus 41882 1009 DB Amsterdam/The Netherlands
DIEPERINK, A.E.L.	K.V.I. Zernikelaan 25 9747 AA Groningen/The Netherlands

DIOSZEGI, I.
Institute of Isotopes of the
Hungarian Academy of Sciences
P.O. Box 77
H-1525 Budapest/Hungary

DORAN, S.M.
Dept. of Physics and Astronomy
Kelvin Laboratory
The University of Glasgow
East Kilbride
Glasgow G75 0QU/England

FOKKE-DE LA BEY, M.
Fysisch Laboratorium
Rijksuniversiteit Utrecht
Postbus 80.000
3508 TA Utrecht/The Netherlands

GARRIDO-BELLIDO, E.
c/o Prof. J.M. Gomez
Dept. Fisica Nuclear
Facultad de Ciencias
E-37008 Salamanca/Spain

GODRE, S.S.
Physics Dept.
Indian Institute of Technology
Kanpur 208016/India

GUNDLACH, J.H.
Nuclear Physics Laboratory, GL-10
University of Washington
Seattle, Wash. 98195/U.S.A.

GUNGOR, F.
Itü, Fen-ed. Fakültesi
Mathematik Bölümü
Maslak-Istanbul/Turkey

HAMMANS, M.
Institut für Physik
Universität Basel
Klingelbergstrasse 82
CH-4056 Basel/Switzerland

HAVEMAN, J.
R. van de Graaff Lab.
Rijksuniversiteit Utrecht
Postbus 80.000
3508 TA Utrecht/The Netherlands

HANSCHEID, H.
Institut für Strahlen- und Kernphysik
Universität Bonn
Nussallee 14-16
D-5300 Bonn/West-Germany

HARAKEH, M.N.
Natuurkundig Laboratorium
Vrije Universiteit
de Boelelaan 1081
1081 HV Amsterdam/The Netherlands

HENNING, H.
Institut für Theoretische Physik
Universität Hannover
Appelstrasse 2
D-3000 Hannover 2/West-Germany

HOFSTEE, M.A.
K.V.I.
Zernikelaan 25
9747 AA Groningen/The Netherlands

JOHANSSEN, L.	Institute of Physics University of Aarhus DK-8000 Aarhus-C/Denmark
JONG, F.E. DE	K.V.I. Zernikelaan 25 9747 AA Groningen/The Netherlands
JONGMAN, J.R.	K.V.I. Zernikelaan 25 9747 AA Groningen/The Netherlands
KAMERMANS, R.	Fysisch Laboratorium Rijksuniversiteit Utrecht Postbus 80.000 3508 TA Utrecht/The Netherlands
KARCZMARCZYK, W.	Nuclear Physics Laboratory Institute of Experimental Physics Warsaw University 69 Hoza Street PL-00681 Warsaw/Poland
KOCH, J.H.	NIKHEF-K Postbus 41882 1009 DB Amsterdam/The Netherlands
KONIJN, J.	NIKHEF-K Postbus 41882 1009 DB Amsterdam/The Netherlands
KRAMER, L.H.	Dept. of Physics Duke University Durham, NC 27706/USA
KUNISZ, K.	Institute of Physics Pedagogical University Lesna 16 25-509 Kielce/Poland
LAAT, C.T.A.M. DE	Buys Ballot Laboratorium Princetonplein 5 3584 CC Utrecht/The Netherlands
LALAZISSIS, G.	Department of Theoretical Physics University of Thessaloniki GR-54006 Thessaloniki/Greece
LEEGTE, H.K.W.	K.V.I. Zernikelaan 25 9747 AA Groningen/The Netherlands
MANDEVILLE, J.B.	Nuclear Physics Lab. University of Illinois 23, Stadium Drive Champaign, Ill. 61820/U.S.A.
MEYER, H.	NIKHEF-K Postbus 41882 1009 DB Amsterdam/The Netherlands

MORAWEK, W.	Institut für Kernphysik Technische Hochschule Darmstadt Schlossgartenstrasse 9 D-6100 Darmstadt/West-Germany
MUELLER, B.	Institut für Theoretische Physik Universität Frankfurt Robert Mayerstrasse 3 - 10 D-6000 Frankfurt 1/West-Germany
MUELLER, U.	Institut für Kernphysik Universität Mainz Postfach 3980 D-6500 Mainz/West-Germany
NECK, D.V.Y. van	Institute for Nuclear Physics Proeftuinstraat 86 B-9000 Gent/Belgium
NEU, R.	Physikalisches Institut Universität Tübingen Auf der Morgenstelle 14 D-7400 Tübingen/West-Germany
ODERKERK, R.P.	NIKHEF-K Postbus 41882 1009 DB Amsterdam/The Netherlands
OGUL, R.	Faculty of Science and Arts, S.U Physics Department Kampus Konya/Turkey
OSKAM-TAMBOEZER, M.	NIKHEF-K Postbus 41882 1009 DB Amsterdam/The Netherlands
PLOMPEN, A.	Natuurkundig Laboratorium Vrije Universiteit De Boelelaan 1081 1081 HV Amsterdam/The Netherlands
PORRAS, I.	Departamento di Fisica Nuclear Faculdad de Ciencias Universidad de Granada E-18071 Granada/Spain
RABEN, H.B.M.	NIKHEF-K Postbus 41882 1009 DB Amsterdam/The Netherlands
RIEDEMAN, D.E.J.	NIKHEF-K Postbus 41882 1009 DB Amsterdam/The Netherlands
RISSE, F.	Institut für Strahlen- und Kernphysik Universität Bonn Nussallee 14-16 D-5300 Bonn/West-Germany

ROESEL, Ch.F.G.	Institut für Strahlen- und Kernphysik Universität Bonn Nussallee 14-16 D-5300 Bonn/West-Germany
SANDULESCU, N.Ch.	Theoretical Physics Department Central Institute of Physics P.O. Box MGG Bucharest/Rumania
SCHAAR, M. VAN DER	NIKHEF-K Postbus 41882 1009 DB Amsterdam/The Netherlands
SCHAGEN, J.P.S. VAN	Natuurkundig Laboratorium Vrije Universiteit de Boelelaan 1081 1081 HV Amsterdam/The Netherlands
SCHERER, S.	Institut für Kernphysik Universität Mainz Postfach 3980 D-6500 Mainz/West-Germany
TAAL, A.	NIKHEF-K Postbus 41882 1009 DB Amsterdam/The Netherlands
TEMPLON, J.A.	Physics Department Indiana University Bloomington, Ind. 47401/U.S.A.
THEUERKAUF, J.	Institut für Kernphysik Universität Köln Zülpicherstrasse 77 D-5000 Köln 41/West-Germany
UCHIYAMA, T.	K.V.I. Zernikelaan 25 9747 AA Groningen/The Netherlands
VARMA, R.	R. van de Graaff Laboratories Department of Physics Indian Institute of Technology Kanpur 208016/India
WITT HUBERTS, P.K.A. DE	NIKHEF-K Postbus 41882 1009 DB Amsterdam/The Netherlands
ZONDERVAN, A.	NIKHEF-K Postbus 41882 1009 DB Amsterdam/The Netherlands

INDEX